# Atrial Fibrillation - Current Management and Practice

*Edited by Richard Schuessler and Chawannuch Ruaengsri*

Published in London, United Kingdom

Atrial Fibrillation - Current Management and Practice
http://dx.doi.org/10.5772/intechopen.1003310
Edited by Richard Schuessler and Chawannuch Ruaengsri

Contributors
Alexandr Glupak, Alexandr Troitsky, Alexandr Zotov, Ali Oto, Allen Ninh, Anna Reichardt, Ashley Diaz, Chawannuch Ruaengsri, Chin-Yu Lin, Christina Golna, Corey E. Tabit, Daniel Bujnowski, Daniel L. Beckles, Dat Tran Cao, Dimitrios Trafalis, Ebru Sahin, Elisabeta Bădilă, Emil Sakharov, Gyanendra K. Sharma, Igor Khamnagadaev, Ilias Gountas, Ioana Cristina Daha, Irina Bulavina, Jakraphan Yu, James Harris Calhoun, Jamil Francis, Jeffrey A. Switzer, Jose Ruiz, Jovany Castro-Lara, Juan Leoni, Konstantinos Vemmos, Kuang-Drew Li, Kyriakos Souliotis, Larissa Kiwakyou, Lauren Chow, Louise Sun, Manuel Alejandro Vera-Fuentes, Manuel Quiroz-Flores, Marc Leon, Marwan M. Refaat, Mehmet Hakan Uzun, Mehmet Ozgeyik, Mei Gao, Mikhil Patel, Mohammad Montaser Atasi, Mustafa Ucar, Myrto Barmpouni, Natalya Mokrysheva, Oleg Shelest, Ozge Turgay Yildirim, Razan Dankar, Robert Khabazov, Rohan M. Goswami, Rohan Sharma, Sandra Sánchez-Cassio, Shriya Sharma, Soham Kulkarni, Vincent J.B. Robinson, Yinglong Hou, Yujiao Zhang, Zhan Li



First published in London, United Kingdom, 2025 by IntechOpen
IntechOpen is the global imprint of INTECHOPEN LIMITED, registered in England and Wales, registration number: 11086078, 167-169 Great Portland Street, London, W1W 5PF, United Kingdom

For EU product safety concerns: IN TECH d.o.o., Prolaz Marije Krucifikse Kozulić 3, 51000 Rijeka, Croatia, info@intechopen.com or visit our website at intechopen.com.

British Library Cataloguing-in-Publication Data
A catalogue record for this book is available from the British Library

Atrial Fibrillation - Current Management and Practice
Edited by Richard Schuessler and Chawannuch Ruaengsri
p. cm.

This title is part of the Cardiology and Cardiovascular Medicine Book Series, Volume 9
Topic: Cardiovascular Electrophysiology
Series Editor: Kaan Kırali
Topic Editor: Karine Guerrier

Print ISBN 978-0-85466-458-0
Online ISBN 978-0-85466-457-3
eBook (PDF) ISBN 978-0-85466-459-7
ISSN 3033-361X

If disposing of this product, please recycle the paper responsibly.

IntechOpen Book Series

# Cardiology and Cardiovascular Medicine

Volume 9

## Aims and Scope of the Series

Today, since molecular science on structural causes of oncological pathologies and their molecular treatments are developing at an unbelievable rate, the primary medical cause of death in the twenty-first century will be cardiovascular disease. Neither pandemics that threaten all humanity nor deterioration in the ecosystem will be able to change this fact. Especially, this century seems poised to witness an incredible struggle against atherosclerotic disease, which develops in the arterial walls and results in narrowing and occlusion of the arterial lumen. In addition to this disease, there has been an increasing prevalence of heart rhythm problems, deterioration of heart valves due to aging, and heart failure. Serious vascular pathologies such as stenosis and occlusion, dissection and rupture, and aneurysmal enlargement are also major concerns. Medical and invasive treatment methods may work to save human lives, but they will never provide a real solution. All kinds of medical, technological, and genetic engineering developments obtained in these processes have not yet been sufficient to alleviate or eliminate cardiovascular disease. This book series, Cardiology and Cardiovascular Medicine, includes three topics. The first, Cardiovascular Diseases and Health, reviews important cardiovascular diseases and the developments in their prognosis. The second topic, Cardiovascular Electrophysiology, illuminates the abnormal functioning of the cardiac conduction system, which is caused by all heart pathologies and negatively affects prognosis. The third topic in this series, Cardiovascular Surgery, details treatment for cardiovascular pathologies and how to regulate normal physiological functions with percutaneous or extracorporeal interventions.

# Meet the Series Editor

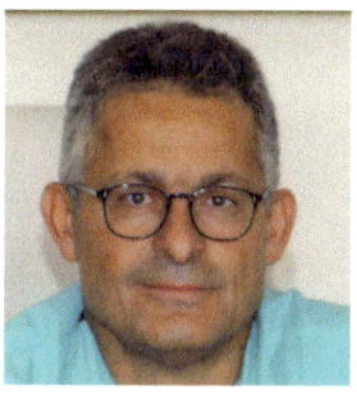

After completing his studies at the Medicine Faculty of Istanbul University in 1990, Prof. Kaan Kırali fulfilled his mandatory medical service and commenced his residency training at Koşuyolu Heart and Research Hospital in 1992. Following five years of assistant education, he pursued further training in England and the USA in 1998. Specializing in laparoscopic and minimally invasive cardiac surgery, he earned the titles of consultant cardiovascular surgeon in 1998, Assistant Professor in 1999, Associate Professor in 2002, and Chief in 2005 at the same hospital. Prof. Kırali also developed an interest in preventive medicine, obtaining an MSc in Public Health from Istanbul University in 2000. Over the past two decades, he has concentrated his scientific pursuits on cardiovascular repairs requiring specialized experience. With his expertise in coronary artery surgery, minimally invasive cardiac surgery, valve repair, and aortic root surgery, he has established new methods for awake coronary bypass revascularization, a new surgical approach for AVR during first and re-operations, aortic valve-sparing procedure, and radiofrequency ablation. Notably, he pioneered awake complete coronary artery bypass grafting (CABG) with bilateral internal mammary arteries (BIMA) and played a crucial role in advancing aortic root surgery with a new aortotomy incision, simplifying aortic valve interventions. Since the year 2000, Prof. Kırali has expanded his interests to heart transplantation, and in recent years, to left ventricular assist devices. He has served as the head of the transplantation department since 2015 and currently continues his work as the director of Koşuyolu High Specialization Education and Research Hospital in Istanbul, Turkey. In his prolific career, he has authored numerous papers in SCI journals, contributed to various book chapters, and served as an editor and reviewer for multiple academic journals. Additionally, he has edited several international books in the field of cardiovascular medicine.

# Meet the Volume Editors

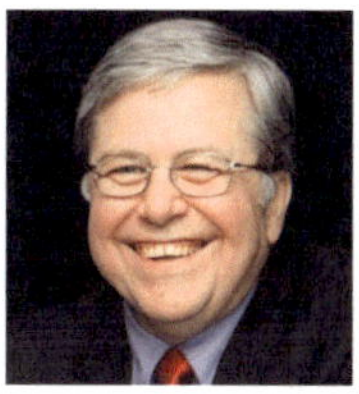

Dr. Richard Schuessler is a distinguished retired Professor of Surgery at Washington University School of Medicine in St. Louis, where he has made significant contributions to cardiovascular research and surgical innovation. With a Ph.D. in Biomedical Engineering, Dr. Schuessler dedicated his career to advancing the understanding of cardiac electrophysiology, atrial fibrillation, and surgical ablation techniques. A member of the Department of Surgery's Cardiothoracic Division and research laboratory director, Dr. Schuessler has collaborated extensively with clinicians and scientists to develop pioneering treatments for heart rhythm disorders. His research has been instrumental in developing and refining the Cox-Maze procedure, a gold-standard surgical treatment for atrial fibrillation. His work combines experimental models with clinical translation, improving patient outcomes worldwide. An accomplished scholar with an H index of 81, Dr. Schuessler has authored numerous peer-reviewed publications and book chapters, earning recognition from prestigious organizations in cardiothoracic surgery and electrophysiology. He is still actively involved in mentoring trainees and fostering interdisciplinary research. Dr. Schuessler's leadership at Washington University drove innovation in cardiac surgery, blending scientific rigor with a commitment to patient care.

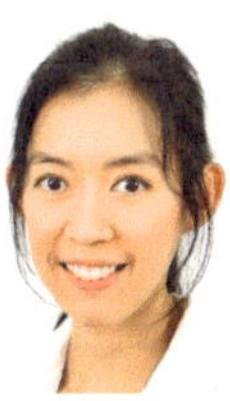

Dr. Chawannuch Ruaengsri is a Clinical Assistant Professor at Stanford University School of Medicine. She obtained her MD at Mahidol University, Bangkok, Thailand. She also did her residency and fellowship in Adult Cardiac Surgery. She also completed a postdoctoral fellowship in Atrial Fibrillation at Washington University, clinical fellowships in Mechanical Circulatory Support and Cardiac Transplant at Washington University, and Minimally Invasive Adult Cardiac Surgery at Emory University. She has a strong background in basic science research, particularly in atrial fibrillation, cardiac electrophysiology, and mitral valve regurgitation, which she studied during her postdoctoral research fellowship. As a co-investigator on an NIH-funded grant, she contributed to a project on atrial fibrillation surgery. In the field of heart and lung transplantation, her work centers on donor-site optimization, innovative transplant techniques, and organ preservation strategies to increase donor organ availability. She has successfully led multiple research projects, collaborating with cardiologists, pediatric and adult cardiac transplant teams, and other researchers, resulting in numerous peer-reviewed publications. Additionally, she has extensive expertise in experimental study design and data analysis. Her present research focuses on heart and lung transplantation, emphasizing developing novel surgical techniques and improving organ preservation methods to expand the donor pool.

# Contents

# Preface

This book provides a comprehensive guide for treating atrial fibrillation (AF). It is accessible to the primary care physician, emergency and urgent care physician, hospitalist, internist, and cardiologist. It moves beyond societal guidelines by providing an international perspective on how various groups have implemented their care programs. It starts with chapter 1 by giving a perspective chapter on the management and practice of atrial fibrillation. The following four chapters address the most significant risks of AF, thrombosis, and stroke and its treatment with the use of left atrial appendage exclusion. Chapters 6 and 7 address the role of heart failure and AF in detail. Chapter 8 provides a unique and practical guide for developing, implementing, and monitoring clinical pathways. The authors provide two examples, one for the emergency room and one for in-hospital AF. Chapter 9 provides guidance and special considerations for anesthesia for surgical or catheter ablation of AF. Chapters 10 through 14 describe ablation techniques, catheter ablation, surgical ablation, and sympathetic renal nerve ablation. Finally, chapter 15 gives insight into factors associated with the recurrence of AF after treatment, and chapter 16 provides insight into the role of exercise in managing AF.

It is unusual for a text like this to be edited by a basic scientist like me. However, I found it very rewarding. I was very fortunate to have worked with James L. Cox, MD, on developing the first treatment of AF that eliminated AF and restored NSR, the Cox-Maze procedure. This surgical procedure was developed in animal models in our research laboratory at Washington University in St. Louis in the late 1980s and then translated to humans. Since then, it has been modified and simplified with the introduction of various ablation devices by Ralph J. Damiano Jr., MD. It became and remains the gold standard for the nonpharmacologic treatment of AF. Following the introduction of the Cox-Maze procedure, clinical electrophysiologists introduced catheter ablation techniques that are less invasive, which have made the treatment available to a wider cohort of patients. It is very rewarding to see how basic research can be translated into a treatment that reduces both the morbidity and mortality caused by AF. Patients receiving these treatments live longer and have a better quality of life.

I would like to thank co-editor Chawannuch Ruaengsri, MD, a Clinical Assistant Professor at Stanford University School of Medicine. Her knowledge of the treatment of atrial fibrillation was invaluable. I would also like to thank Nina Miocevic, Publishing Process Manager for IntechOpen. Her help and gentle reminders help bring this project to the finish line.

Finally, I would like to dedicate this book to my high school biology teacher, Mr. Roy Pfund. He taught me the scientific method, which has served me well over my 45+ year career. Not only did I have a great time doing science, but our research team has helped advance the treatment of AF, prolonging and providing many patients with a high quality of life.

**Richard B. Schuessler**
Washington University School of Medicine,
St. Louis, Missouri, USA

**Chawannuch Ruaengsri**
Division of Cardiothoracic Surgery,
Stanford University,
Stanford, California, USA

Chapter 1

# Perspective Chapter: Management and Practice for Atrial Fibrillation

*Dat Tran Cao and Chin-Yu Lin*


## Abstract

Atrial fibrillation (AF) is a prevalent arrhythmia projected to affect millions of people worldwide, increasing the risk of stroke, myocardial infarction, and cardiac death. Effective management strategies for AF focus on a comprehensive approach that addresses the disease as a whole rather than isolating individual aspects. The three main pillars of AF management are stroke prevention, symptom management, and risk factor modification. Stroke prevention remains paramount, utilizing anticoagulation therapy and left atrial appendage occlusion (LAAO) for patients intolerant to novel oral anticoagulants (NOACs). Symptom management prioritizes rhythm control, particularly through catheter ablation, which is effective in maintaining sinus rhythm and improving patient outcomes. Risk factor modification involves managing obesity, hypertension, diabetes, alcohol consumption, and smoking cessation, as well as promoting physical activity to reduce AF incidence and recurrence. This holistic approach, integrating advanced diagnostic tools and personalized treatment plans, aims to mitigate the multifaceted impact of AF and enhance long-term prognosis.


**Keywords:** atrial fibrillation, rhythm control, catheter ablation, management strategy, risk factor modification

## 1. Introduction

Atrial fibrillation (AF) is being increasingly diagnosed worldwide as the global population ages. It is estimated that, by 2030, there will be over 12 million patients with AF in the USA alone [1]. The lifetime incidence of the disease varies, being highest among white individuals (30–40%) and lowest among Asian groups, who have an estimated risk of 15% [2, 3]. Atrial fibrillation also increases the risks of stroke, myocardial infarction, and cardiac death by 1.5 to 2 times. In one observational study, death accounted for 19.5% of the adverse outcomes in patients with AF over 5 years, while heart failure was the second most common outcome at 13.7% [4]. Furthermore, AF progresses over time, with an annual conversion rate from paroxysmal to persistent AF of around 11% within 3 years. As the disease progresses, patient's prognosis worsens. Consequently, AF has placed a significant burden on patients, and the management of this disease has also advanced significantly over the last decade, thanks to advancements in the field of electrophysiology. While in the previous decade, valvular heart disease was demonstrated to be associated with atrial fibrillation, this concept has been refuted in recent years as electrophysiologists have begun to see AF as a separate disease entity with the pathophysiology completely different from those that involved valvular heart disease. Furthermore, the concepts of valvular and non-valvular AF were deemed from studies examining the efficacy of different anticoagulants but not truly related to the disease nature as for that, these terms have been deemed obsolete in the current era. Lone AF was also found to be irrelevant in this course of time, as this term was referred to single out those AF in younger patients without structural heart disease. As pointed out by recent guidelines, the term itself limited the spectrum of AF and the effective management of the disease [5].

## 2. Diagnosis

The definite diagnosis of atrial fibrillation is based on documented episodes of atrial fibrillation that last for more than 30 seconds [5]. Other than this, several other methods, especially those implementing advances in technology such as smartwatches, have also been recognized for their role in diagnosing AF [6].

Moreover, even though it remained unpopular in the past, the implantable loop recorder (ILR), which was initially intended to be an extended monitoring device for any bradycardia, can actually also be used to unveil the early form of paroxysmal AF. Similar to the ILR, pacemakers, besides their main function as a bradycardia treatment method, also have monitoring capabilities. As such, atrial high-rate episodes (AHRE) documented by these devices have become issues of interest in the last couple of years. Of course, these episodes cannot be translated into AF since, even if organized, regular or not, they are the tracings of one single endocardial lead, and this kind of signal might very well be recorded in both true AF and other atrial tachycardias. However, regardless of the methods utilized, the true problem is whether AF truly occurs or not, and our limitation is the currently available methods to detect AF, especially those paroxysmal forms. Multiple ambulatory ECG monitors could be suggested for documenting those episodes of arrhythmias. However, it is needless to say that the probability is still limited. Some of the smart devices on the market these days have allowed us to better screen for AF, but the definite diagnosis still needs to be confirmed by doctors. Although the role of AHRE is still unclear, some studies suggest that the risk of stroke should not be overlooked [7, 8].

As pointed out in the early part of this chapter, valvular atrial fibrillation as well as lone AF are terms that have been written out of the recent approach and management as these would have reflected the true nature of atrial fibrillation.

## 3. Classification

The current and most applicable classification is the duration-based system (**Table 1**) [8, 9]. Atrial fibrillation that occurs for less than 7 days is defined as paroxysmal, and these episodes could terminate spontaneously or with intervention. AF that sustains for more than 7 days is classified as persistent. Long-standing AF refers to AF that persists for more than 1 year. Lastly, if the clinician determines to abstain from any rhythm control strategies, long-standing AF should be classified as permanent [5]. Several other methods have also been proposed; however, this remains the standard classification system to simplify the initial impression for initiation of the management.

More sustained forms of AF (persistent, long-standing) imply that atrial remodeling has already occurred, which affects the management of these groups of patients.

| Terminology | Definition |
|---|---|
| First detected AF | The first documentation of AF, regardless of previous symptoms |
| Paroxysmal atrial fibrillation | AF that is intermittent and terminates within ≤7 d of onset |
| Persistent atrial fibrillation | AF that is continuous and sustains for >7 d and requires intervention. Of note, patients with persistent AF who, with therapy, become paroxysmal should still be defined as persistent as this reflects their original pattern and is more useful to predict outcomes and define substrate. |
| Early persistent atrial fibrillation | Persistent AF that lasted less than 3 months |
| Long-standing atrial fibrillation | AF that is continuous for >12 months in duration |
| Permanent atrial fibrillation | A term that is used when the patient and clinician make a joint decision to stop further attempts to restore and/or maintain sinus rhythm Acceptance of AF represents a therapeutic decision and does not represent an inherent pathophysiological attribute of AF |
| Subclinical atrial fibrillation | Subclinical atrial fibrillation is short-lasting and asymptomatic and can usually be detected only by long-term continuous monitoring with pacemakers or defibrillators. |

**Table 1.**
*Classification of AF based on the duration of the disease.*

However, viewing AF in this way only indicates the current stage of the atrial substrate and does not paint the whole picture. The extent of the substrate and its relation to the patient's response to AF ablation remains controversial when based solely on duration. Cases with extensive remodeling in the myocardium of patients with only paroxysmal AF have been reported. Furthermore, it is not rare to see early persistent AF with minimal substrate respond quite well to pulmonary vein isolation (PVI) alone [10].

## 4. Management strategies

Atrial fibrillation, together with its complex pathophysiology and natural disease progression, has facilitated changes in management strategies over the past decade [11]. It is now known that to effectively treat AF, one must consider all aspects of the disease as well as the stage of the arrhythmia while also considering the prevention of complications. **Figure 1** illustrates the three main pillars clinicians must address in the management of AF [12]: stroke prevention, symptom management, and risk management.

## 5. Concomitant factors managements

AF management should currently be assessed thoroughly in the same way we treat hypertension [9, 12]. Extensive and numerous studies have concluded the correlation between multiple factors and the incidence of AF. Although some factors may not have been detailed regarding their pathophysiology, current evidence still urges us to address these concomitant issues as a crucial part of the overall AF management strategy. Among these risk factors, obesity, smoking, excessive alcohol consumption, diabetes mellitus, hypertension, and physical inactivity have been demonstrated to be independent risk factors for AF. Managing thoroughly these factors would bring about the potential benefits, that is reducing the incidence and the recurrence of AF.

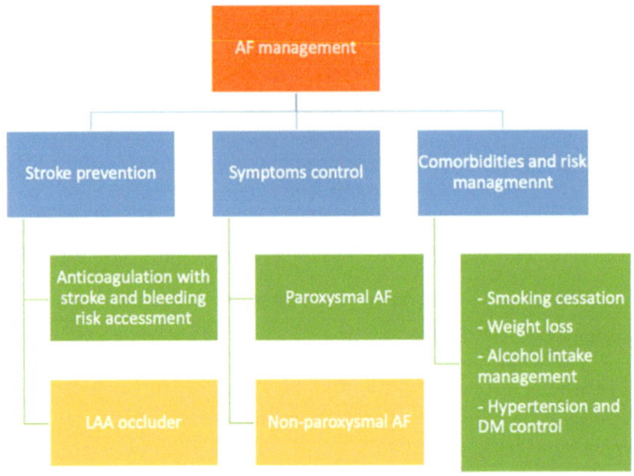


**Figure 1.**
*Management of atrial fibrillation in current practice.*

### 5.1 Obesity

It has been shown that obese patients with high BMI would have higher chances of developing AF compared with those without this issue. Furthermore, weight loss of at least 10% in this group of patients would also reduce the recurrence rate after AF ablation [13]. Keeping the BMI less than 27 also helps decrease the risk of AF recurrence. However, this effect seems to be limited to the paroxysmal group [14]. For those with AF for an extended amount of time, weight loss does not reduce the recurrence rate. The correlation between obesity and AF might come from the number of adipose tissues around the left atrium. The abundance of some of those translates to increased heterogeneity of the LA substrate, while in patients with persistent AF, these abnormal zones might have already developed extensively, and weight loss might not exert any effect on the recurrence rate after AF ablation.

### 5.2 Alcohol consumption

Excessive consumption of alcohol has been shown to increase the risk of AF. Alcohol slows down conduction and shortens the refractory period of the atrium, facilitating abnormal conduction within the chamber [15]. Autonomic changes caused by alcohol also affect the heart, and the increase of the fatty acids, which are products of alcohol, is arrhythmogenic. All of these mechanisms and clinical evidence render alcohol consumption a factor facilitating AF. Reducing alcohol intake to less than 3 standard drinks per week decreases the incidence of AF [16].

### 5.3 Hypertension

It has already been established that hypertension is the independent risk factor for AF. Even in the very initial study, the prevalence of AF was determined in the patients with hypertension and hypertension can increase the risk of AF up to 2 times. In the AF groups, up to 60–70% of the patients will also have concomitant high blood pressure. The increased load on the LV would also put more pressure on the left atrium and then this process can eventually lead to AF as evidenced by countless studies, these two conditions are more than common co-exist and facilitate the formation of each other.

### 5.4 Diabetes mellitus

Diabetes mellitus has also been shown to increase the risk of AF, as this condition facilitates several changes in the myocardium, including gap junction remodeling and fibrotic processes that promote the heterogeneity of conduction in the atrium and the formation of AF [17]. Furthermore, several studies have shown that poor control of DM results in a higher recurrence rate of AF post-ablation. This includes both pre-ablation glycemic conditions and management after the procedure. Patients with an HbA1c level of more than 9% have a higher chance of recurrence compared to those with a controlled level of less than 7% [18].

### 5.5 Physical inactivity

People who remain inactive have a higher risk of developing AF, while moderate exercise has been shown to reduce this incidence [19]. This condition is usually found in people with metabolic syndrome, and physical inactivity might increase the risk of obesity, all of which are precursors for AF. Furthermore, it is also found that this condition affects the recurrence rate of AF patients after catheter ablation. Patients who enrolled in a cardiac-exercise program after the procedure had a lower chance of AF recurrence compared to those who did not [20]. Therefore, 210 minutes of moderate exercise per week is recommended to reduce the risk of AF as well as the risk of recurrence after ablation.

### 5.6 Smoking cessation

Smoking has been demonstrated to facilitate worse outcomes in patients with AF, including increased risks of heart failure, hospitalization, and death [21]. This effect has been shown to be reversible once patients stop smoking. Hence, in patients with AF, it is recommended to take the initiative to prevent smoking, which entails both behavior modification and medication if necessary.

## 6. Stroke preventions

### 6.1 Anticoagulation

Even with our extensive work on finding new management strategies for AF, the most crucial component remains the prevention of strokes, as this outcome is the most burdensome to patients. It is estimated that AF increases the risk of stroke up to 8 times. Furthermore, in patients with documented ischemic strokes, it is estimated that 15% have undetected AF, which is only elucidated after the adverse event.

The use of anticoagulant agents has been proven effective, and the current regimen remains the cornerstone treatment for stroke prevention. The $CHA_2DS_2$-VASc score considers all risk factors that increase the risk of stroke in patients with AF [22]. Hence, it is reasonable to use this scoring system in clinical practice to guide blood-thinner therapy. Female patients with a score of more than 2 or male patients with a score of more than 3 should be prescribed anticoagulants. In those patients at risk for strokes who do not meet the qualification for initiation of anticoagulants, other stroke risk factors need to be considered [23]. However, current evidence does not specify the exact number of additional factors to consider before starting medication. In these

| | Dabigatran | Apixaban | Edoxaban | Rivaroxaban |
|---|---|---|---|---|
| Standard dose | 150 mg BD | 5 mg BD | 60 mg daily | 20 mg daily |
| Reduced dose | 110 mg BD if any 1 of the following<br>• Age ≥ 80<br>• Concomitant verapamil<br>Consider<br>• Age: 75–80<br>• Increased bleeding risk | 2.5 mg if any 2 of the following<br>• Age ≥ 80<br>• BW ≤ 60 kg<br>• Serum creatinine >133 umol/L | 30 mg daily if any 1 of the following<br>• BW ≤ 60 kg<br>• Concomitant ciclosporin, dronedarone, erythromycin or ketoconazole | |
| Renal dose | CrCl 30–50 ml/min<br>• 110 mg BD<br>Contraindicated if CrCl <30 ml/min | CrCl 15–30 ml/min<br>• 2.5 mg BD<br>Contraindicated if CrCl<15 ml/min | CrCl 15–50 ml/min<br>• 30 mg daily<br>Contraindicated if CrCl<15 ml/min | CrCl 15–50 ml/min<br>• 15 mg daily<br>Contraindicated if CrCl<15 ml/min |

**Table 2.**
*Dosing of anticoagulants for stroke prophylaxis in AF patients.*

situations, it falls upon our experience to judge whether our patients would benefit from this therapy.

Furthermore, clinical bleeding risk scores have been developed to identify patients with a higher propensity for adverse effects from anticoagulants. These scores typically consider the function of other organs such as the liver or kidneys, and patients with abnormal function of these organs have a higher chance of bleeding if placed on anticoagulants [24]. Even with high-risk profiles, no definite alternative treatment therapies or discontinuation of anticoagulants are recommended. Additional attempts to reduce the risk of adverse effects, such as withdrawing any co-administered antiplatelets, NSAIDs, or using LAA occlusion, should be taken in these groups of patients.

Novel oral anticoagulants are mostly recommended these days for patients with AF, except for those with mechanical heart valves or severe mitral stenosis (**Table 2**). In these latter situations, warfarin should be used, aiming to maintain an INR of 2-3. It is also important to note the limits of renal function for each type of NOAC. It is suggested that a lower dosage of apixaban would be safe in patients with renal dysfunction down to an eGFR of 15 ml/min. Furthermore, when considering bleeding risks, a lower dosage of dabigatran provides the same preventive effect while also having lower bleeding risks compared with other anticoagulants.

### 6.2 LAA occluder

In AF patients, 90% of the thrombus would be formed in the left atrial appendage. As for that, one of the additional treatments that has been considered in recent years is the use of the LAA occluder that would prevent the development within this structure and hence, reduce the risk of stroke. LAAO is mainly recommended in AF patients who do not tolerate NOAC or have contraindications to NOAC. The efficacy and safety of the procedure have been tested out in several studies [25, 26]. However, current evidence is still conflicting regarding the use of anticoagulants post-implantation. As for that, it is still recommended that we should continue this therapy after the device is implanted.

Other than device intervention, several recent studies have also been carried out for the concomitant closure of the LAA during surgery for other cardiovascular diseases that require operative intervention [27]. While this additional clipping or closure of the LAA would prove the benefit over the following period in those studies, this indication is self-limited as it requires the patients to go under other cardiac surgery in order to have LAA isolation which would not be the sole target for primary prevention. That is, we could not consult the patient to have an operation just to have his LAA clipped.

## 7. Symptoms managements

In patients with AF, symptoms and sequelae arise from the fast and irregular heart rate. Current management targeting this condition is divided into two main strategies. Rhythm control aims at restoring the normal sinus rhythm of the patient, while rate control focuses on keeping the ventricular response at an acceptable rate. Both approaches have their pros and cons, and choosing the appropriate therapy requires clinicians to take into account different patient characteristics. In general, rhythm control is more favored in younger groups of patients who are more symptomatic and have a shorter duration of AF and less atrial remodeling. Even though studies have demonstrated the safety and efficacy of AF ablation in patients over 80 years of age, whether or not to ablate these groups of older patients are at the discrete of the electrophysiologists rather than one fixed arbitrary threshold above which catheter ablation would not bring additional benefit. Furthermore, as for the shorter duration of AF, it is because of the nature of the disease that would lead to the ultimate atrial remodeling and this condition would significantly reduce the efficacy of catheter ablation. The classification of AF is the cornerstone of this approach. Patients with paroxysmal AF to early persistent AF would benefit the most from catheter ablation. Conversely, in patients at the more advanced stage of AF, especially those with atrial cardiomyopathy (ACM), rate control seems to be a more applicable method (**Figure 2**).

## 7.1 Rhythm control

### *7.1.1 Medication strategies*

One of the interesting features of the study was that the ratio of catheter ablation took up only 7 to 15% of the rhythm control group in the EAST-AFNET trial (initial and cross-over cohort) while the remaining would benefit from the medical treatment for rhythm control [28]. However, the result of that study still favored the rhythm control approach with lower mortality and hospitalization. **Table 3** lists the medication for rhythm control. However, one of the problems with medication is the bradycardia effect which should be tailored carefully in elder patients, in which AF would be also prevalent. Even though the long-term outcome of these medications has been proven to be effective and safe in AF patients. After almost 5 years on medication, 82–88% of patients would still maintain sinus rhythm and these medications even including sodium channel blockers would prove to be safe in AF patients [29]. As for that, rhythm management with medication would be one of the simple but yet safe and effective for the long-term management of AF. In clinical practice, an initial trial for 1 month with AAD would be attempted for spontaneous returning to sinus rhythm. If the patient remains in AF even on these medications, electrical cardioversion would be helpful as the initial trigger and after successful reversion to sinus rhythm, maintenance therapy with AAD is also required thereafter. The choice of the medication would mostly depend on the availability of the drugs and the concomitant heart disease. While amiodarone is relatively safe in patients with structural heart disease (stable heart failure and ischemic heart disease), flecainide

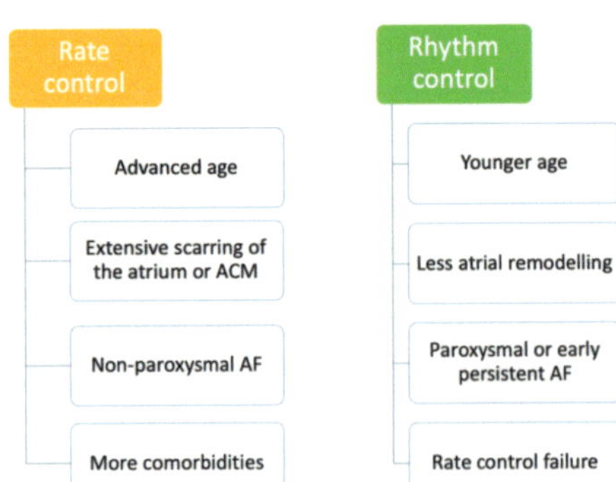


**Figure 2.**
*Factors for strategies consideration for symptom management in AF patients.*

| Drug | Oral dose |
|---|---|
| Amiodarone | 200 mg thrice daily for 4 weeks<br>Then 200 mg thereafter |
| Dronedarone | 400 mg twice a day |
| Flecainide | 100–200 mg twice daily OR<br>200 mg (slow-release form) once a day |
| Propafenone | 150–300 mg thrice daily |
| Disopyramide | 100–400 mg 2–3 times a day<br>Max: 800 mg/24 h |
| Sotalol | 80–160 mg twice a day |

**Table 3.**
*Antiarrhythmia medication for rhythm control in AF patients.*

should not be indicated in these groups of patients. While recent studies have demonstrated a relatively safe profile of flecainide in stable ischemic heart disease (complete revascularized), the current recommendation is still based on the previous strategic outcomes of the CAST study which showed significant adverse outcomes with the usage of flecainide in patients with structural heart disease [30].

### *7.1.2 Electrical cardioversion*

Electrical cardioversion would be one of the simple but yet underappreciated treatments of AF. This treatment has demonstrated its safety profile over a wide range of patients. Cardioversion should be considered for symptomatic AF patients in whom rhythm control is desired. Stepping up from 50 J up to 150 J, delivery of electric shock could successfully restore the sinus rhythm in up to 96% of patients. The success rate, however, decreased in patients with longer and more sustainable AF and older patients. In patients over the age of 80, the efficacy of cardioversion decreased to 68% [31]. Another group of patients that should also be taken into account is heart failure patients. Repeated shock to the depressed heart might result in unfavorable outcomes. Furthermore, AF patients who are on optimal anticoagulant treatment would still exhibit a residual risk of strokes, and electrical cardioversion might be the trigger for such catastrophic events. As for that, a transesophageal echocardiogram might offer one simple but useful pre-procedural preparation. Patients who were found to have thrombi in the left atrial appendage should be withheld from electrical cardioversion as these shocks would mobilize the thrombi in situ and embolism might occur.

Another advancement in recent years is the usage of the dual current cardioversion. AF and obesity often co-exist and the latter would usually facilitate the former. Extra weight also poses a hindrance to effective energy delivery. Dual current cardioversion has been demonstrated to be one of the effective solutions in those situations. Dual energy delivery is more effective than single current shock not only in obese patients but also in patients in whom the traditional cardioversion failed, dual energy delivery could successfully terminate the AF [32].

### *7.1.3 Catheter ablation*

Perhaps one of the fastest advancements in the last decades in the field of cardiology is the management of AR as we have revisited and reappreciated what has been done wrong in the past. The controversy of rhythm and rate management dates back more than 10 years ago with the final straw of the AFFIRM study that led to the equality of both strategies which was then translated into 15 years of clinical practice [33]. However, it was not until the recent EAST-AFNET trial that the importance of carefully selecting patients for early intervention was highlighted, leading to a renewed recognition of the potential benefits of the rhythm control strategy [28]. Rhythm control would reduce the mortality and the rehospitalization rate which was hindered due to failure to maintain sinus rhythm in the AFFIRM study. Furthermore, with the continuation of the anticoagulants, adverse events were evened out between the two groups. The updated consensus and clinical trials suggested catheter ablation is superior to medication in selected patients (**Figure 3**) [9]. It is then without doubt that catheter ablation would present as one effective method for rhythm control of AF. Furthermore, as the way we access the outcomes after ablation is changing. In the previous time, we were focusing on maintaining the sinus rhythm as the main target after ablation. However, the burden of AF seemed to be more relevant to the ultimate outcome of the patients. With the decrease of arrhythmia burden, the quality of life seemed to be ameliorated while the mortality was also reduced. As for that even with persistent AF, catheter ablation would still be one of the options if one considers it as a method of reducing AF burden. With that to say, there are still some other parameters that would pinpoint the high recurrence rate of AF such as the presence of atrial cardiomyopathy, or dilated left atrium. However, it is also of great importance that even though these clinical factors have been proven to be the prognostic factors for AF recurrence, it is also vary from study to study and there is no concrete universal predictor. One can say ablation in AF patients with a left atrial diameter of more than 45 mm would result in a high likelihood of AF relapse, the number itself is arbitrary and different from other findings. The current consensus would not recommend one specific number for LA diameter above which catheter ablation is contraindicated.

### *7.1.4 Preprocedural preparation*

With the patients who are opted for ablation, the medical treatment periprocedural should be taken into account. As we are trying to reverse the normal contraction function of the atrium, the exclusion of any prior thrombus is a must. In patient with the $CHA_2DS_2$-VASc score of 1 for male and 2 for female, continuation of anticoagulants for 3 weeks before the ablation was recommended for thrombus formation prevention. Transesophageal echocardiography or cardiac CT could also be performed in these groups of patients to rule out the thrombus. As for the day of the procedure, current evidence seemed to be conflicting regarding whether we would do a minimal interruption by stopping only one single dose of NOAC on the day of ablation or continuation without interruption. Major adverse effects were not different between the two groups. As for that, based on the doctor's discretion, we might utilize either approach.

### *7.1.5 Ablation strategies*

Catheter ablation for atrial fibrillation has witnessed quite extensive changes over the past decades. From the cornerstone of PVI, we have also incorporated different ablation strategies and energies in order the enhance the outcomes of the procedure. The aim of PVI was to create the complete electrical dissociation between the four pulmonary veins and the left atrium. This target would be confirmed by the entrance block (with no remaining signal from the atrium in the pulmonary vein) and the exit

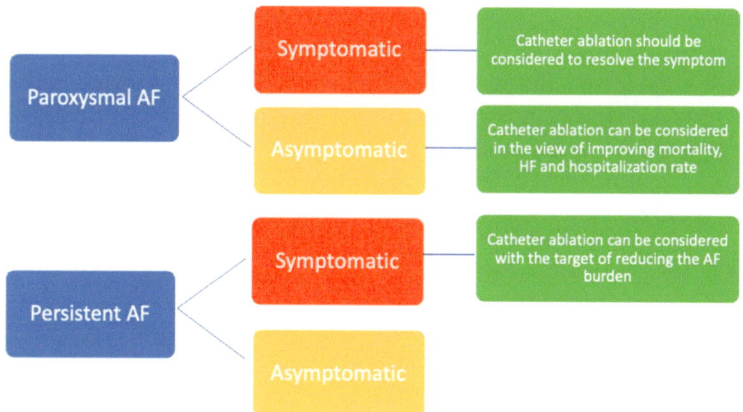


**Figure 3.**
*Role of catheter ablation in AF management.*

block (with the signal documented in the atrium when pacing from the pulmonary veins) [34, 35]. However, as one needs to take into account the epicardial conduction [36], we can sometimes only achieve a unidirectional block and even though in theory, this result might have been less promising than the two direction blocks. Clinical data did not show the superiority of one target over the other. Regarding the strategy for PVI, circumferential ablation remains to be the standard approach in current practice with consideration of adequate lesion formation and the risks of causing collateral tissue damage [37].

One of the applications of the new technology that has helped to ameliorate the efficacy of catheter ablation in recent years is the usage of the contact force together with the ablation index (AI) which might represent the lesion's depth and extent. AI-based ablation has then helped to decrease the recurrence rate dramatically [37]. Studies have also shown that a distance between lesions of less than 6 mm would create adequate lesion density [38]. With the traditional ablation approach of normal energy and long duration. However, ablation with high power and short-duration lesions would significantly reduce the procedure time and in turn, improve the efficacy of the procedure. Furthermore, lesions formed in this way would be more extensive on the endocardium while maintaining adequate depth for the durability of the circumferential lines. Head-to-head studies compared between these two ablation strategies had been conducted extensively all of which would reach the same conclusion of the superiority of the latter approach in both lesion size in vivo and long-term recurrence rate.

Another key feature that has a pivotal role in the success of reducing AF recurrence is the application of the high power-short duration set-up. Lesions created by this strategy would be wider in both size and depth and hence, therefore, they would be more durable over time. Together with the guarantees of sufficient contact with the myocardium and the ablation duration, we have achieved a higher first pass rate and less chances of AF returning [38]. Furthermore, with such technology, the concern of collateral organ damages (esophagus or the bronchi, lung) would also be secured as if we modified the optimal index, we would be able to achieve adequate lesion while sparing other structures.

Due to the different nature of the pathophysiology which would have a direct effect on the ablation outcomes, we would classify the recommendation based on the AF types.

### 7.1.6 Paroxysmal AF

For paroxysmal forms, the current guidelines would favor ablation in the scenarios of symptomatic AF. However, current evidence also pointed to the groups of asymptomatic groups as a potential candidate for ablation. As suggested in the EAST-AFNET trial, early intervention would result in improved cardiovascular outcomes not only the symptoms (**Figure 4**).

### 7.1.7 Persistent AF

With regards to the current approach for persistent AF ablation, there have yet to be the best strategies that would secure a similar recurrence rate as PAF. Traditional strategies for managing AF can be divided into two groups. The first group targets the anatomical structures of the left atrium (LA) that are believed to facilitate or maintain AF. The second group focuses on the functional aspects of the LA that also contribute to the development and persistence of AF. Among all of these, posterior wall isolation in combination with PVI seemed to be the most promising so far, however; the benefit of such a method might be limited down to those patients with rapid electrical activities at the posterior wall of LA [39]. It is also worth mentioning that, AF recurrence was most likely due to PV reconnection and so that, it is not the LA substrate is the sole reason for our failure [40]. It is also the effective energy penetration that led to the conduction gap whether in the endocardium or transmurally. We tend to use LA size as a parameter for predicting to response of patients to RF ablation but the changes in the LA myocardium itself would not lead to the reconnection. In our opinion, in order to enhance our efficacy in dealing with persistent AF switching to other energy sources might be a more reasonable approach as compared with modifying our ablation sites.

The main difference between PAF and those non-paroxysmal forms would not only be limited to the formation of the LA substrate but also the prognosis. Persistent AF would experience significantly higher mortality and stroke rates compared with those who experience AF intermittently [41]. However, the current approach for persistent AF ablation could not achieve quite as good outcomes as those paroxysmal forms which might stemmed from the substrate and our inadequate lesions formation in the scarred atrium. However, there are also some interesting features of persistent AF that would intrigue further research.

Other strategies for those with persistent forms of AF include anatomic ablation or substrate modification or driver ablation. Anatomic ablation refers to those approaches that target anatomical landmarks in the LA and deliver some additional linear ablation

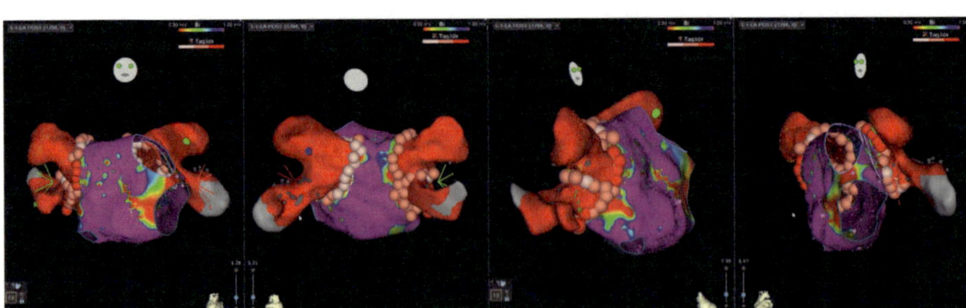

**Figure 4.**
*Circumferential ablation of the four pulmonary veins.*

lines over these areas. This strategy has been applied for more than a decade; its efficacy remains to be equivocal to PVI alone. Substrate modification includes ablation of those of complex atrial activity and driver ablation. Multiple advanced modules have been developed in order to elucidate these areas of interest. However, even though prior extensive studies also pointed toward the effectiveness of these extra ablation lesions, the recurrent rate of persistent AF remains to be high. In one study that actually compared all of these ablation strategies, an extensive approach including both anatomic and functional ablation would result in the least recurrence rate [42]. These findings in turn actually conflict with other studies pointing out that the more lines we create in the LA, the more chances of a stiff atrium and atypical atrial flutter.

Even with PVI, we might have actually already achieved some conceivable outcomes with persistent AF. As compared with those that occupied the heart entire day and night, catheter ablation would reduce the AF burden quite significantly and this would translate to better outcomes for the patients [43]. Furthermore, one of the advancements in the current era is the use of different energy sources which would lead to better and more homogenous lesion formation, especially in the anatomic and electric remodeled LA.

Adjunctive driver-guided ablation in addition to PVI has been proposed as a strategy to improve procedural success and outcomes for various populations with AF. Phase mapping appears to be superior to electrogram-based driver mapping in PerAF ablation in the meta-analysis [44]. The recent RCT demonstrated the waveform similarity and recurrence pattern derived from high-density mapping might provide an improved guiding approach for ablation of persistent AF [45]. Further studies were required for the driver-based approach.

#### *7.1.8 Non-PV triggers*

Up until now, the two nature of AF remains in some part, a mystery. That is even though in the majority of cases, the firing of the electrical activities from the pulmonary veins could initiate AF but the fact that we cannot achieve a 100% successful rate in treating AF by ablation of the PVs has led us to re-think about AF and its formation. One of the proposed mechanisms is the non-PV triggers [46]. A step-wise systematic approach was described as the Taipei Approach in 2006 by Chen SA et al. [46]. Electrical impulses from areas other than the PVs could actually initiate or "triggers" this kind of arrhythmia. The most common ectopic beat would originate from the superior vena cava, the crista terminalis, or the ligament of Marshalls. Indeed, scanning and targeting these triggers can help reduce the recurrence rate of AF to 18.5% [47]. With the advanced 3D technologies that we have currently including the high-density mapping catheters, revealing these ectopic by activation maps would become a feasible and crucial approach [48], especially in circumstances where there is durable PV isolation and AF still recurring.

#### *7.1.9 Patients with heart failure*

Arrhythmia-induced cardiomyopathy has become quite recognizable in the last decades. And indeed, with successful management of the rhythm, heart function would ameliorate which is the golden criterion for diagnosis of this kind of cardiomyopathy.

One of the indications for rhythm control is the co-existence of heart failure and AF. Whether it is the reason that deteriorates the heart function or the facilitating factor, AF would pose an unfavorable hemodynamic condition to the failing heart which in turn renders even non-responsive to HF medical therapy. And in line with our hypothesis, the evidence we have at hand also points toward the role of rhythm control of AF in patients with heart failure. Furthermore, what would be even more interesting is that while in the general population, catheter ablation and medical management for rhythm control would have the same benefits, in those with HF and reduced EF, ablation would seem to be superior to medicine in terms of outcomes (all-cause mortality and hospitalization) [9, 49, 50]. It is then also understandable that because most of the medications that we usually use for rhythm control would assert some inotrope or negative effect on the heart contraction function which is why catheter ablation would be more beneficial in this group. In selected patients, the severe functional mitral regurgitation (MR) could be reversible after ablation for AF [51]. The remodeling of MR also improves effective cardiac output. The effect of catheter ablation in the spectrum of patients with heart failure has also been studied. It is demonstrated that catheter ablation would potentially bring about the benefit of reducing cardiovascular death in patients with reduced EF compared with patients with persevered EF [52]. Additional effects in the latter groups might need more extensive study and review.

Interestingly, catheter ablation would bring about the effect in a quite fragile group of heart failure patients. In the past, patients with EF < 25% were considered inappropriate for any AF intervention such as catheter ablation and this number has remained one of the considerations for the adverse argument against catheter intervention. CASTLE-HTx however begged on the difference. With the effect of reducing mortality in even end-stage heart failure patients, catheter ablation has been considered one of the pivotal treatments in heart failure patients with AF [53].

#### *7.1.10 Other ablation energy*

##### *7.1.10.1 Cryoablation*

A recent advance in electrophysiology was the application of different energy sources. Of which cryo-energy prevails as a relatively safe and effective choice. Using the cryo-balloon for AF ablation has had to reduce the procedure time while it still maintains equivocal efficacy and safety (**Figure 5**). Furthermore, with the new generation of the balloon comes a variety of sizes and ablation options for electrophysiology. Time to isolation, which is an important parameter directly related to the recurrence rate of AF, could be documented more frequently in the newer version of the cryo-balloon and it might affect the ablation strategy as a whole. The minimal dosing for cryo-energy delivery was the TTI plus 120 seconds or 150 seconds and more TTI documentation would result in a better dosing regimen while avoiding the complication.

The FIRE AND ICE trial compared energy modalities for AF ablation, randomizing 762 patients with drug-refractory PAF to treatment with either the second-generation cryo-balloon or conventional RF ablation using a prospective multicenter design [54]. The study demonstrated that cryo-balloon ablation was non-inferior to RF ablation in terms of its primary endpoints of efficacy and safety. Secondary analyses suggested a possible reduction in re-hospitalization or re-ablation. Phrenic nerve injury was the most commonly reported complication at discharge in the cryo-balloon ablation group (2.7%), with permanent PN palsy occurring in 0.3% of patient. The CIRCA-DOSE trial evaluated contemporary approaches to PVI using the latest generation technology in both the cryo-balloon ablation and RF ablation arms,

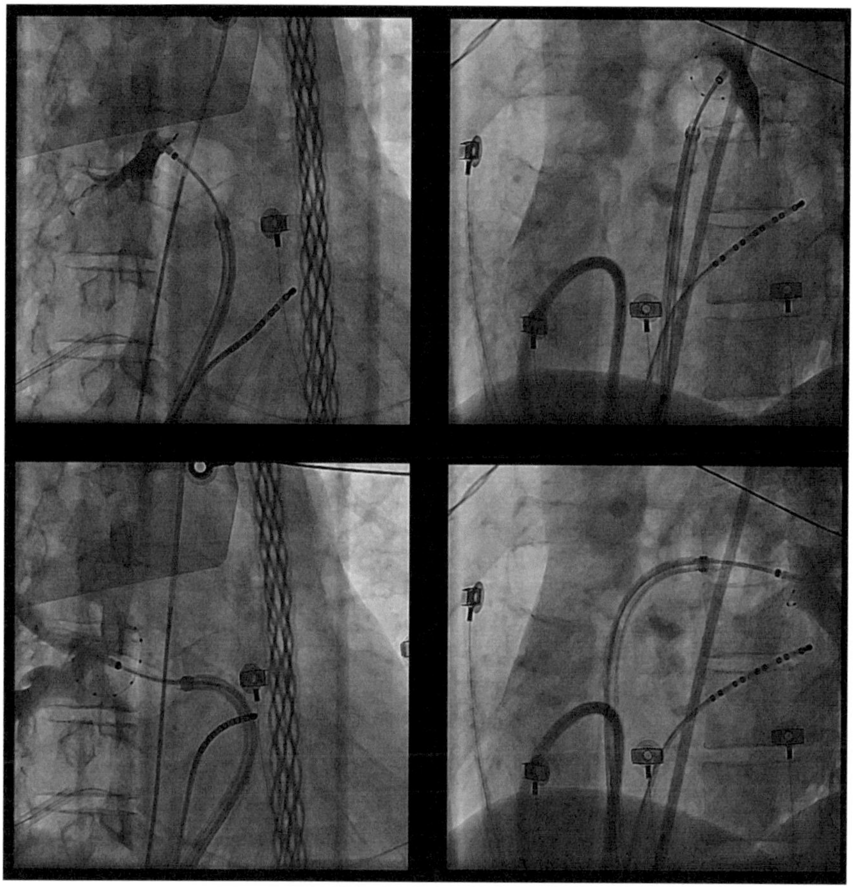

**Figure 5.**
*Cryoablation of the four pulmonary veins with the PolarX balloon catheter.*

utilizing an ICM for post-ablation rhythm monitoring [55]. The trial found no difference in 1-year efficacy (freedom from atrial tachyarrhythmia) between the compared groups. Continuous monitoring showed a median AF burden reduction of over 99% with both ablation technologies.

### *7.1.10.2 Pulse field ablation*

Perhaps one of the most promising tools in the field of EP would be the novel energy source. Pulse field ablation induces the electroporation of the myocardium which results in irreversible injury to the targeted cells while sparing the adjacent organs. As for this, every viable tissue, even those buried deep in the scarred myocardium would be affected by this source of energy and this, in turn, will create transmural damage to the entire myocardium. While it would be quite strong energy, cells in different organs would have different membrane characteristics which render them invulnerable to the selected field frequency. Pulse field ablation, therefore, should be the safest choice for ablation. Current evidence has demonstrated the non-inferiority of PFA regarding both efficacy and safety, especially when we observed its results in the short to mid-term [56]. The long-term recurrence rate remains to be the same as other ablation methods due to the lack of a prolonged monitoring study. Furthermore, even though this source of energy might create a whole different process of tissue healing over the antral of the PVs, reconnection and then recurrence of AF still happened. As for that, we might need to have more evidence especially focusing on the dosing and the recurrence pattern of these groups of patients before figuring out the best application of this novel energy.

### 7.2 Rate control

One of the other treatment methods for symptomatic AF is the use of AV node-blocking agents to control the ventricular rates [57]. The cut-off for the target of the average ventricular response rate is less than 110 bpm and a more tightly managed target of less than 80 bpm would not bring any additional benefits. This treatment strategy remains valuable in those with long-standing and permanent AF during this time when atrium cardiomyopathy is still one hindrance for electrophysiologists. The choice of drugs for rate control depends on the patient's condition as AF would usually come with comorbidities. In patients with EF < 40%, beta-blockers or digoxin should be used to control the heart rate while in patient with normal ejection fraction, other medications such as calcium channel blockers could also be considered.

Recently, ablate and pace approach has regained its value as one of the solutions for patients with persistent AF and reduced ejection fraction [57]. Current evidence has demonstrated that with optimal bi-ventricular pacing or even more advanced now, conduction system pacing together with AV nodal ablation or modification would ameliorate the outcomes as well as the clinical course of patients with heart failure.

## 8. Conclusion

The management of AF has witnessed some drastic changes over the past decades alongside the new pathophysiological findings of the disease as well as the application of different novel technologies. AF has become somewhat a metabolic change that requires a wholesome and intensified approach in order to achieve the best outcomes and to avoid adverse and devastating sequelae. Management of the risk factors together with stroke prevention and most importantly early rhythm control might yield better outcomes for AF patients so that AF might 1 day become a curable disease rather than an incessant sickness burden.

## Acknowledgements

This work was supported by the Biosense Webster IIS (C2304900), Ministry of Science and Technology (MOST 110-2314-B-A49A-541-MY3, MOST 111-2314-B-075-007-MY3); and Taipei Veterans General Hospital (grant no. C19-027). The funders did not involve the design of this study. C-YL was the recipient of the funding award. The funders had no role in the study design, data collection and analysis, decision to publish, or manuscript.

## Conflict of interest

None.

## Data availability statement

Authors can confirm that all relevant data are included in the article.

## Author details

Dat Tran Cao[1,2] and Chin-Yu Lin[1,3]*

1 Heart Rhythm Center, Taipei Veteran General Hospital, Taipei, Taiwan

2 Arrhythmia Treatment Department, Cho Ray Hospital, Vietnam

3 Department of Medicine, National Yang-Ming University, Taipei, Taiwan

*Address all correspondence to: clouaa@gmail.com

## References

[1] Colilla S, Crow A, Petkun W, Singer DE, Simon T, Liu X. Estimates of current and future incidence and prevalence of atrial fibrillation in the US adult population. The American Journal of Cardiology. 2013;**112**(8):1142-1147

[2] Mou L, Norby FL, Chen LY, et al. Lifetime risk of atrial fibrillation by race and socioeconomic status: ARIC study (atherosclerosis risk in communities). Circulation: Arrhythmia and Electrophysiology. 2018;**11**(7):e006350

[3] Chao T-F, Liu C-J, Tuan T-C, et al. Lifetime risks, projected numbers, and adverse outcomes in Asian patients with atrial fibrillation: A report from the Taiwan nationwide AF cohort study. Chest. 2018;**153**(2):453-466

[4] Piccini JP, Hammill BG, Sinner MF, et al. Clinical course of atrial fibrillation in older adults: The importance of cardiovascular events beyond stroke. European Heart Journal. 2014;**35**(4):250-256

[5] Joglar JA, Chung MK, Armbruster AL, et al. 2023 ACC/AHA/ACCP/HRS guideline for the diagnosis and management of atrial fibrillation: A report of the American College of Cardiology/American Heart Association joint committee on clinical practice guidelines. Circulation. 2024;**149**(1):e1-e156

[6] Wasserlauf J, Vogel K, Whisler C, et al. Accuracy of the apple watch for detection of AF: A multicenter experience. Journal of Cardiovascular Electrophysiology. 2023;**34**(5):1103-1107

[7] Yamada S, Lin CY, Chang SL, et al. Risk of stroke in patients with short-run atrial tachyarrhythmia. Stroke. 2017;**48**(12):3232-3238. DOI: 10.1161/STROKEAHA.117.018475

[8] Healey JS, Lopes RD, Granger CB, et al. Apixaban for stroke prevention in subclinical atrial fibrillation. The New England Journal of Medicine. 2024;**390**(2):107-117. DOI: 10.1056/NEJMoa2310234

[9] Tzeis S, Gerstenfeld EP, Kalman J, et al. European heart rhythm association/Heart Rhythm Society/Asia Pacific Heart Rhythm Society/Latin American Heart Rhythm Society expert consensus statement on catheter and surgical ablation of atrial fibrillation. Europace. 2024;**26**(4):euae043. DOI: 10.1093/europace/euae043

[10] Lin CY, Lin YJ, Lo MT, et al. Efficacy of patient-specific strategy: Catheter ablation strategy of persistent atrial fibrillation based on morphological repetitiveness by periodicity and similarity. Circulation. Arrhythmia and Electrophysiology. 2021;**14**(5):e009719. DOI: 10.1161/CIRCEP.121.009719

[11] Staerk L, Sherer JA, Ko D, Benjamin EJ, Helm RH. Atrial fibrillation: Epidemiology, pathophysiology, and clinical outcomes. Circulation Research. 2017;**120**(9):1501-1517

[12] Chao TF, Joung B, Takahashi Y, et al. 2021 focused update of the 2017 consensus guidelines of the Asia Pacific Heart Rhythm Society (APHRS) on stroke prevention in atrial fibrillation. Journal of Arrhythmia. 2021;**37**(6):1389-1426. DOI: 10.1002/joa3.12652

[13] Aldaas OM, Lupercio F, Han FT, et al. Meta-analysis of effect of modest (≥ 10%) weight loss in management of overweight and obese patients with atrial

fibrillation. The American Journal of Cardiology. 2019;**124**(10):1568-1574

[14] Al-Kaisey AM, Kalman JM. Obesity and atrial fibrillation: Epidemiology, pathogenesis and effect of weight loss. Arrhythmia & Electrophysiology Review. 2021;**10**(3):159

[15] Jiang H, Mei X, Jiang Y, et al. Alcohol consumption and atrial fibrillation risk: An updated dose-response meta-analysis of over 10 million participants. Frontiers in Cardiovascular Medicine. 2022;**9**:979982

[16] Conen D, Tedrow UB, Cook NR, Moorthy M, Buring JE, Albert CM. Alcohol consumption and risk of incident atrial fibrillation in women. Journal of the American Medical Association. 2008;**300**(21):2489-2496

[17] Leopoulou M, Theofilis P, Kordalis A, et al. Diabetes mellitus and atrial fibrillation-from pathophysiology to treatment. World Journal of Diabetes. 2023;**14**(5):512

[18] Papazoglou AS, Kartas A, Samaras A, et al. Prognostic significance of diabetes mellitus in patients with atrial fibrillation. Cardiovascular Diabetology. 2021;**20**:1-11

[19] Sanchis-Gomar F, Lavie CJ. Protecting against sedentary lifestyle, left atrial enlargement and atrial fibrillation. Archives of Disease in Childhood. 2022;**9**:e001962

[20] Elliott AD, Verdicchio CV, Mahajan R, et al. An exercise and physical activity program in patients with atrial fibrillation: The ACTIVE-AF randomized controlled trial. Clinical Electrophysiology. 2023;**9**(4):455-465

[21] Chamberlain AM, Agarwal SK, Folsom AR, et al. Smoking and incidence of atrial fibrillation: Results from the atherosclerosis risk in communities (ARIC) study. Heart Rhythm. 2011;**8**(8):1160-1166

[22] Ibdah R, Obeidat O, Khader Y, et al. Validation of CHA2DS2 VASc score predictability of stroke and systemic embolization in a middle eastern population with AF: The Jordan atrial fibrillation (JoFib) study. Vascular Health and Risk Management. 2023;**19**:255-264

[23] Komen JJ, Pottegård A, Mantel-Teeuwisse AK, et al. Oral anticoagulants in patients with atrial fibrillation at low stroke risk: A multicentre observational study. European Heart Journal. 2022;**43**(37):3528-3538

[24] Goel N, Jain D, Haddad DB, Shanbhogue D. Anticoagulation in patients with end-stage renal disease and atrial fibrillation: Confusion, concerns and consequences. Journal of Stroke. 2020;**22**(3):306

[25] Davtyan KV, Kalemberg AA, Topchyan AH, Simonyan GY, Bazaeva EV, Shatahtsyan VS. Left atrial appendage occluder implantation for stroke prevention in elderly patients with atrial fibrillation: Acute and long-term results. Journal of Geriatric Cardiology: JGC. 2017;**14**(9):590

[26] Lakkireddy D, Thaler D, Ellis CR, et al. Amplatzer amulet left atrial appendage occluder versus watchman device for stroke prophylaxis (amulet IDE): A randomized, controlled trial. Circulation. 2021;**144**(19):1543-1552

[27] Zheng Y, Rao C-F, Chen S-P, He L, Hou J-F, Zheng Z. Surgical left atrial appendage occlusion in patients with atrial fibrillation undergoing mechanical heart valve replacement. Chinese Medical Journal. 2020;**133**(16):1891-1899

[28] Kirchhof P, Camm AJ, Goette A, et al. Early rhythm-control therapy in patients with atrial fibrillation. New England Journal of Medicine. 2020;**383**(14):1305-1316

[29] Rillig A, Eckardt L, Borof K, et al. Safety and efficacy of long-term sodium channel blocker therapy for early rhythm control: The EAST-AFNET 4 trial. Europace. 2024;**26**:euae121

[30] Epstein AE, Hallstrom AP, Rogers WJ, et al. Mortality following ventricular arrhythmia suppression by encainide, flecainide, and moricizine after myocardial infarction: The original design concept of the cardiac arrhythmia suppression trial (CAST). Journal of the American Medical Association. 1993;**270**(20):2451-2455

[31] Bonfanti L, Annovi A, Sanchis-Gomar F, et al. Effectiveness and safety of electrical cardioversion for acute-onset atrial fibrillation in the emergency department: A real-world 10-year single center experience. Clinical and Experimental Emergency Medicine. 2019;**6**(1):64

[32] Aymond JD, Sanchez AM, Castine MR, et al. Dual vs single cardioversion of atrial fibrillation in patients with obesity: A randomized clinical trial. JAMA Cardiology. 2024;**9**(7):641-648

[33] Investigators AFF-uIoRM. A comparison of rate control and rhythm control in patients with atrial fibrillation. New England Journal of Medicine. 2002;**347**(23):1825-1833

[34] Chen S, Meng W, SHENG HE D, et al. Blocking the pulmonary vein to left atrium conduction in addition to the entrance block enhances clinical efficacy in atrial fibrillation ablation. Pacing and Clinical Electrophysiology. 2012;**35**(5):524-531

[35] Gurevitz O, Friedman PA. Pulmonary vein exit-block during radio-frequency ablation of paroxysmal atrial fibrillation. Circulation. 2002;**105**(17):e124-e125

[36] Vroomen M, Maesen B, Luermans JL, et al. Epicardial and endocardial validation of conduction block after thoracoscopic epicardial ablation of atrial fibrillation. Innovations. 2020;**15**(6):525-531

[37] Sousa PA, Barra S, Saleiro C, et al. Ostial vs. wide area circumferential ablation guided by the ablation index in paroxysmal atrial fibrillation. Europace. 2023;**25**(6):euad160

[38] Di Cori A, Parollo M, Gentile F, et al. Short and long-term outcomes of lesion index-guided high-power short-duration approach for atrial fibrillation ablation. Journal of Clinical Medicine. 2023;**12**(15):4986

[39] Segan L, Chieng D, Prabhu S, et al. Posterior wall isolation improves outcomes for persistent AF with rapid posterior wall activity: CAPLA substudy. Clinical Electrophysiology. 2023;**9**(12):2536-2546

[40] Darby AE. Recurrent atrial fibrillation after catheter ablation: Considerations for repeat ablation and strategies to optimize success. Journal of Atrial Fibrillation. 2016;**9**(1):1427

[41] Proietti R, Hadjis A, AlTurki A, et al. A systematic review on the progression of paroxysmal to persistent atrial fibrillation: Shedding new light on the effects of catheter ablation. JACC: Clinical Electrophysiology. 2015;**1**(3):105-115

[42] Li K, Xu C, Zhu X, et al. Multi-Centre, prospective randomized comparison of three different substrate ablation strategies for

persistent atrial fibrillation. Europace. 2023;**25**(5):euad090

[43] O'Neill L, Almorad A, El Haddad M, et al. Impact of catheter ablation on arrhythmia burden in patients with shock-resistant persistent atrial fibrillation. Clinical Electrophysiology. 2023;**9**(10):2071-2081

[44] Lin CY, Lin YJ, Narayan SM, et al. Comparison of phase mapping and electrogram-based driver mapping for catheter ablation in atrial fibrillation. Pacing and Clinical Electrophysiology. 2019;**42**(2):216-223. DOI: 10.1111/pace.13573

[45] Lin CY, Lin YJ, Higa S, et al. Catheter ablation with morphologic repetitiveness mapping for persistent atrial fibrillation. JAMA Network Open. 2023;**6**(11):e2344535. DOI: 10.1001/jamanetworkopen.2023.44535

[46] Higa S, Tai CT, Chen SA. Catheter ablation of atrial fibrillation originating from extrapulmonary vein areas: Taipei approach. Heart Rhythm. 2006;**3**(11):1386-1390. DOI: 10.1016/j.hrthm.2006.09.006

[47] Higa S, Lo L-W, Chen S-A. Catheter ablation of paroxysmal atrial fibrillation originating from non-pulmonary vein areas. Arrhythmia & Electrophysiology Review. 2018;**7**(4):273

[48] Matsunaga-Lee Y, Egami Y, Matsumoto S, et al. Electrophysiological characteristics of non-pulmonary vein triggers excluding origins from the superior vena cava and left atrial posterior wall: Lessons from the self-reference mapping technique. PLoS One. 2022;**17**(4):e0263938

[49] Packer DL, Piccini JP, Monahan KH, et al. Ablation versus drug therapy for atrial fibrillation in heart failure: Results from the CABANA trial. Circulation. 2021;**143**(14):1377-1390

[50] Siow YK, Lin CY, Chung FP, et al. Catheter ablation in patients with atrial fibrillation and dilated cardiomyopathy. Frontiers in Cardiovascular Medicine. 2024;**11**:1305485. DOI: 10.3389/fcvm.2024.1305485

[51] Bautista JAL, Lin CY, Lu CT, et al. Clinical significance of substrate characteristics and ablation outcomes in patients with atrial fibrillation and significant functional mitral regurgitation. Frontiers in Cardiovascular Medicine. 2023;**10**:1265890. DOI: 10.3389/fcvm.2023.1265890

[52] Oraii A, McIntyre WF, Parkash R, et al. Atrial fibrillation ablation in heart failure with reduced vs preserved ejection fraction: A systematic review and meta-analysis. JAMA Cardiology. 2024;**9**(6):545-555

[53] Sohns C, Fox H, Marrouche NF, et al. Catheter ablation in end-stage heart failure with atrial fibrillation. New England Journal of Medicine. 2023;**389**(15):1380-1389

[54] Kuck K-H, Brugada J, Fürnkranz A, et al. Cryoballoon or radiofrequency ablation for paroxysmal atrial fibrillation. New England Journal of Medicine. 2016;**374**(23):2235-2245

[55] Andrade JG, Champagne J, Dubuc M, et al. Cryoballoon or radiofrequency ablation for atrial fibrillation assessed by continuous monitoring: A randomized clinical trial. Circulation. 2019;**140**(22):1779-1788

[56] Reddy VY, Gerstenfeld EP, Natale A, et al. Pulsed field or conventional thermal ablation for paroxysmal atrial fibrillation. New England Journal of Medicine. 2023;**389**(18):1660-1671

[57] Alobaida M, Alrumayh A. Rate control strategies for atrial fibrillation. Annals of Medicine. 2021;**53**(1):682-692

**Chapter 2**

# How Does Atrial Fibrillation Cause Development of Atrial Thrombosis and Subsequent Thromboembolism?

*Vincent J.B. Robinson, Gyanendra K. Sharma, Rohan Sharma, Lauren Chow, James Harris Calhoun, Mikhil Patel, Soham Kulkarni, Kuang-Drew Li and Jeffrey A. Switzer*

## Abstract

Atrial fibrillation is the most common arrhythmia and carries a substantial risk for embolic stroke which can be significantly mitigated by anticoagulant therapy. In this chapter, we review the epidemiology of atrial fibrillation and the biologic antecedents leading to atrial fibrillation. We then comment on the interaction between atrial fibrillation and atrial cardiopathy. We will explore the question of whether atrial cardiopathy alone can produce embolic stroke. We hope the reader will then focus on the expanding surge of atrial fibrillation closely aligned with the increasing burden of embolic stroke. There are additional cardioembolic strokes that appear to occur in the presence of atrial cardiopathy without the onset of atrial fibrillation. Promising new markers are available for predicting atrial cardiopathy and hence guiding treatment for initiation of DOACs. This has the potential to prevent many embolic strokes before they occur. Another missed clinical opportunity is aggressively targeting diastolic dysfunction with ACE-I, AT2 blockers, and MRAs to prevent the development of advanced atrial cardiopathy and subsequent embolic stroke and atrial fibrillation.

**Keywords:** left atrial cardiopathy, cardiac thromboembolism, embolic stroke, atrial fibrillation, diastolic dysfunction, $CHA_2DS_2$-VAsc score, plasma D-dimer, brain natriuretic peptide (BNP), N-terminal pro b-type natriuretic peptide (NT-proBNP), dilated left atrium, embolic stroke of undetermined source (ESUS), inflammation

## 1. Introduction

Atrial fibrillation (AF) is the most common arrhythmia, occurring with increasing frequency in the aging population. The incidence of AF is approximately 17% in patients over the age of 85 [1]. AF also afflicts younger individuals who have heart failure and other causes of diastolic dysfunction. What makes AF so important for clinicians is the associated risk of cardioembolic stroke, which has one of the highest rates of recurrence out of all ischemic stroke subtypes [2]. Some studies have sought to link the likelihood of embolic stroke to the duration of AF [3]. Although this seems to be an intuitive approach, more recent studies have shown that atrial thrombosis and subsequent thromboembolism can occur with atrial cardiopathy even in the absence of AF [4, 5]. In this chapter, we will review the epidemiology of AF and its pathophysiological correlates, the different theories for the development of AF, the conditions that lead to the formation of left atrial (LA)/left atrial appendage (LAA) thrombus, and finally we will show that risk scores applied equally are predictive of stroke in patients with and without AF. This may lead us to consider whether atrial cardiopathy is the underlying cause of embolic stroke and precursor of (trigger/perpetuation) AF. In this chapter, we will take an in-depth look at atrial cardiopathy and the relationship between AF and cardioembolic stroke.

## 2. Epidemiological studies on the prevalence of atrial fibrillation

AF is the most ubiquitous arrhythmia in humans. The lifetime risk of AF is estimated between 20 and 33% varying based on race [6]. The risk of AF also increases with age. The overall prevalence of AF in the Rotterdam study was 5.5%, with 0.7% in subjects 55–59 years of age, increasing up to 17.8% in subjects aged 85 and older [1]. However, many individuals do not follow this trajectory because of other risk factors of AF such as valvular heart disease, pulmonary embolism, chronic obstructive pulmonary disease (COPD), and obesity.

In the Framingham Heart Study ($n = 4731$), 562 subjects developed AF during the 38 year follow-up period [7]. The risk for AF increased with each decade of age (2.1 for men and 2.2 for women, $p < 0.0001$), however, men had an overall 1.5 times increased risk for AF compared to women when adjusting for age and multiple risk factors [7]. In both men and women, diabetes, hypertension, congestive heart failure and valve disease were risk factors significantly associated with AF. In the Rotterdam study, the lifetime risk of AF for men was 23.8% and for women was 22.2% at 55 years of age [1]. After age 75, the lifetime risk decreased for men and women. In Olmstead county, subject data ($n = 4618$) suggested the incidence of AF was 3.68 per 1000 person-years (95% CI, 3.42–3.95, $p = 0.008$ for trend) in the year 2000 [8]. However, more recent data from electronic medical records of over 500,000 patients suggests that the incidence may be increasing. The incidence of AF per 1000 person-years increased significantly from 4.74 in 2006 (95% CI, 4.58–4.90) to 6.82 in 2018 (95% CI, 6.65–7.00) ($p < 0.001$) [9]. This may be due to the increase in the prevalence of risk factors like hypertension, obesity (BMI $\geq$ 30), and diabetes [9].

Beyond demographic descriptors, investigators have developed antecedent biologic conditions which are associated with the development of new AF. These fall into three groups as described below.

## 3. Antecedents of AF

### 3.1 Diastolic dysfunction

Epidemiologic studies of populations that develop AF have routinely identified markers of diastolic dysfunction and associated LA enlargement (LAE) as predictors for AF beyond increasing age. Echocardiographic data from the Framingham Heart

Study (n = 1924) by Vaziri et al. revealed that atrial and ventricular abnormalities predict nonrheumatic AF [10]. The subjects (59–90 years old) underwent echocardiography and were assessed during follow-up visits for a mean time of 7.2 years and had an overall incidence of 8% of developing AF. After adjustment for clinical characteristics, three echocardiographic predictors; LA size (HR per 5 mm increment, 1.39; 95% CI, 1.14–1.68; p = 0.001), left ventricular fractional shortening (HR per 5% decrement, 1.34; 95% CI, 1.08–1.66; p = 0.007) and left ventricular wall thickness (HR per 4 mm increment, 1.28; 95% CI, 1.03–1.60, p = 0.028), displayed both a dose-response relationship and an additive relationship for AF. There was a 4.6-fold age-adjusted increase in risk for developing AF when two or more of the highest-quartile echocardiographic predictors were present. Vaziri acknowledged that the presence of these risk markers "does not necessarily imply causality" and that "these features may simply be markers for unidentified factors that are causally related to the development of atrial fibrillation" [10]. What was clear from their study was the increased risk of AF in populations with cardiac structural abnormalities generally associated with worsening diastolic function.

A retrospective study by Tsang et al. confirmed that LAE is predictive of AF [11]. This retrospective cohort study (n = 1655) used transthoracic echocardiogram (TTE) data from subjects aged 65 and older with no history of AF. Development of AF occurred in 11.4% of the cohort and these subjects were more likely to be older and have more comorbidities. Risk stratification by quartiles of LA diameter and volume suggested that volume may be a more sensitive variable within the lowest quartile of dimension for AF. LA volume quartiles predicted risk at 3%, 12%, 15%, and 26% respectively for AF in a Cox 5-year cumulative risk model. After adjusting for clinical characteristics, a 30% increase in LA volume was associated with a 43% increased risk for AF. [11]. Tsang suggested that aging patients with cardiovascular risks are likely to develop diastolic dysfunction leading to increased LA filling pressures, atrial stretch, and atrial enlargement, increasing the risk for AF. Significant baseline clinical predictors of AF in their multivariate clinical model included age, hypertension, valvular heart disease, myocardial infarction, and congestive heart failure. There is a clear overlap between diseases associated with diastolic dysfunction and those significantly associated with the development of AF. LA volume was a significantly strong predictor for the development of AF and may be valuable if incorporated into risk prediction models for AF.

Tiwari et al. conducted a prospective study (n = 2406) and found that LA size was a significant predictor for the development of AF in both sexes [12]. Echocardiographic and mitral Doppler parameters were used as surrogates for diastolic dysfunction. In a multivariate analysis, a moderately enlarged LA (2.2–2.79 cm/$m^2$) compared to normal-sized LA (<2.2 cm/$m^2$) was significantly associated with the risk for AF (HR 1.6, 95% CI, 1.2–2.0, p linear trend <0.001). The risk for developing AF increased in the subjects with severely enlarged LA (≥2.8 cm/$m^2$) compared to normal-sized LA (HR 4.2, 95% CI 2.7–6.5, p linear trend <0.0001). There was no association between mitral Doppler indices of diastolic dysfunction and AF independent of LA size, however, abnormal mitral Doppler flow had a 30% (95% CI, 1.0–1.6, p = 0.034) increased risk of AF when adjusted for LA size compared to subjects with normal flow. Mitral Doppler indices are a more acute measurement of diastolic dysfunction compared to LA size which is a more stable, chronic representation of diastolic dysfunction and subsequent atrial remodeling.

Edwards et al. also found a significant association between LAE and the risk of future AF [4]. In a cohort of 32,454 subjects aged 65 and older, LAE and excessive atrial ectopy (markers of atrial cardiopathy) were measured, and subjects were followed to determine associations between these markers and patient outcomes (ischemic stroke, incident AF, and death). LAE measured by 10 mm increases was significantly associated with the development of AF at 2 and 5 years ($p < 0.0001$).

The prevalence of AF is consistently linked to enlargement of the LA in populations regardless of age. Left ventricular diastolic dysfunction has negative implications on the mechanics of the LA via increased afterload, atrial stretching, and stress on the wall, all of which alter cellular mechanisms of the atria which can lead to AF [13]. Studies of populations that develop AF are pointing towards a common factor, atrial cardiopathy. This is what Vaziri alluded to regarding LA and ventricular abnormalities possibly being markers of an unknown factor that increases the risk of developing AF [10].

Many diseases are associated with development of AF, and linked to diastolic dysfunction and subsequent atrial remodeling, thus leading to atrial cardiopathy. This concept will be investigated further in this chapter, however we will first discuss other causes of AF, besides diastolic dysfunction, as AF is a heterogenous disease and the multitude of factors that can cause AF may also play a role in the pathogenesis of thrombus formation.

### 3.2 Inflammation

While many inflammatory conditions have been correlated with AF and thromboembolic stroke, the exact mechanism behind this relationship is not well understood, and is a major focus of recent research. Sogaard and Skjoth showed a correlation between the inflammation caused by pneumonia and new-onset AF, ultimately leading to an increased risk of thromboembolism and all-cause mortality [14]. Xiao and Chen investigated how sepsis is related to AF, providing evidence that inflammation from sepsis causes myocardial necrosis and electrical instability in myocytes. Specifically, the study found the rate of new-onset AF varied from 1.9% for mild sepsis to 46% for septic shock [15]. This difference can be explained by the correlation of severity of sepsis, and inflammation. Additionally, new-onset AF is well known to occur in post-operative patients due to the high inflammatory burden. In a meta analysis, Baker et al. showed that reducing inflammation with N-acetylcysteine leads to a significant decrease in the number of patients developing new-onset AF after cardiothoracic surgery [16].

Recent studies have aimed to identify the myocardial biochemical and structural changes caused by inflammation. Guadino showed that Interleukin-6 (IL-6) is linked with postoperative AF while C-reactive protein (CRP) is linked with post and non-postoperative AF [17]. Schnabel identified a relationship between a multitude of inflammatory markers and AF [18]. Ways to reduce inflammation have also been a focus of recent studies. For instance, utilizing N-acetylcysteine to reduce inflammation and oxidative stress from cardiac surgery has been shown to significantly reduce the incidence of AF [16, 19].

The anti-inflammatory drug colchicine has also been investigated for atrial fibrillation prevention. In a recent meta-analysis of subjects 18 years of age and older, colchicine, compared to placebo, was shown to prevent AF (RR: 0.75, 95% CI: 0.68–0.83, $P < 0.001$) [20]. The study population included patients who were post-pulmonary vein isolation (PVI) or ablation, post-cardiac surgery, post non-cardiac thoracic surgery, and patients with myocardial infarction or coronary disease. Of the patients who received colchicine, 6.6% had AF whereas 9% of those receiving the placebo had AF. Colchicine was effective in all age groups in the study and was effective for first-onset of AF and recurrent AF ((RR:0.79, 95% CI:0.64–0.97) and (RR: 0.66, 95% CI:0.54–0.81) respectively) [20]. No data was provided on the efficacy of colchicine based on sex, which may be a limitation of the meta-analysis lacking access to individual patient data.

Although there are not many randomized prospective clinical trials on inflammation as an antecedent of AF, the available data clearly points out that inflammation can facilitate the development of AF in most patients. Adjunctive therapy to counteract inflammatory-derived AF has not been delineated but colchicine and N-acetylcysteine show promise.

### 3.3 Catecholamine surges

Catecholamine surges may induce AF in some patients. The mechanism is likely through the α- and β-adrenergic, dopamine receptor agonist [21]. Catecholamine surges have implications on calcium levels however the exact mechanisms are still unclear, specifically which mechanism is the leading cause of AF [22]. Post-operative AF is a common complication of cardiac surgery and the mechanisms that induce arrhythmia in these patients are likely different from the mechanisms in the general population. Many of the studies on catecholamine-induced AF are acute studies with small cohorts, so overall data is limited.

Higher intrinsic catecholamines (adrenergic tone) levels before surgery are predictive of post-op AF. Anderson et al. studied plasma monoamine oxidase (MAO-B), dopamine (DE), epinephrine (EPI), and norepinephrine (NE) levels in 324 pre-op patients who were scheduled to have coronary artery bypass grafting or aortic valve surgery with cardiopulmonary bypass and were monitored for AF [23]. There was a significant, positive association between plasma NE (unadjusted RR: 2.0; $p = 0.0006$) and EPI (unadjusted RR: 1.5; $p = 0.047$) in the fourth quartiles. Dopamine had an inverse relationship (unadjusted RR: 2.2; $p = 0.0034$) significant to post-op AF in the fourth quartile. After controlling for clinical characteristics, patients with plasma NE levels in the fourth quartile were most likely to have post-operative AF, and patients with DE levels in the fourth quartile were least likely to develop post-operative AF. These parameters, when combined, were significantly associated with a four-fold increase in post-op AF (adjusted $p = 0.0001$). The inverse relationship observed with DE was unexpected but may be explained by the rapid conversion of NE in some patients leading to a low level of DA, differing rates of re-uptake in some patients, or a higher rate of metabolism of DA than NE. Notably, catecholamines induce oxidative stress as a result of their inotropic effect, which may link the catecholamine surge hypothesis of post-operative AF to the inflammatory surge hypothesis.

There is also evidence that an extrinsic source of catecholamine surge from IV medication may induce AF. A randomized controlled trial enrolled patients with vasoplegic shock to receive either vasopressin ($n = 149$) or norepinephrine ($n = 153$) [24]. Incident AF was measured as a secondary outcome at the end of 30 days, and Hajjar et al. found that the patients who received vasopressin had a lower incidence of AF than those who received norepinephrine (95 [63.8%] vs. 124 [82.1%]; adjusted OR, 0.37; 95% CI, 0.22–0.64; $p = 0.0004$). If norepinephrine increases atrial ectopic activity and adrenergic stimuli, thus inducing AF, then this pathway is a possible trigger for AF. It may be that catecholamine surges provide additional oxidative stress and inflammation in post-operative situations. Hence, catecholamine surges may be part of the inflammatory hypothesis.

## 4. Atrial cardiopathy

### 4.1 Description of atrial cardiopathy

We have reviewed epidemiological studies of AF, which consistently showed that LAE, a result of diastolic dysfunction, is a significant, independent predictor for the development of AF. The term atrial cardiopathy has been used to describe various atrial-specific changes that occur before the onset of atrial fibrillation. Atrial cardiopathy (cardiomyopathy) is defined as: "Any complex of structural, architectural, contractile or electrophysiological changes affecting the atria with the potential to produce clinically-relevant manifestations" [25]. In other words, atrial cardiopathy is any structural or electrical remodeling of the atria that may precede a clinically relevant diagnosis such as AF. Atrial cardiopathy, by definition, is a seemingly heterogeneous condition that may be caused by diastolic dysfunction, aging, hypertension, obesity, diabetes, valvular heart diseases like mitral stenosis, mitral regurgitation, and obstructive sleep apnea (OSA), many of which also are associated with AF [25]. These factors cause an increase in LA pressure and LA size, even in patients with OSA which initially was thought to only affect right-sided heart structures [26]. Therefore, LAE and associated structural changes such as fibrosis, as a result of remodeling, is the primary lesion of atrial cardiopathy.

The EHRAS histological classification may be used to explain the underlying cause/causes of atrial cardiopathy. The 4 classes differentiate between 1) primarily cardiomyocyte dependent (lone AF and diabetes mellitus), 2) primarily fibroblast dependent (aging and cigarette smoking), 3) mixed cardiomyocyte-fibroblast dependent (Congestive heart failure and valvular disease), and 4) primarily non-collagen deposit cardiopathy (isolated atrial amyloidosis and granulomatosis) [25]. This classification scheme may help to determine the pathology of the cardiopathy, however, the challenge with a histological classification is that it requires an invasive procedure to obtain a biopsy. Other critiques include the likelihood of overlap between the classes and that there is no clinical endpoint in terms of how the patient should be managed based on their histology [27]. We acknowledge that the contributions of histological tissue type are useful in predicting the onset and perpetuation of AF in different patients; however, histology is difficult to access, especially in a clinical situation. In contrast, the onset and development of diastolic dysfunction can be easily assessed by LA size or LA pressure.

There are currently no standardized diagnostic criteria for atrial cardiopathy. A variety of diagnostic techniques and imaging modalities have been used to evaluate patients for atrial cardiopathy, and coupled with the fact that the availability of these diagnostic tools is resource-dependent, there are many different markers used in current research. Markers of atrial cardiopathy can be categorized as electrical, structural/mechanical, and biochemical [28, 29]. Common ECG parameters include P-wave terminal force in lead V1 (PTFV1) [30] (which is associated with atrial enlargement in patients with valvular disease [31], ischemic stroke [32, 33] and left ventricular diastolic dysfunction [34]) and P-wave duration (increased in patients with obesity [35] and associated with ischemic stroke [36]). Serum biomarkers can be used to assess inflammation and myocyte stretch. Echocardiographic markers including increased LA volume and diameter, as previously discussed in this chapter, are associated with risk for AF. Epidemiologically, one common pathway among many of these markers for atrial cardiopathy is increased LA pressure and subsequent increased LA size.

The prevalence of atrial cardiopathy in the general population without AF may be better understood if measured with more specific biomarkers. A cohort study by Johnson et al. (n = 385) evaluated subjects free of AF for the presence of atrial cardiopathy by either P-wave duration, LA volume index (LAVi), or premature atrial contractions (PAC) frequency [37]. Results showed that 42% of the subjects had at least one marker present, but despite the high prevalence, only 9% of the population had 2 markers present and 0.3% had 3 markers present. Clinical correlates associated with PACs were current smoking, systolic blood pressure, diabetes, and coronary artery disease, whereas increased physical activity was associated with LAVi and BMI was associated with P-wave duration. Limitations of this study include a relatively young population (average age of 57 years old) and a low rate of heart failure in the population (less than 1%). More research is needed to understand the relationship between the presence of these markers and the incidence of future AF. However, Johnson's study did show that each marker was associated with different clinical correlates, therefore based on these comorbidities, most of the patients likely had some degree of diastolic dysfunction. An editorial comment on this study remarked on how due to the high prevalence of at least one atrial cardiopathy marker in the healthy population, the criteria for defining atrial cardiopathy may have been too lenient [38]. On the other hand, citing the Framingham data, the risk of AF in the general population is 37%, meaning that Johnson's data may not be too far from illustrating the risk of AF in the general population [38]. Johnson's study appears to identify populations who would be at risk for atrial cardiopathy and subsequent development of AF. Prospective follow-up of the population to see if AF occurs in a significant number would be important to confirm. Given the easy availability of Brain natriuretic peptide (BNP) and N-terminal pro b-type natriuretic peptide (NT-proBNP) at this point, any future prospective evaluation for atrial cardiopathy must include serum biomarkers such as these measures, however their limitations will also be reviewed in this chapter. The current gold standard for measuring LA size is the echocardiographic bi-plane method, however, future research is needed to assess if any improvement is provided by tomographic methods [39].

Atrial cardiopathy is a term used to describe atrial remodeling and evidence suggests that it is present before the onset of AF in most patients. Histological typing to determine the pathophysiologic cause of atrial cardiopathy may be clinically relevant but is not very accessible for the day-to-day management of the patient. There are many different markers used in current studies to evaluate atrial cardiopathy. Many of these markers are surrogates for LAE. Biomarkers to assess LA pressure are available and will be reviewed later in this chapter.

### 4.2 Atrial cardiopathy in recurrence and maintenance of atrial fibrillation

Diastolic dysfunction resulting in atrial cardiopathy appears to be a main cause of developing AF. It is also likely that atrial cardiopathy is a primary mechanism for sustaining the arrhythmia. The pulmonary veins are a common source of AF triggers, however other arrhythmias and the autonomic nervous system may also be sources of triggers [40]. Once the trigger fires and the arrhythmia is established, abnormalities in the atria maintain the rhythm. Mechanisms include atrial remodeling, electrical remodeling, fibrosis, inflammation and oxidative stress [40]. The common pathway among many of these mechanisms is atrial cardiopathy. Atrial cardiopathy as the maintenance mechanism for AF may explain the recurrence of AF post-catheter ablation and associated with hospitalization.

A systematic review and meta-analysis investigated LA stiffness as a predictor for AF recurrence after catheter ablation [41]. In the three articles used in the final analysis, LA stiffness was a significant independent predictor of AF (HR = 3.55, 95% CI 1.75–4.73, p = 0.0002). This was a small meta-analysis that only used observational studies and more research is needed to determine the relationship between LA stiffness and AF development and recurrence. However, the results of this study suggest that if LA stiffness could be measured non-invasively in patients before ablation, then clinicians may be able to determine the likelihood of arrhythmia recurrence.

Atrial fibrosis is another characteristic of atrial cardiopathy and a possible substrate for AF. The DECAAF study by Marrouche et al. investigated the relationship between atrial fibrosis and catheter ablation outcomes in patients with AF [42]. All subjects (n = 260) received delayed enhancement MRI scans before undergoing first-time ablation for AF. The quantity of fibrosis was categorized into stages based on the percentage of atrial wall that was fibrosed. Patients were monitored at 3, 6, and 12 months from the time of ablation. Of the demographic and clinical factors studied, only percent of atrial fibrosis (per 1% increase: (HR 1.06, 95% CI, 1.03–1.08; P < 0.001) and history of mitral valve disease (HR 3.45, 95% CI, 1.78–6.68; P < 0.001) were statistically significant to recurrent AF [42]. The quantity of fibrosis may be used to evaluate which patients will benefit from ablation, and predict which patients are most likely to experience recurrent arrhythmia.

However, treating this fibrosis as attempted in the DECAAF II study, did not result in any improvement in clinical endpoints and could worsen patient outcomes [43]. The DECAAF II study evaluated pulmonary vein isolation (PVI) versus PVI plus MRI-guided fibrosis ablation for the treatment of AF. There was no significant difference between the two groups for AF recurrence. The PVI plus fibrosis-guided ablation group experienced significantly higher safety events (9 [2.2%] vs. 0 in the PVI group; P = 0.001). One possible explanation for the higher rate of ischemic stroke in the fibrosis-guided group is the increased injury due to ablation and overall increased procedure time which may increase the risk for overall complications. Results from the DECAAF study demonstrate the association between fibrosis and the likelihood of recurrent arrhythmia, however, the results from DECAAF II currently do not support targeting fibrosis directly as a way to prevent AF recurrence. An important clinical implication of this information is consideration for an early intervention for rhythm control before progression of fibrosis and worsening atrial cardiopathy.

LAE may also be a predictor for AF recurrence. A study by McIntyre et al. investigated AF occurring transiently with stress in hospitalized patients and the risk for recurrent AF [44]. Patients who experienced transient new-onset AF during hospitalization for either noncardiac surgery (n = 69) or medical illness (n = 70) were included and matched to patients hospitalized for either surgery or illness who did not experience transient AF. After one year, recurrent AF occurred in 33.1% (95% CI, 25.3% to 40.9%) of the patients who experienced transient AF in the hospital, and 5.0% (CI, 1.4% to 8.7%) of matched control participants. McIntyre and colleagues make an important note about their findings, "this study has important implications for management of patients who have a first presentation of AF that is concurrent with a reversible physiologic stressor. An AF recurrence risk of 33.1% at 1 year is neither low enough to conclude that transient new-onset AF in the setting of another illness is benign nor high enough that all such transient new-onset AF can be assumed to be paroxysmal AF. Instead, these results call for risk stratification and follow-up in these patients" [44]. The only clinical feature that this study identified as being associated with risk for AF recurrence in the follow-up was LA size. The primacy of atrial cardiopathy, as evidenced by LA size, was the main predictor for AF recurrence. Meta-analyses have also found that LAE, measured by LA volume, is a predictor for AF recurrence after ablation [45, 46].

In patients with atrial cardiopathy, fibrosis and increased LA size are substrates for the arrhythmia and are predictive of AF recurrence. Atrial cardiopathy is not only a predictor for AF, but also a mechanism to perpetuate the arrhythmia.

### 4.3 Atrial fibrillation as a cause of diastolic dysfunction

There is a clear association between diastolic dysfunction as a precursor for atrial cardiopathy and AF. Additionally, diastolic function can also worsen as a result of AF. Patients who have gradual increases in diastolic dysfunction may develop adaptive atrial responses where with atrial hypertrophy increasing amounts of stroke volume are attributed to LA contraction. The normal contribution of LA contraction to stroke volume is 20% which can increase to closer to 60% in patients with severe aortic stenosis or mitral stenosis [47]. At the same time, atrial cardiopathy is increasing in severity with increasing LA size, stretch, and fibrosis. When these patients develop AF, there is a sudden loss of the atrial contribution to stroke volume and diastolic function worsens acutely. This generally leads to severe clinical deterioration in the patient's condition with reduced left ventricular ejection fraction (LVEF), hypotension, and pulmonary edema.

Patients with mitral or aortic stenosis and concomitant AF experience worsening hemodynamics and a decrease in diastolic function leading to worse outcomes. Laenens et al. investigated whether AF is the cause of cardiac remodeling in patients with aortic stenosis or if LV diastolic dysfunction plays a significant role [48]. In this study on patients with aortic stenosis ($n = 2849$), 24.1% had a history of AF. After 10 years, the mortality rate in the AF group was significantly greater than those with aortic stenosis in sinus rhythm (46.8% vs. 36.8%; log-rank $P < 0.001$). Multivariate models were created to then determine the independent prognostic value of AF with patient mortality. Laenens determined that "AF is independently associated with outcomes when correcting for age, comorbidities, LV systolic function, LV mass, and RV systolic function. However, when additionally correcting for LV diastolic function (using E/e', LAVI, or both), AF is no longer an independent prognostic marker. These findings imply that AF is a surrogate for LV diastolic function" [48]. Clinical implications of diastolic dysfunction in these patients include the increased likelihood of cardiac remodeling which may warrant further work-up. In another study with patients who have rheumatic mitral stenosis, LA strain (OR 7.53 [4.47–12.69], $p < 0.001$) was significantly associated with atrial fibrillation [49]. LA strain is an indirect measure of diastolic function [50].

AF can lead to tachycardia-induced left ventricular cardiomyopathy [51]. This condition is treatable with pharmacological intervention and rate and rhythm control [51]. In a small study, BNP was found to have significantly decreased in patients with AF after undergoing successful cardioversion ($p < 0.05$) [52]. Another small study found that restoration to sinus rhythm after cardioversion improves LA reservoir strain ($p < 0.0001$) via restoring LA active strain ($p < 0.0001$) [53].

Hence, it can be implied from the above studies that onset of AF is a marker for acute deterioration of diastolic function. AF can lead to LV dysfunction and worsening diastolic function which can be corrected with cardioversion.

### 4.4 Which comes first, atrial fibrillation or atrial cardiopathy?

Left atrial cardiopathy and AF are closely related, but there is a controversy on whether AF is merely a marker of atrial cardiopathy. Atrial cardiopathy can predispose individuals to AF by altering atrial tissue properties. Structural abnormalities such as fibrosis and dilation in the atrium create a substrate that facilitates the initiation and perpetuation of abnormal electrical impulses, thereby increasing the risk of AF. Bamen et al. acknowledged that "identification of atrial cardiopathy and its features carry clinical implications, including elevating a patient's risk for development of AF, as well as associations with outcomes related to catheter-based and surgical AF ablation" [54]. The presence of incidental AF found on monitoring devices (subclinical AF), particularly a higher burden, is significantly correlated with an increased thromboembolic risk [55]. Therefore, the presumption exists that subclinical AF may be an early manifestation of atrial cardiopathy with increased risk of stroke and not the underlying cause of thromboembolic events [55]. "Lone" AF is also discussed as a possible marker of an existing atrial cardiopathy. "Lone" AF is diagnosed when there is no underlying explanation and other facilitating comorbidities [25].

On the other hand, AF leads to AF and thus most likely promotes atrial cardiopathy, as AF per se can also cause atrial remodeling due to changes in ion channels and the development of atrial fibrosis. This mechanism conversely leads to the perpetuation of AF and progression from lower to higher AF burden. Whereas very brief AF episodes do not alter the degree of fibrosis, longer-lasting AF episodes may cause AF-induced atrial cardiopathy [25]. AF and atrial cardiopathy are closely related conditions, but their exact relationship, and which comes first, can vary depending on individual cases, and can be bidirectional and complex as illustrated in **Figure 1** [28]. There are also worsening hemodynamic effects due to preexisting diastolic dysfunction in the presence of AF, especially with uncontrolled ventricular rates [56]. Tachycardia induced cardiomyopathy and the lack of synchronized atrial contribution to stroke volume results in ever increasing LA pressures and hence acceleration of atrial

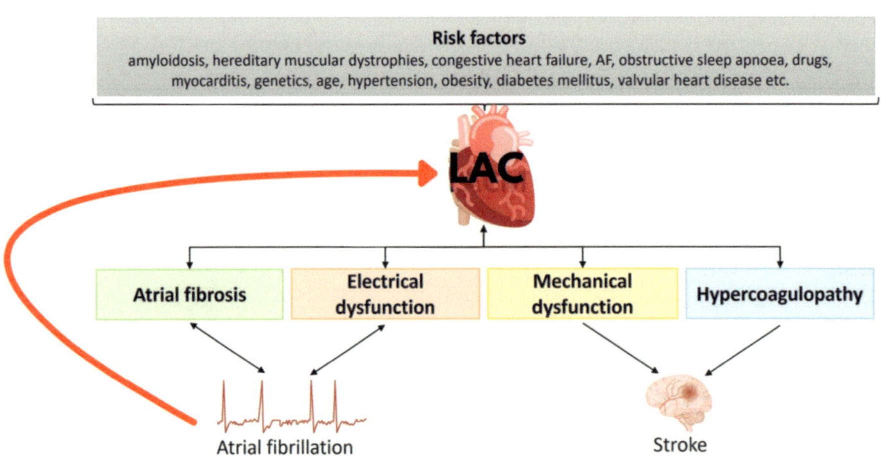


**Figure 1.**
*Adapted and modified from Kreimer F, Gotzmann M. Left Atrial Cardiomyopathy – A Challenging Diagnosis. Front Cardiovasc Med. 2022. CC-BY. Figure illustrates the relationship between risk factors, left atrial cardiopathy (LAC), and AF and stroke. The red arrow pointing from AF to left atrial cardiopathy demonstrates the feedback loop from AF that causes worsening and progression of atrial cardiopathy caused by AF.*

cardiopathy [57]. Presence of risk factors resulting in diastolic dysfunction will lead to atrial cardiopathy. This process is accelerated in the presence of AF with or without uncontrolled ventricular response.

LA cardiopathy is a significant precursor to AF. Early recognition and intervention can prevent the progression to AF and its associated complications. Advances in imaging and diagnostic techniques are crucial for the timely identification and management of atrial cardiopathy, ultimately improving patient outcomes. The advent of BNP measurements as a reliable marker of elevated LA pressure provides a precise target for lowering BNP to prevent subsequent atrial cardiopathy.

## 5. Can we prevent atrial fibrillation and does this also reduce stroke incidence?

### 5.1 The role of pharmacologic therapy on atrial fibrillation prevention and mitigation of atrial fibrillation-related embolic stroke

We have now established that atrial cardiopathy is a likely precursor for AF in most patients, and additionally, that atrial cardiopathy can develop or worsen as a result of AF. Angiotensin II is an important factor in the regulation of blood pressure, cardiac hypertrophy, and fibroblast proliferation, all of which can lead to increased risk for AF via direct Angiotensin II's effects. Angiotensin Converting Enzyme-inhibitors (ACE-I) and Angiotensin Receptor Blockers (ARBs) can suppress AF, particularly in those patients with congestive heart failure and left ventricular dysfunction and/or hypertrophy by reducing LA pressure [58, 59]. In particular, increased levels of ACE and Angiotensin II are the result of atrial remodeling, and studies have shown ACE-I and ARBs may directly reduce fibroblast growth [60]. Therefore, ACE-I and ARBs can be used clinically to prevent new-onset AF and recurrence of existing AF [59].

Current medical treatments for AF include combinations of anticoagulation and anti-arrhythmic medications (rate or rhythm control) in addition to lifestyle modifications. However, such interventions are prescribed after the onset of AF. Many recent trials have proven the importance of the use of ACE-I and ARBs in the prevention and reduction of the incidence of AF clinically. One Taiwanese study utilizing over 25,000 patient records found users of ACE-I (adjusted HR: 0.53, 95% CI 0.47–0.59, $P < 0.001$) and ARBs (adjusted HR: 0.51, 95% CI 0.44–0.58, $P < 0.001$) had lower rates of new-onset AF compared with non-users [61]. Furthermore, the use of ACE-I and ARBs can be targeted to patients with an increased risk of developing AF. One meta-analysis with 56,000 patients found that ACE-I and ARBs significantly reduced the relative risk of AF, particularly among those patients with heart failure (relative risk reduction [RRR] = 44%, $p = 0.007$) [62]. The CHARM trials also found a reduction in rates of AF when Candesartan (ARB) was used in patients with symptomatic congestive heart failure (95% CI 0.650–0.990, $P = 0.039$) [58].

One major adverse event associated with AF is the development of LA appendage (LAA) thrombosis and the occurrence of subsequent thromboembolic stroke. While current guidelines recommend the use of anticoagulation to prevent thromboembolic stroke after occurrences of AF, the use of certain medications, such as ACE-I and ARBs to prevent the onset of AF-related conditions such as AF-related embolic stroke is not well studied. One study from China ($n = 199$) found a significant association between ACE-I and ARB use and a lower risk of LAA thrombosis ($OR = 0.222$, 95% CI 0.084–0.585, $p = 0.002$) in patients with AF suggesting ACE-I and ARBs may potentially reduce the risk of thrombus formation and subsequent embolic stroke [63]. Another study (n = 131) found users of ACE-I and ARBs were associated with increased LAA emptying flow velocity (LAA eV) and LA peak systolic strain relative to nonusers (p = 0.032, p = 0.005, respectively) while also showing lower D-dimer and fibrinogen levels (p = 0.004, p = 0.018, respectively) when compared with nonusers [64]. LA peak systolic strain tends to decrease with LAE and increased age. As a result, the LA peak systolic strain has potential to be a reliable marker for LAA dysfunction and thrombus formation in AF patients [65]. Thus, through inhibition of the renin-angiotensin-aldosterone system, ACE-I and ARBs can reduce atrial blood flow stasis and formation of thrombi via a reduction in atrial stretch and fibrosis [66, 67]. Usage of ACE-I and ARBs can therefore theoretically provide a mechanism by which to prevent LA stretch, LAA stasis, and thrombus formation. However, a retrospective cross-sectional analysis based on the results of the SPORTIF III and V trials (n = 7329) found no significant difference in ACE-I/ARB use and stroke/systemic embolic events (adjusted HR = 0.95, 95% CI 0.68–1.32, p = 0.76) in patients with AF [68]. Since ACE-I and ARB use is associated with reduced risk of AF, further research and large-scale trials into the use of ACE-I and ARBs for the prevention of embolic stroke in patients with AF may prove to be an intriguing and worthwhile area of study.

In addition to ACE-I and ARBs, Mineralocorticoid Receptor Antagonists (MRAs) were also found to potentially reduce the risk of AF. One meta-analysis (n = 11,356 patients) found that MRAs did not reduce new-onset AF (RR 0.84, 95% CI 0.61 to 1.16, p = 0.28) but did reduce the risk of recurrent AF (RR 0.73, 95% CI 0.59 to 0.90, p = 0.004) [69]. Furthermore, additional meta-analyses (n = 21,791) found MRAs reduced AF/atrial flutter events (risk ratio = 0.76, 95% CI: 0.67–0.87) in patients with and without prior history of AF [70]. However, MRAs were not found to reduce the risk of stroke (17 RCTs, 30,393 participants; RR = 0.94, 95% CI: 0.81–1.09) [70]. While MRAs were found to be beneficial in the prevention of AF, given the stronger relationship in AF risk reduction with ACE-I/ARB use, ACE-I and ARBs may prove to be superior in the prevention of AF and AF-related adverse events.

While anticoagulation has been a mainstay of treatment to prevent stroke in patients with AF, evidence has shown the power of ACE-I, ARBs, and MRAs on AF prevention and risk reduction. Furthermore, there may be evidence to suggest that ACE-I and ARBs in particular may reduce the risk of AF-induced thromboembolic stroke. Therefore, the addition of ACE-I, ARBs, and/or MRAs to the current treatment regimen of patients, especially those with high-risk for AF (such as post-operative AF patients found in the study [44]) may prove useful in delaying the onset of AF and reducing the adverse effects associated with AF.

### 5.2 Anticoagulation to prevent stroke

Antithrombotic treatment for prevention of primary and recurrent ischemic strokes in patients is well established. Selection of the most appropriate agent, either anticoagulant or antiplatelet, is heavily dependent on the etiology of stroke. Antiplatelet therapy is the recommended treatment for patients with ischemic stroke of non-cardioembolic origin, such as large artery atherosclerosis and small vessel disease, whereas anticoagulant treatment is recommended for cardioembolic strokes which are commonly caused by AF [71].

It has been well established that patients with AF benefit from anticoagulant treatment, compared to antiplatelet treatment, to prevent cardioembolic stroke. A pooled meta-analysis using data from 6 randomized controlled trials (n = 4052) involving patients with AF randomly assigned to anticoagulants or aspirin concluded that oral anticoagulants significantly decreased the risk of stroke [72]. The patients assigned to oral anticoagulants experienced a significantly lower risk of any stroke type (2.4 vs. 4.5 events per 100 patient-years; hazard ratio [HR], 0.55; 95% confidence interval [CI], 0.43–0.71), and lower risk of ischemic stroke (HR, 0.48; 95% CI, 0.37–0.63). Despite the benefit of anticoagulants to decrease the risk of stroke, there was an increased risk of bleeding in these patients. The primary anticoagulant of choice among these studies was warfarin, which led to further studies investigating the efficacy and safety of warfarin versus direct-acting oral anticoagulants (DOACs).

In 4 large randomized controlled trials, warfarin was tested against dabigatran (RE-LY trial), rivaroxaban (ROCKET AF trial), apixaban (ARISTOTLE trial), and edoxaban (ENGAGE AF trial) for efficacy and safety of preventing stroke in patients with AF [73–76]. The RE-LY trial determined that dabigatran significantly decreased the risk of ischemic stroke and that 150 mg of dabigatran was more effective than warfarin in preventing strokes and embolism, and 110 mg of dabigatran had less associated major bleeding compared to warfarin [73]. The ROCKET AF trial found that rivaroxaban was non-inferior to warfarin for stroke prevention, however the rivaroxaban group overall had significantly fewer incidences of intracranial hemorrhage (0.5% vs. 0.7%, P = 0.02) and fatal bleeding (0.2% vs. 0.5%, P = 0.003) [74]. Patients who took apixaban in the ARISTOTLE trial had a 21% reduced risk of stroke compared to patients who took warfarin and significantly reduced intracranial and major bleeding [75]. Results from the ENGAGE AF trial showed that edoxaban was non-inferior to warfarin and that both high- and low- doses of exodaban had significantly lower rates of major bleeding compared to warfarin [76].

These treatment trials prove the pathophysiology of cardioembolic strokes and the improved safety profile provides evidence to support use of DOACs for prevention of cardioembolic stroke.

### 5.3 A critical review of recent treatment trials with ESUS

As mentioned, it is understood that atrial cardiopathy causes atrial thrombosis and subsequent embolism with or without the presence of AF. While most AF progresses from atrial cardiopathy, patients with atrial cardiopathy without (or have yet to develop) AF still have a risk of embolic stroke. Embolic stroke of undetermined source (ESUS) is a type of cryptogenic stroke, a classification of patients who suffered from an infarction with brain imaging characteristics of an embolic source but due to an obscure or unknown origin despite a comprehensive diagnostic evaluation [71]. Up to one-third of patients with ESUS are found to have AF after prolonged cardiac monitoring, however, method and duration of monitoring impact this estimation [77]. Other possible covert causes of ESUS may include valvular diseases, cancer (causing hypercoagulability or tumors), arteriogenic embolism (from nonstenotic atherosclerotic plaques) and paradoxical embolism (via patent foramen ovale or atrial septal defect) [78, 79].

The ARCADIA Trial studied patients with ESUS and atrial cardiopathy [5]. The trial sought to determine whether there was a benefit from anticoagulant (apixaban) treatment over antiplatelet (aspirin) treatment. The rationale is that a stroke with cardiac thrombus etiology precipitated from atrial cardiopathy would benefit more from anticoagulants than antiplatelets, which are more suitable for strokes caused by atherosclerosis or a ruptured plaque. Patients were eligible for the trial if they were determined to have atrial cardiopathy by any of the following; PTFV1 > 5000 μV × ms, serum NT-proBNP >250 pg./mL, or LA diameter index ≥3 cm/m2. ARCADIA trial results were not significant to support apixaban over aspirin to prevent recurrent stroke. There were 40 recurrent strokes in each treatment group (HR, 1.00 [95% CI, 0.64–1.55]; P value for log-rank test = 0.99).

Anticoagulant use in AF patients is well known for its prevention of thrombus formation, subsequent embolism and thromboembolic stroke [80, 81]. The deficits of the ARCADIA trial lie not with a failure to prove anticoagulant efficacy, but to identify patients who are truly at risk of atrial thrombosis and may benefit from anticoagulants. In the ARCADIA trial, only 11.7% of consented patients had any LAE, and only 1.6% of the patients had severely enlarged (LA diameter index ≥3.0 cm/m2) LA. This is surprising as entry into the study was due to atrial cardiopathy being present. It allows us to speculate that some of the markers for atrial cardiopathy may not be strongly associated with LA dilation, which appears to be the highest risk for thromboembolism.

Atrial cardiopathy is a highly heterogeneous diagnosis and may contribute to stroke risk in some but not all ESUS patients. The trial results may have been confounded by such mixed etiologies. Ultimately, the diagnostic method for atrial cardiopathy used in the trial would have benefitted from stricter selective criteria that detect more severe forms of atrial cardiopathy that contribute directly to thromboembolism. Biomarkers for atrial cardiopathy with higher specificity should be included in further treatment trials. Future studies may want to determine what degree of atrial cardiopathy is required for anticoagulation to benefit. Without adequate stratification or scoring of atrial cardiopathy, it is possible that only a few atrial cardiopathy cases are severe enough to cause stroke without AF. Furthermore, patients at lower stratification with milder atrial cardiopathy and lower thromboembolic risk may have diluted the benefits of anticoagulation therapy.

For example, a secondary analysis on the NAVIGATE ESUS trial (which did not find a reduction in recurrent stroke with rivaroxaban use versus aspirin use in ESUS patients) used the HAVOC score and known predictors of AF to identify patients with atrial cardiopathy, stratify severity, and estimate the risk of atrial thrombosis in this subset of patients [82]. This secondary study by Healey et al. found that in patients who have enlarged LA diameter (>4.6 cm), the rivaroxaban group had lower rates of ischemic stroke versus the aspirin group (1.7% per year vs. 6.5% per year, HR, 0.26, 95% CI, 0.07–0.94, P for interaction = 0.02) [82]. This subset of patients (9% of the study population) with severe atrial cardiopathy significantly benefited from anticoagulant treatment.

The ARCADIA trial provides insight into how future trials studying ESUS patients with atrial cardiopathy would have to factor for the heterogenous etiology and severity when selecting their experimental groups. Diagnostic methods must have robust specificity when selecting atrial cardiopathy criteria or biomarkers that possess strong associations with thromboembolism risk to reduce confounding results from mixed etiologies. If adequate research remains unavailable for such criteria, care must be taken to stratify patients' risk for thromboembolism. Considerations may be put towards improving $CHA_2DS_2VASc$ scores with additional criteria as a tool to stratify atrial cardiopathy risk factors pertinent to cardioembolic stroke. To assess the efficacy of different treatments in the prevention of atrial thrombosis and subsequent embolism, more consideration needs to be put into diagnostic criteria for atrial cardiopathy and risk stratification must be established.

## 6. Predicting the risk of thromboembolism

### 6.1 Strengths and limitations of the current CHA2DS2-VASc score

What causes atrial thrombosis in patients with AF? To answer this question, we must critically evaluate the $CHA_2DS_2$-VASc score and current studies on AF burden. The $CHA_2DS_2$-VASc scoring system is used to estimate the annual risk of thromboembolism in patients with AF. However, many investigators have sought to determine the duration of AF needed to estimate thromboembolic risk, so that the $CHA_2DS_2$-VASc score can be applied appropriately to determine treatment. In a study of patients with implantable electronic devices and not on anticoagulation ($n = 21,768$), increasing duration of AF and increasing $CHA_2DS_2$-VASc scores were each significantly ($p < 0.001$) associated with the endpoint of stroke and systemic embolism [83]. The investigators determined that "stroke risk crossed an actionable threshold defined as >1%/y in patients with a $CHA_2DS_2$-VASc score of 2 with >23.5 hours of AF, those with a $CHA_2DS_2$-VASc score of 3 to 4 with >6 minutes of AF, and patients with a $CHA_2DS_2$-VASc score ≥5 even with no AF" [83]. While this study did not provide echocardiographic data on the subjects, considering the high-risk subjects who experienced stroke even with no AF, the CHA2DS2-VASc of 5 or greater suggests that it is likely that these patients would have had evident atrial cardiopathy if examined. Meta-analysis data showed similar discrimination of $CHA_2DS_2$-VASc in patients with non-valvular AF (NVAF) compared to patients without NVAF for predicting ischemic stroke [84].

Increasing $CHA_2DS_2$-VASc scores have been linked to worsening diastolic function. In a study with 4180 subjects with NVAF, patients were grouped by $CHA_2DS_2$-VASc score and TTE data was used to determine a relationship between the scores and structural/functional characteristics of the heart [85]. Diastolic parameters (LAVI and E/E') were increased significantly with higher $CHA_2DS_2$-VASc scores ($P < 0.001$). Left ventricular hypertrophy (HR, 3.609; CI, 2.426–5.369; $p < 0.001$), E/E′ (HR, 1.087; CI, 1.054–1.121; $p < 0.001$) and left ventricular end-diastolic diameter (HR; 0.887; CI, 0.860–0.915; $p < 0.001$) were predictors of a $CHA_2DS_2$-VASc score of 2 or greater. This study supports the theory that diastolic dysfunction is the underlying mechanism for increasing $CHA_2DS_2$-VASc scores and thus increases the risk for thromboembolism. Increased LA pressure results in the blood stasis in the LAA leading to spontaneous echo contrast and subsequent thrombus formation.

If $CHA_2DS_2$-VASc is a surrogate for diastolic dysfunction, then adding more direct measures of diastolic function would improve stroke risk prediction, whether or not the patient has atrial fibrillation. Edwards et al. evaluated the $CHA_2DS_2$-VASc score in patients with atrial cardiopathy but without AF, and found that adding parameters for LAE and excessive atrial ectopy increased the stroke risk prediction significantly [4]. In a subset of their study subjects, adding both parameters to the $CHA_2DS_2$-VASc increased the 2-year C-statistic from 0.68 (using the $CHA_2DS_2$-VASc alone) to 0.75 ($P = 0.008$) and the 5-year C-statistic from 0.70 to 0.76 ($P = 0.003$). This study demonstrated that in a large cohort, the $CHA_2DS_2$-VASc plus measures of atrial cardiopathy were predictive of ischemic stroke. Other studies have evaluated the predictive value of the $CHA_2DS_2$-VASc with additional markers. Tiwari et al. determined that adding LA size to $CHA_2DS_2$-VASc ≥1 increased the risk prediction of stroke, even in patients without AF [86].

It may be that atrial cardiopathy is the primary cause of atrial thrombosis and subsequent thromboembolism and in such cases, one would expect that markers of atrial cardiopathy may be just as potent for the prediction of thromboembolism and stroke in patients who do not have AF.

### 6.2 Best markers of atrial cardiopathy to predict risk of thromboembolism

Atrial cardiopathy has been increasingly studied as a strong predictor of thromboembolic stroke events. Numerous markers exhibit potential in stratifying patients by risk. Edwards et al. determined that for every 10 mm increase in LA diameter, the adjusted cause-specific stroke risk increased (the 2-year HR, 1.72; $P = 0.007$; the 5-year HR, 1.87; $P < 0.0001$) [4]. Conversely, excessive atrial ectopy was not significantly associated with ischemic stroke at either the 2 or 5-year mark after adjustment for AF. In this study, LAE is a stronger predictor for ischemic stroke.

A meta-analysis of 6 prospective cohort studies that included a total of 66,007 patients and 3549 stroke events sought to evaluate the relationship between LAE and stroke [87]. Conducting a literature search of databases such as PubMed, EMBASE, Web of Science, and the Cochrane Library, the authors found that patients with LAE displayed an increased risk of stroke (adjusted HR 1.68, 95% CI 1.36–2.07). Furthermore, they elucidated that there existed a graded association with stroke relating to LAE and stratified LAE into three groups: mild (adjusted HR 1.50, 95% CI 0.98–2.28), moderate (adjusted HR 1.40, 95% CI 1.12–1.75), and severe (adjusted HR 1.59, 95% CI 1.33–1.90). In addition, this paper stated that every increase of 1 cm in LA diameter was shown to increase the stroke risk by 24% (adjusted HR 1.24, 95% CI 1.03–1.50).

Commonly studied, LAA velocity (LAAV) has been determined to predict LAA thrombus in patients with AF [88]. A study from 2020 that included transesophageal echocardiography (TEE) data from 1476 consecutive AF patients before direct current cardioversion or ablation aimed to highlight the risk factors for decreased LAAV with respect to LAA thrombus formation. There were two groups that consisted of 1405 patients with LAAV ≥20 cm/s and 71 patients with LAAV <20 cm/s. The group with LAAV <20 cm/s was seen to have more advanced age, non-paroxysmal AF, and comorbidities (hypertension, diabetes, vascular disease, and heart failure) with a higher median CHA2DS2-VASc score (3 [2–4] vs. 2 [1–3], $p < 0.001$) and lower GFR. Additionally, LAA thrombus was found more frequently in those with LAAV <20 cm/s (20% vs. 4.6%, $p < 0.001$). Within the LAAV <20 cm/s group, the authors found no difference in the prevalence of LAA thrombus between patients on vitamin K antagonists as opposed to those treated with DOAC. In contrast, there was an observed benefit of DOAC therapy in those with LAAV ≥20 cm/s. After multivariate logistic regression, it was shown that those aged≥65 years, heart failure, and non-paroxysmal AF predicted LAA thrombus as well as LAAV <20 cm/s.

The use of the biomarker NT-proBNP has been exceedingly studied in the diagnosis and differentiation of various cardiac conditions, most notably heart failure. A prospective observational study analyzed serum NT-proBNP levels from patients hospitalized due to stroke to determine its predictive capabilities [89]. 207 patients experiencing their first ischemic stroke were included in the study where serum

NT-proBNP levels were measured from blood samples on admission. It was determined that serum NT-proBNP levels were significantly higher ($p < 0.001$) in the cardioembolic stroke group (2069 pg./mL ± 488.5). ROC curves demonstrated that a NT-proBNP value >499 pg./mL was the optimum value for diagnosing ischemic stroke (sensitivity 82%, specificity 80%). Moreover, the authors found that serum NT-proBNP levels >499 pg./mL were independently associated with cardioembolic stroke (OR 9.881, $p = 0.001$). A threshold of NT-proBNP >1500 pg./mL was also seen to be useful in predicting 90-day mortality (sensitivity 70%, specificity 93%).

Notably, the ARCADIA trial eligibility criteria included patients with NT-proBNP levels greater than 250 pg./mL, and the median NT-proBNP level of the subjects who completed the full duration of follow-up was 300 pg./mL [5]. NT-proBNP levels were minimally elevated and hence the ARCADIA trial did not interrogate the value of NT-proBNP readings usually associated with severe atrial cardiopathy. At the biomarker threshold set in ARCADIA, NT-proBNP was not predictive, however, the levels were lower than other studies which showed better prediction for embolic stroke [89].

The ability to predict cardioembolic stroke has become a promising search as various markers have been studied as of late. LA diameter, LAE, LAAV, and NT-proBNP all have shown potential in improving risk stratification for cardioembolic stroke among many others. Such studies are needed to enable early detection.

### 6.3 Role of inflammation

On a clinical level, we have reviewed inflammatory events such as sepsis and surgical procedures as possible provoking factors for AF, and on a cellular level, inflammation is a key component in Virchow's triad contributing to thrombosis. The biomarker high sensitivity C-reactive protein (Hs-CRP) is an inflammatory marker linked to cardiovascular risk [90]. Hs-CRP has been found to be significantly associated with ischemic strokes [91, 92]. IL-6 is a biomarker related to inflammation and is tightly regulated, with levels elevated during periods of infection, stress, ischemia and reperfusion [93]. Meta-analysis data shows that in patients with AF, IL-6 was an independent risk factor for predicting stroke (HR 3.81; 95% CI, 1.11–13.05; $p = 0.033$) and mortality (HR = 3.11; 95% CI, 1.25–7.72; $p = 0.015$), and when added to the $CHA_2DS_2$-VASc score, AUC increased from 0.81 to 0.88 ($p = 0.006$) [94].

### 6.4 Role of microthrombi

Microthrombi is also a cause of atrial thrombosis. We discussed the use of D-dimer for the detection of thrombi in several case studies [95–97]. In our single-center study ($n = 59$), we evaluated patients with AF, atrial flutter, or acute stroke for the presence of atrial thrombus. We determined that with a cutoff value of D-dimer ≥200 ng/mL, the D-dimer assay had a 100% sensitivity, 26.9% specificity, 100% negative predictive value (NPV), and 15.6% positive predictive value (PPV) for detecting thrombus [98]. We also noted that in patients with a positive D-dimer test (≥200 ng/mL), those with LAA thrombus had a significantly decreased LAAV compared to those who did not have a thrombus (Positive D-dimer and LAA thrombus: 22.4 ± 8.4 cm/s [95% CI, 14.7–30.2], Positive D-dimer and no thrombus: 44.4 ± 25.1 cm/s [95%CI, 36.3–55.6], $P = 0.0024$). We proposed a decision algorithm for predicting thrombus using D-dimer and hemodynamic parameters (LAAV and LVEF). Meta-analysis data also supports using D-dimer as a rule-out marker for LAA thrombus [99]. In patients with NVAF who had ischemic strokes, increases in D-dimer levels were significantly associated with LAE [100]. In a study on predicting ischemic stroke in patients with NVAF, a combined model with D-dimer, NT-proBNP and LA diameter had a sensitivity of 77.2% and specificity of 76.4% compared to $CHA_2DS_2$-VASc which had a sensitivity of 69.1% and specificity of 61.2% for patients with stroke [101].

## 7. Conclusion

We have elaborated the concept of atrial cardiopathy to understand the risks of thromboembolism in patients with atrial fibrillation (**Figure 2**). We have reviewed in detail the bi-directional relationship between atrial cardiopathy and atrial fibrillation. Current evidence supports that it is the severity of diastolic dysfunction leading to atrial cardiopathy that increases risk for thromboembolism, not just the presence of atrial arrhythmia.

If atrial cardiopathy is the cause for embolic stroke and AF, then one would expect patients with a high $CHA_2DS_2$-VASc score even in the absence of AF to be at high risk for embolic stroke [4]. The precision for this prediction would be increased as the severity of atrial cardiopathy increases, measured by LAE.

Given the primacy of atrial cardiopathy in the pathogenesis of cardioembolic stroke, biomarkers capable of detecting atrial cardiopathy, with or without diagnostic imaging, should be able to improve the prediction of stroke in patients with or without AF. Preliminary studies have shown that LAAV measured by TEE is a potent predictor of thromboembolic stroke/LA thrombus, but this measure is acquired semi-invasively. In the future, non-invasive biomarkers with appropriate thresholds may be used to predict left atrial cardiopathy to then select patients for further TEE interrogation, whether or not they have AF, to obtain LAAV and other high-risk markers of thromboembolism.

The cornerstone for the development and perpetuation of atrial fibrillation appears to be atrial cardiopathy. There are robust studies showing that atrial cardiopathy alone in the absence of AF is associated with increased ischemic stroke risk.

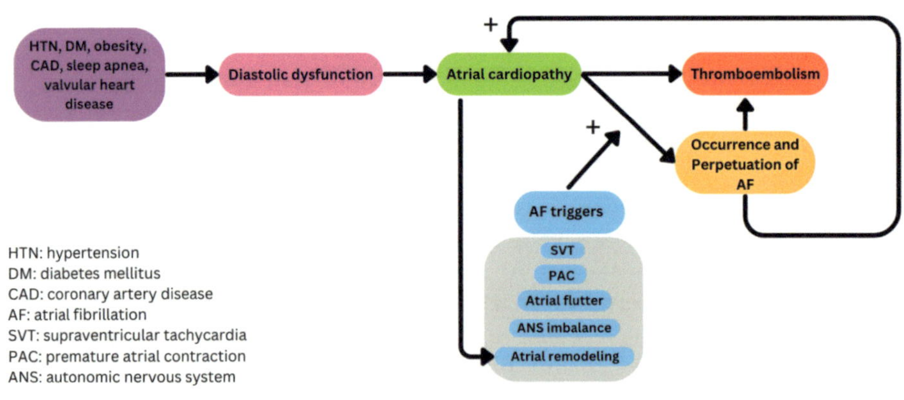


**Figure 2.**
*Illustrates the relationship between atrial cardiopathy, AF and thromboembolism. Risk factors including HTN, DM, and obesity can cause diastolic dysfunction which can cause atrial cardiopathy. Atrial cardiopathy can cause atrial remodeling, which is one of many triggers for AF. The presence of atrial cardiopathy and AF triggers (relationship represented with "+" in the diagram) combined can cause the occurrence and perpetuation of AF. Presence of AF exacerbates atrial cardiopathy (relationship represented with a "+" in the diagram). Thromboembolism may be caused by atrial cardiopathy directly, or by AF (which can be caused by atrial cardiopathy or inflammation).*

It would appear that a concerted effort to treat diastolic dysfunction using BNP and nt-proBNP targets could result in a significant reduction of embolic stroke in patients with or without atrial fibrillation.

## Glossary of terms

| | |
|---|---|
| AF | atrial fibrillation |
| LA | left atrium |
| EHRAS | Acronym to represent the European Heart Rhythm Association (EHRA), the Heart Rhythm Society (HRS), the Asian Pacific Heart Rhythm Society (APHRS), and Sociedad Latino Americana de Estimulacion Cardiaca y Electrofisiologia (SOLAECE) |
| LAA | left atrial appendage |
| LAE | left atrial enlargement |
| LAAV | left atrial appendage velocity |
| COPD | chronic obstructive pulmonary disease |
| MAO-B | plasma monoamine oxidase |
| DE | dopamine |
| EPI | epinephrine |
| NE | norepinephrine |
| PTFV1 | P-wave terminal force in lead V1 |
| LAVi | left atrial volume index |
| PAC | premature atrial contractions |
| BNP | brain natriuretic peptide |
| NT-proBNP | N-terminal pro-B-type natriuretic peptide |
| IL-6 | interleukin-6 |
| CRP | C-reactive protein |
| TTE | transthoracic echocardiogram |
| TEE | transesophageal echocardiogram |
| LVEF | left ventricular ejection fraction |
| ACE-I | angiotensin converting enzyme-inhibitors |
| ARB | angiotensin receptor blocker |
| MRA | mineralocorticoid receptor antagonists |
| ESUS | embolic stroke of undetermined source |
| NVAF | non-valvular atrial fibrillation |
| DOAC | direct-acting oral anticoagulant |

## Author details

Vincent J.B. Robinson[1*], Gyanendra K. Sharma[1], Rohan Sharma[2], Lauren Chow[3*], James Harris Calhoun[3], Mikhil Patel[3], Soham Kulkarni[3], Kuang-Drew Li[3] and Jeffrey A. Switzer[4]

1 Division of Cardiology, Department of Medicine, Medical College of Georgia at Augusta University, Augusta, GA, USA

2 Department of Medicine, Medical College of Georgia at Augusta University, Augusta, GA, USA

3 Medical College of Georgia at Augusta University, Augusta, GA, USA

4 Department of Neurology, Medical College of Georgia at Augusta University, Augusta, GA, USA

*Address all correspondence to: vrobinso@augusta.edu and lchow@augusta.edu

## References

[1] Heeringa J, van der Kuip DAM, Hofman A, Kors JA, van Herpen G, Stricker BHC, et al. Prevalence, incidence and lifetime risk of atrial fibrillation: The Rotterdam study. European Heart Journal. 2006;**27**(8):949-953

[2] Kolmos M, Christoffersen L, Kruuse C. Recurrent ischemic stroke – A systematic review and meta-analysis. Journal of Stroke and Cerebrovascular Diseases. 2021;**30**(8):105935

[3] Leung M, Van Rosendael PJ, Abou R, Ajmone Marsan N, Leung DY, Delgado V, et al. The impact of atrial fibrillation clinical subtype on mortality. JACCL: Clinical Electrophysiology. 2018;**4**(2):221-227

[4] Edwards JD, Healey JS, Fang J, Yip K, Gladstone DJ. Atrial Cardiopathy in the absence of atrial fibrillation increases risk of ischemic stroke, incident atrial fibrillation, and mortality and improves stroke risk prediction. Journal of the American Heart Association. 2020;**9**(11):e013227

[5] Kamel H, Longstreth WT Jr, Tirschwell DL, Kronmal RA, Marshall RS, Broderick JP, et al. Apixaban to prevent recurrence after cryptogenic stroke in patients with atrial Cardiopathy: The ARCADIA randomized clinical trial. Journal of the American Medical Association. 2024;**331**(7):573-581

[6] Kornej J, Börschel CS, Benjamin EJ, Schnabel RB. Epidemiology of atrial fibrillation in the 21st century. Circulation Research. 2020;**127**(1):4-20

[7] Benjamin EJ, Levy D, Vaziri SM, D'Agostino RB, Belanger AJ, Wolf PA. Independent risk factors for atrial fibrillation in a population-based cohort. The Framingham Heart Study. JAMA. 1994;**271**(11):840-844

[8] Miyasaka Y, Barnes ME, Gersh BJ, Cha SS, Bailey KR, Abhayaratna WP, et al. Secular trends in incidence of atrial fibrillation in Olmsted County, Minnesota, 1980 to 2000, and implications on the projections for future prevalence. Circulation. 2006;**114**(2):119-125

[9] Williams BA, Chamberlain AM, Blankenship JC, Hylek EM, Voyce S. Trends in atrial fibrillation incidence rates within an integrated health care delivery system, 2006 to 2018. JAMA Network Open. 2020;**3**(8):e2014874

[10] Vaziri SM, Larson MG, Benjamin EJ, Levy D. Echocardiographic predictors of nonrheumatic atrial fibrillation. The Framingham heart study. Circulation. 1994;**89**(2):724-730

[11] Tsang TSM, Barnes ME, Bailey KR, Leibson CL, Montgomery SC, Takemoto Y, et al. Left atrial volume: Important risk marker of incident atrial fibrillation in 1655 older men and women. Mayo Clinic Proceedings. 2001;**76**(5):467-475

[12] Tiwari S, Schirmer H, Jacobsen BK, Hopstock LA, Nyrnes A, Heggelund G, et al. Association between diastolic dysfunction and future atrial fibrillation in the Tromsø study from 1994 to 2010. Heart. 2015;**101**(16):1302-1308

[13] Rosenberg MA, Manning WJ. Diastolic dysfunction and risk of atrial fibrillation. Circulation. 2012;**126**(19):2353-2362

[14] Søgaard M, Skjøth F, Nielsen PB, Smit J, Dalager-Pedersen M, Larsen TB,

et al. Thromboembolic risk in patients with pneumonia and new-onset atrial fibrillation not receiving anticoagulation therapy. JAMA Network Open. 2022;**5**(5):e2213945

[15] Xiao FP, Chen MY, Wang L, He H, Jia ZQ, Kuai L, et al. Outcomes of new-onset atrial fibrillation in patients with sepsis: A systematic review and meta-analysis of 225,841 patients. The American Journal of Emergency Medicine. 2021;**42**:23-30

[16] Baker WL, Anglade MW, Baker EL, White CM, Kluger J, Coleman CI. Use of N-acetylcysteine to reduce post-cardiothoracic surgery complications: A meta-analysis. European Journal of Cardio-Thoracic Surgery: Official Journal of European Association of Cardiovascular-Thoracic Surgeons. 2009;**35**(3):521-527

[17] Gaudino M, Andreotti F, Zamparelli R, Di Castelnuovo A, Nasso G, Burzotta F, et al. The -174G/C interleukin-6 polymorphism influences postoperative interleukin-6 levels and postoperative atrial fibrillation. Is atrial fibrillation an inflammatory complication? Circulation. 2003;**108**(Suppl. 1):II195-II199

[18] Schnabel RB, Larson MG, Yamamoto JF, Kathiresan S, Rong J, Levy D, et al. Relation of multiple inflammatory biomarkers to incident atrial fibrillation. The American Journal of Cardiology. 2009;**104**(1):92-96

[19] Zhao J, Li M, Tan C. Efficacy of N-acetylcysteine in preventing acute kidney injury and major adverse cardiac events after cardiac surgery: A meta-analysis and trial sequential analysis. Frontiers in Medicine. 2022;**9**:795839

[20] Tian X, Zhang N, Korantzopoulos P, Bazoukis G, Letsas KP, Tse G, et al. Efficacy and safety of colchicine for atrial fibrillation prevention: An updated meta-analysis of randomized controlled trials. International Journal of Cardiology. 2024;**406**:132068

[21] Lefkowitz RJ, Rockman HA, Koch WJ. Catecholamines, cardiac β-adrenergic receptors, and heart failure. Circulation. 2000;**101**(14):1634-1637

[22] Workman AJ. Cardiac adrenergic control and atrial fibrillation. Naunyn-Schmiedeberg's Archives of Pharmacology. 2010;**381**(3):235-249

[23] Anderson EJ, Efird JT, Kiser AC, Crane PB, O'Neal WT, Ferguson TB, et al. Plasma catecholamine levels on the morning of surgery predict post-operative atrial fibrillation. JACC: Clinical Electrophysiology. 2017;**3**(12):1456-1465

[24] Hajjar LA, Vincent JL, Barbosa Gomes Galas FR, Rhodes A, Landoni G, Osawa EA, et al. Vasopressin versus norepinephrine in patients with Vasoplegic shock after cardiac surgery: The VANCS randomized controlled trial. Anesthesiology. 2017;**126**(1):85-93

[25] Goette A, Kalman JM, Aguinaga L, Akar J, Cabrera JA, Chen SA, et al. EHRA/HRS/APHRS/SOLAECE expert consensus on atrial cardiomyopathies: Definition, characterization, and clinical implication. EP Europe. 2016;**18**(10):1455-1490

[26] Holtstrand Hjälm H, Fu M, Hansson PO, Zhong Y, Caidahl K, Mandalenakis Z, et al. Association between left atrial enlargement and obstructive sleep apnea in a general population of 71-year-old men. Journal of Sleep Research. 2018;**27**(2):252-258

[27] Guichard JB, Nattel S. Atrial cardiomyopathy: A useful notion in cardiac disease management or a passing

fad? Journal of the American College of Cardiology. 2017;**70**(6):756-765

[28] Kreimer F, Gotzmann M. Left atrial cardiomyopathy – A challenging diagnosis. Frontiers in Cardiovascular Medicine [Internet]. 2022;**9**:1-20. Available from: https://www.frontiersin.org/articles/10.3389/fcvm.2022.942385

[29] Sajeev JK, Kalman JM, Dewey H, Cooke JC, Teh AW. The atrium and embolic stroke: Myopathy not atrial fibrillation as the requisite determinant? JACC: Clinical Electrophysiology. 2020;**6**(3):251-261

[30] Chen LY, Ribeiro ALP, Platonov PG, Cygankiewicz I, Soliman EZ, Gorenek B, et al. P wave parameters and indices: A critical appraisal of clinical utility, challenges, and future research—A consensus document endorsed by the International Society of Electrocardiology and the international society for Holter and noninvasive Electrocardiology. Circulation. Arrhythmia and Electrophysiology. 2022;**15**(4):e010435

[31] Morris JJ, Estes EH, Whalen RE, Thompson HK, Mcintosh HD. P-wave analysis in Valvular heart disease. Circulation. 1964;**29**(2):242-252

[32] Kwon Y, McHugh S, Ghoreshi K, Lyons GR, Cho Y, Bilchick KC, et al. Electrocardiographic left atrial abnormality in patients presenting with ischemic stroke. Journal of Stroke and Cerebrovascular Diseases. 2020;**29**(9):105086

[33] Kamel H, Hunter M, Moon YP, Yaghi S, Cheung K, Di Tullio MR, et al. Electrocardiographic left atrial abnormality and risk of stroke. Stroke. 2015;**46**(11):3208-3212

[34] Fukuda Y, Nitta K, Morita Y, Higashihara T, Takeda A, Nakano T, et al. P-wave terminal force V1 is associated with left ventricular diastolic function in patients with No significant perfusion abnormality: Assessment by myocardial perfusion single-photon emission computed tomography. International Heart Journal. 2022;**63**(2):299-305

[35] Vaidean GD, Manczuk M, Magnani JW. Atrial electrocardiography in obesity and hypertension: Clinical insights from the polish-Norwegian study (PONS). Obesity. 2016;**24**(12):2608-2614

[36] He J, Tse G, Korantzopoulos P, Letsas KP, Ali-Hasan-Al-Saegh S, Kamel H, et al. P-wave indices and risk of ischemic stroke. Stroke. 2017;**48**(8):2066-2072

[37] Johnson LS, Platonov PG, Conen D, Kennbäck C, Jujic A, Healey JS, et al. Markers of atrial myopathy in the general population: Prevalence, predictors, and inter-relations. JACC: Clinical Electrophysiology. 2023;**9**(11):2240-2249

[38] Nattel S. Atrial cardiomyopathy manifestations in the general population: The tip or the iceberg?*. JACC: Clinical Electrophysiology. 2023;**9**(11):2250-2252

[39] Lang RM, Badano LP, Mor-Avi V, Afilalo J, Armstrong A, Ernande L, et al. Recommendations for cardiac chamber quantification by echocardiography in adults: An update from the American Society of Echocardiography and the European Association of Cardiovascular Imaging. European Heart Journal - Cardiovasc Imaging. 2015;**16**(3):233-271

[40] Olshansky B, Arora R. Mechanisms of atrial fibrillation. In: Connor RF, editor. UpToDate. Wolters Kluwer. Available from: https://www.wolterskluwer.com/en/solutions/uptodate/resources/educator-resources [Accessed: May 30, 2024]

[41] de Correia ETO, dos Barbetta LMS, da Silva OMP, Mesquita ET. Left atrial stiffness: A predictor of atrial fibrillation recurrence after radiofrequency catheter ablation - a systematic review and meta-analysis. Arquivos Brasileiros de Cardiologia. 2019;**112**(5):501-508

[42] Marrouche NF, Wilber D, Hindricks G, Jais P, Akoum N, Marchlinski F, et al. Association of atrial tissue fibrosis identified by delayed enhancement MRI and atrial fibrillation catheter ablation: The DECAAF study. Journal of the American Medical Association. 2014;**311**(5):498-506

[43] Marrouche NF, Wazni O, McGann C, Greene T, Dean JM, Dagher L, et al. Effect of MRI-guided fibrosis ablation vs conventional catheter ablation on atrial arrhythmia recurrence in patients with persistent atrial fibrillation: The DECAAF II randomized clinical trial. Journal of the American Medical Association. 2022;**327**(23):2296-2305

[44] McIntyre WF, Vadakken ME, Connolly SJ, Mendoza PA, Lengyel AP, Rai AS, et al. Atrial fibrillation recurrence in patients with transient new-onset atrial fibrillation detected during hospitalization for noncardiac surgery or medical illness. Annals of Internal Medicine. 2023;**176**(10):1299-1307

[45] Njoku A, Kannabhiran M, Arora R, Reddy P, Gopinathannair R, Lakkireddy D, et al. Left atrial volume predicts atrial fibrillation recurrence after radiofrequency ablation: A meta-analysis. EP Europe. 2018;**20**(1):33-42

[46] Zhuang J, Wang Y, Tang K, Li X, Peng W, Liang C, et al. Association between left atrial size and atrial fibrillation recurrence after single circumferential pulmonary vein isolation: A systematic review and meta-analysis of observational studies. Europace, European Pacing Arrhythm Card Electrophysiology Journal of Work Groups Card Pacing Arrhythmia Card Cell Electrophysiology European Society of Cardiology. 2012;**14**(5):638-645

[47] Xanthopoulos A, Starling RC, Triposkiadis F. Mitral valve stenosis: Still a clinical challenge? Cardiology. 2018;**140**(1):45-46

[48] Laenens D, Stassen J, Galloo X, Ewe SH, Singh GK, Ammanullah MR, et al. The impact of atrial fibrillation on prognosis in aortic stenosis. European Heart Journal - Quality of Care and Clinical Outcomes. 2023;**9**(8):778-784

[49] Pourafkari L, Ghaffari S, Bancroft GR, Tajlil A, Nader ND. Factors associated with atrial fibrillation in rheumatic mitral stenosis. Asian Cardiovascular & Thoracic Annals. 2015;**23**(1):17-23

[50] Nagueh SF, Khan SU. Left atrial strain for assessment of left ventricular diastolic function: Focus on populations with Normal LVEF. JACC: Cardiovascular Imaging. 2023;**16**(5):691-707

[51] Huizar JF, Ellenbogen KA, Tan AY, Kaszala K. Arrhythmia-induced cardiomyopathy. Journal of the American College of Cardiology. 2019;**73**(18):2328-2344

[52] Vinch CS, Rashkin J, Logsetty G, Tighe DA, Hill JC, Meyer TE, et al. Brain natriuretic peptide levels fall rapidly after cardioversion of atrial fibrillation to sinus rhythm. Cardiology. 2004;**102**(4):188-193

[53] von Roeder M, Blazek S, Rommel KP, Kresoja KP, Gioia G, Mentzel L, et al. Changes in left atrial function in patients undergoing cardioversion for atrial fibrillation: Relevance of left atrial strain in heart failure. Clinical Research in Cardiology. 2022;**111**(9):1028-1039

[54] Baman JR, Cox JL, McCarthy PM, Kim D, Patel RB, Passman RS, et al. Atrial fibrillation and atrial cardiomyopathies. Journal of Cardiovascular Electrophysiology. 2021;**32**(10):2845-2853

[55] Kreimer F, Mügge A, Gotzmann M. How should I treat patients with subclinical atrial fibrillation and atrial high-rate episodes? Current evidence and clinical importance. Clinical Research Cardiology: Official Journal of Geriatrics Card Society. 2022;**111**(9):994-1009

[56] Shinbane JS, Wood MA, Jensen DN, Ellenbogen KA, Fitzpatrick AP, Scheinman MM. Tachycardia-induced cardiomyopathy: A review of animal models and clinical studies. Journal of the American College of Cardiology. 1997;**29**(4):709-715

[57] Báez Cabanillas MV, Colque R, Tibaldi MÁ, Kaplinsky E, Perrone S, Barbagelata A. Emerging concepts in heart failure management and treatment: Focus on tachycardia-induced cardiomyopathy. Drugs Context. 2023;**12**:2022-8-4

[58] Ducharme A, Swedberg K, Pfeffer MA, Cohen-Solal A, Granger CB, Maggioni AP, et al. Prevention of atrial fibrillation in patients with symptomatic chronic heart failure by candesartan in the candesartan in heart failure: Assessment of reduction in mortality and morbidity (CHARM) program. American Heart Journal. 2006;**152**(1):86-92

[59] Anis RR. Role of angiotensin-converting enzyme inhibitors and angiotensin receptor blockers in the management of atrial fibrillation. Experimental and Clinical Cardiology. 2009;**14**(1):e1-e7

[60] Tang L, Both K, Taylor R. ACE inhibition and fibroblast growth factor in cultured human vascular smooth muscle. Vascular medicine (London, England). 1999;**4**(3):129-134

[61] Hsieh YC, Hung CY, Li CH, Liao YC, Huang JL, Lin CH, et al. Angiotensin-receptor blocker, angiotensin-converting enzyme inhibitor, and risks of atrial fibrillation: A Nationwide cohort study. Medicine (Baltimore). 2016;**95**(20):e3721

[62] Healey JS, Baranchuk A, Crystal E, Morillo CA, Garfinkle M, Yusuf S, et al. Prevention of atrial fibrillation with angiotensin-converting enzyme inhibitors and angiotensin receptor blockers: A meta-analysis. Journal of the American College of Cardiology. 2005;**45**(11):1832-1839

[63] Suo Y, Zhang Y, Wang Y, Yuan M, Kariyawasam S, Tse G, et al. Renin-angiotensin system inhibition is associated with reduced risk of left atrial appendage thrombosis formation in patients with atrial fibrillation. Cardiology Journal. 2018;**25**(5):611-620

[64] Suo Y, Zhang Z, Fu H, Zhang Y, Yuan M, Wang Y, et al. Inhibition of renin-angiotensin axis reduces the risk of thrombus formation in the left atrial appendage in patients with hypertension complicated by atrial fibrillation. Journal of Renin-Angiotensin-Aldosterone System JRAAS. 2018;**19**(2):1470320318782623

[65] Morris DA, Takeuchi M, Krisper M, Köhncke C, Bekfani T, Carstensen T, et al. Normal values and clinical relevance of left atrial myocardial function analysed by speckle-tracking echocardiography: Multicentre study. European Heart Journal Cardiovascular Imaging. 2015;**16**(4):364-372

[66] Doukky R, Garcia-Sayan E, Gage H, Nagarajan V, Demopoulos A, Cena M, et al. The value of diastolic function parameters in the prediction of left

atrial appendage thrombus in patients with nonvalvular atrial fibrillation. Cardiovascular Ultrasound. 2014;**12**:10

[67] Nakashima H, Kumagai K. Reverse-remodeling effects of angiotensin II type 1 receptor blocker in a canine atrial fibrillation model. Circulation Journal Official Journal of the Japanese Circulation Society. 2007;**71**(12):1977-1982

[68] Lip GYH, Frison L, Grind M. Angiotensin converting enzyme inhibitor and angiotensin receptor blockade use in relation to outcomes in anticoagulated patients with atrial fibrillation. Journal of Internal Medicine. 2007;**261**(6):577-586

[69] Fatima K, Asad D, Shaikh N, Ansari SA, Kumar G, Rehman HA, et al. A systematic review and meta-analysis on effectiveness of mineralocorticoid receptor antagonists in reducing the risk of atrial fibrillation. The American Journal of Cardiology. 2023;**199**:85-91

[70] Oraii A, Healey JS, Kowalik K, Pandey AK, Benz AP, Wong JA, et al. Mineralocorticoid receptor antagonists and atrial fibrillation: A meta-analysis of clinical trials. European Heart Journal. 2024;**45**(10):756-774

[71] Kleindorfer DO, Towfighi A, Chaturvedi S, Cockroft KM, Gutierrez J, Lombardi-Hill D, et al. 2021 guideline for the prevention of stroke in patients with stroke and transient ischemic attack: A guideline from the American Heart Association/ American Stroke Association. Stroke. 2021;**52**(7):e364-e467

[72] van Walraven C, Hart RG, Singer DE, Laupacis A, Connolly S, Petersen P, et al. Oral anticoagulants vs aspirin in Nonvalvular atrial fibrillation an individual patient meta-analysis. Journal of the American Medical Association. 2002;**288**(19):2441-2448

[73] Connolly SJ, Ezekowitz MD, Salim Y, John E, Jonas O, Amit P, et al. Dabigatran versus warfarin in patients with atrial fibrillation. The New England Journal of Medicine. 2009;**361**(12):1139-1151

[74] Patel MR, Mahaffey KW, Jyotsna G, Guohua P, Singer DE, Werner H, et al. Rivaroxaban versus warfarin in Nonvalvular atrial fibrillation. The New England Journal of Medicine. 2011;**365**(10):883-891

[75] Granger CB, Alexander JH, McMurray John JV, Lopes RD, Hylek EM, Michael H, et al. Apixaban versus warfarin in patients with atrial fibrillation. The New England Journal of Medicine. 2011;**365**(11):981-992

[76] Giugliano RP, Ruff CT, Eugene B, Murphy SA, Wiviott SD, Halperin JL, et al. Edoxaban versus warfarin in patients with atrial fibrillation. The New England Journal of Medicine. 2013;**369**(22):2093-2104

[77] Bhat A, Mahajan V, Chen HHL, Gan GCH, Pontes-Neto OM, Tan TC. Embolic stroke of undetermined source: Approaches in risk stratification for Cardioembolism. Stroke [Internet]. 2021;**52**(12):e820-e836. Available from: https://www.ahajournals.org/doi/10.1161/STROKEAHA.121.034498

[78] Ntaios G, Papavasileiou V, Milionis H, Makaritsis K, Manios E, Spengos K, et al. Embolic strokes of undetermined source in the Athens stroke registry: A descriptive analysis. Stroke. 2015;**46**(1):176-181

[79] Kamel H, Merkler AE, Iadecola C, Gupta A, Navi BB. Tailoring the approach to embolic stroke of undetermined

source: A review. JAMA Neurology. 2019;**76**(7):855-861

[80] Ahmad Y, Lip GY. Anticoagulation in atrial fibrillation. Arrhythmia & Electrophysiology Review. 2012;**1**(1):12-16

[81] Kapil N, Datta YH, Alakbarova N, Bershad E, Selim M, Liebeskind DS, et al. Antiplatelet and anticoagulant therapies for prevention of ischemic stroke. Clinical and Applied Thrombosis. 2017;**23**(4):301-318

[82] Healey JS, Gladstone DJ, Swaminathan B, Eckstein J, Mundl H, Epstein AE, et al. Recurrent stroke with rivaroxaban compared with aspirin according to predictors of atrial fibrillation: Secondary analysis of the NAVIGATE ESUS randomized clinical trial. JAMA Neurology. 2019;**76**(7):764-773

[83] Kaplan RM, Koehler J, Ziegler PD, Sarkar S, Zweibel S, Passman RS. Stroke risk as a function of atrial fibrillation duration and CHA2DS2-VASc score. Circulation. 2019;**140**(20):1639-1646

[84] Siddiqi TJ, Usman MS, Shahid I, Ahmed J, Khan SU, Ya'qoub L, et al. Utility of the CHA2DS2-VASc score for predicting ischaemic stroke in patients with or without atrial fibrillation: A systematic review and meta-analysis. European Journal of Preventive Cardiology. 2022;29(4):625-631

[85] Jang AY, Yu J, Park YM, Shin MS, Chung WJ, Moon J. Cardiac structural or functional changes associated with CHA2DS2-VASc scores in Nonvalvular atrial fibrillation: A cross-sectional study using echocardiography. Journal of Cardiovascular Imaging. 2018;**26**(3):135-143

[86] Tiwari S, Løchen ML, Jacobsen BK, Hopstock LA, Nyrnes A, Njølstad I, et al. $CHA_2DS_2$-VASc score, left atrial size and atrial fibrillation as stroke risk factors in the Tromsø study. Open Heart. 2016;**3**(2):e000439

[87] Xu Y, Zhao L, Zhang L, Han Y, Wang P, Yu S. Left atrial enlargement and the risk of stroke: A meta-analysis of prospective cohort studies. Frontiers in Neurology. 2020;**11**:26

[88] Gawałko M, Budnik M, Uziębło-Życzkowska B, Krzesiński P, Scisło P, Kochanowski J, et al. Decreased left atrial appendage emptying velocity as a link between atrial fibrillation type, heart failure and older age and the risk of left atrial thrombus in atrial fibrillation. International Journal of Clinical Practice. 2020;**74**(11):e13609

[89] García-Carmona JA, Conesa-García E, Vidal-Mena D, González-Morales M, Ramos-Arenas V, Sánchez-Vizcaíno-Buendía C, et al. Increased plasma levels of N-terminal pro-B-type natriuretic peptide as biomarker for the diagnosis of cardioembolic ischaemic stroke. Neurología [Internet]. 2022;**39**(6):496-504. Available from: https://www.sciencedirect.com/science/article/pii/S0213485321002814

[90] Bassuk SS, Rifai N, Ridker PM. High-sensitivity C-reactive protein: Clinical importance. Current Problems in Cardiology. 2004;**29**(8):439-493

[91] Chaudhuri JR, Mridula KR, Umamahesh M, Swathi A, Balaraju B, Bandaru VCS. High sensitivity C-reactive protein levels in acute ischemic stroke and subtypes: A study from a tertiary care center. Iranian Journal of Neurology. 2013;**12**(3):92-97

[92] Rost NS, Wolf PA, Kase CS, Kelly-Hayes M, Silbershatz H, Massaro JM, et al. Plasma concentration of C-reactive protein and risk of ischemic

stroke and transient ischemic attack. Stroke. 2001;**32**(11):2575-2579

[93] Su JH, Luo MY, Liang N, Gong SX, Chen W, Huang WQ, et al. Interleukin-6: A novel target for cardio-cerebrovascular diseases. Frontiers in Pharmacology [Internet]. 2021;**12**:1-13. Available from: https://www.frontiersin.org/articles/10.3389/fphar.2021.745061

[94] Jia X, Cheng X, Wu N, Xiang Y, Wu L, Xu B, et al. Prognostic value of interleukin-6 in atrial fibrillation: A cohort study and meta-analysis. Anatolian Journal of Cardiology. 2021;**25**(12):872-879

[95] Sazonova IY, Pondicherry-Harish R, Kadle N, Sharma GK, Figueroa RE, Robinson VJB. Embolic stroke diagnosed by elevated D-dimer in a patient with negative TEE for Cardioembolic source. Journal of Investigative Medicine High Impact Case Reports. 2014;**2**(4):2324709614560907

[96] Ibebuogu UN, Salah AK, Malhotra S, Calkins JB, Thornton JW, Mandawat M, et al. The D-dimer assay: A possible tool in the evaluation of atrial thrombosis. The Canadian Journal of Cardiology. 2008;**24**(6):517-519

[97] Chen PH, Schwade M, Sharma G, Robinson VJB. Value of D-dimer in risk stratification for thromboembolism in patients with atrial fibrillation and low CHA2DS2-VASc score. Journal of Investigative Medicine High Impact Case Reports. 2023;**11**:23247096231165740

[98] Ibebuogu UN, Schafer JH, Schwade MJ, Waller JL, Sharma GK, Robinson VJB. Useful indices of thrombogenesis in the exclusion of intra-cardiac thrombus. Echocardiography (Mount Kisco, N.Y.). 2020;**37**(1):86-95

[99] Casula M, Fortuni F, Frassica R, Coccia MG, Magrini G, Fabris F, et al. D-dimer for the prediction of left atrial appendage thrombosis: Daydream or reality? A meta-analysis. European Heart Journal. 2020;**41**(Suppl. 2):ehaa946.0635

[100] Kim TW, Song IU, Chung SW, Kim JS, Koo J, Lee KS. Serum D-dimer levels are proportionally associated with left atrial enlargement in patients with an acute ischemic stroke due to non-valvular atrial fibrillation. Internal Medicine. 2016;**55**(11):1447-1452

[101] Shen Z, Chen D, Cheng H, Tan F, Yan J, Deng H, et al. N-terminal pro-B-type natriuretic peptide and D-dimer combined with left atrial diameter to predict the risk of ischemic stroke in nonvalvular atrial fibrillation. Clinical Cardiology. 2023;**46**(1):41-48

Chapter 3

# Atrial Fibrillation (AF) Screening to Prevent Stroke: A Public Health Impact Analysis among Adults Aged 65–74 in Greece

*Kyriakos Souliotis, Christina Golna, Ilias Gountas, Dimitrios Trafalis, Myrto Barmpouni and Konstantinos Vemmos*

**Abstract**

Atrial fibrillation (AF) is associated with an increased risk of ischemic stroke and may be difficult to diagnose because of its intermittent nature. The feasibility of screening for undiagnosed AF has been demonstrated in several populations. This study aims to model the impact of screening on AF detection and incidence of stroke between 2020 and 2030 versus background diagnosis only, as well as estimate the cost per averted stroke in each screening scenario. A discrete time, stochastic, individual-based model was developed to assess the efficacy of different screening strategies to diagnose AF among adults aged 65–74 in Greece. Two screening approaches were evaluated: a once-off screening with a 12-lead ECG (electrocardiograph) or a 48-hour Holter monitoring followed by a 12-lead ECG. The clinical event for all scenarios was ischemic stroke. Each scenario was assessed (a) in the total undiagnosed population and (b) in high-risk people only ($CHA_2DS_2$-VASc score $\geq 3$ or 4). Both screening strategies led to better health outcomes (i.e., additional AF cases detected, and strokes avoided) compared to background diagnosis only, across all populations tested, at a manageable cost to the health care system.

**Keywords:** public health, atrial fibrillation, ischemic stroke, screening, prevention, impact analysis

## 1. Introduction

Atrial fibrillation (AF) is the most common cardiac arrhythmia and is associated with an increased risk of ischemic stroke and systemic embolism [1]. The most feared complication in AF patients is ischemic stroke, a risk independent of the nature of AF [2]. In addition, AF may be difficult to diagnose because of its intermittent nature. A risk factor assessment ($CHA_2DS_2$-VASc score) is used to identify the risk of ischemic stroke in individuals with AF [3]. The $CHA_2DS_2$-VASc score considers congestive heart failure, hypertension, age, diabetes mellitus, previous stroke/transient ischemic attack (TIA), vascular disease, and female sex. Oral anticoagulant (OAC) treatment in diagnosed AF patients reduces the risk of ischemic stroke by 64–70%, but under-treatment remains a significant clinical problem [2].

Of all strokes with an established cause, over 85% are ischemic strokes, and the association of AF with ischemic strokes of cardioembolic origin is well recognized. Apart from its morbidity and mortality burden, stroke carries an equally substantial economic burden. In EU27, the total economic burden of stroke was estimated at €27 billion, of which 68.5% accounted for direct and 31.5% for indirect costs. In Greece, in 2015, direct health care and indirect stroke costs were estimated at €356.1 million and €249.7 million, respectively [4].

It is estimated that approximately 15–30% of individuals with AF are asymptomatic or undiagnosed [5] and thus at higher risk for a thromboembolic event. Screening and linking these individuals to care (OAC treatment), particularly the higher-risk ones among them, is expected to minimize their risk of suffering a stroke and result in substantial savings in terms of both morbidity and mortality and direct and indirect costs to patients, their families, and the health system [6]. Studies suggest that, when screening is performed, undiagnosed AF is present in around 1% of the screened general population, rising to 1.4% for those aged at least 65 years. The prevalence of silent AF is even higher in patients with additional risk factors (e.g., patients with heart failure, diabetes mellitus, etc.). Prolonged monitoring of patients with hypertension and an implanted cardiac device showed subclinical atrial arrhythmia in at least 10%, and these patients had a 2.5-fold increased risk of stroke or systemic embolism [7].

The feasibility of screening for silent AF has been demonstrated in several populations. Current practice indicates that the preferred screening methods for silent AF in patients with rhythm control by pharmacological therapy are the 12-lead ECG at outpatient visits and periodical 24- or 48-h Holter recordings [8, 9]. The World Health Organization lists 10 conditions that should be fulfilled to justify mass screening [10]. AF meets all these criteria [2]. In screening for AF, there is an instantaneous indication for initiating OAC treatment in individuals at risk for thromboembolic events, which can then minimize stroke risk by up to 70%. This is particularly highlighted in a very recent discussion by Duncker and Svennberg [11], who stress that "to avoid unwanted downstream consequences from atrial fibrillation, not only does atrial fibrillation need to be detected, but it should also be ensured that stroke-protective treatment is initiated for those with newly detected atrial fibrillation".

This study aims to model the impact of mass screening for AF among people aged 65–74 in Greece on the actual incidence of stroke over the next 10 years (2020–2030) versus maintaining the current screening paradigm, of background diagnosis only, i.e., screening only if, when, and as a physician sees fit, according to his clinical opinion. The study predicts the impact of screening on two population groups: the total undiagnosed Greek population aged 65–74 and the estimated Greek population aged 65–74 with a $CHA_2DS_2$-VASc score $\geq 3$ or $CHA_2DS_2$-VASc score $\geq 4$ (high-risk). Further, the study estimates the cost per ischemic stroke avoided by adopting one of the two screening approaches evaluated versus maintaining the current background diagnosis and linkage to care paradigm.

## 2. Methods

A discrete time, stochastic, individual-based model was developed in language C++ to assess the efficacy of different screening strategies to diagnose AF among

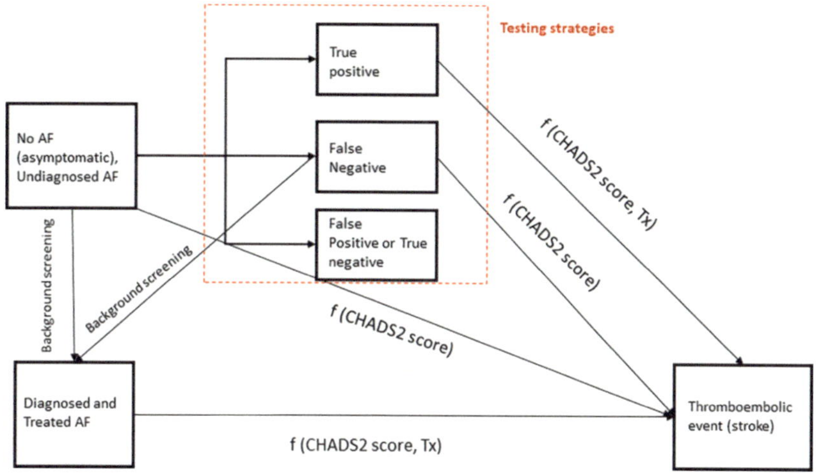


**Figure 1.**
*Simplified schematic of the decision process in the screening model. Parameters: Tx represents the Treatment.*

adults aged 65–74 in Greece (**Figure 1**). A total of 1.230.000 pseudo individuals were created, representing the total Greek population aged 65–74 in 2020 (**Table 1**, [12]). The probability of a stroke event is associated with patient's $CHA_2DS_2$-VASc score [9]. To estimate the baseline score risk, we stratified the population per characteristic (e.g., sex, AF status, diagnosis, stroke risk factors) using data from the EMENO study [13] (**Table 1**). Every year, individuals exit the various states through background deaths. Background general mortality was based on Greek life tables [14]. For patients with AF, a hazard ratio was applied to background mortality rates, reflecting the increased risk of mortality versus the general population after accounting for events

| Parameter | Estimate |
|---|---|
| Total Greek population aged 65–74 in 2020 | 1,230,000 (Males: 578 K) |
| Total atrial fibrillation population in Greece aged 65–74 | 5.73% (Males 4.29%, Females 6.82%) |
| Diagnosed population | 86%* |
| Background mortality | 1.6% |
| Standardized mortality rate for the AF population | Female: 2.3 / Male: 1.5 |
| Bleeding risk | 2.13% |
| *Stroke risk factors among the target population* | |
| Hypertension | 75.8% |
| Diabetes Mellitus | 26.4% |
| Myocardial infarction | 7.8% |

*(*) According to IQVIA data on sales of NOACs and VKAs for 2019, total sales of oral anticoagulants in days of treatment (DOTs) in Greece in 2019 amount to 84,343,623 DOTs. We are assuming a compliance rate of 335 days a year for Novel Oral Anticoagulants (NOACs) and 300 for VKAs. This results in a diagnosed and on-treatment population of 256,835 patients. Of these, 23.25% are aged 65–74. Therefore, diagnosed patients aged 65–74 on treatment for AF are 256,835*23.25% = 59,714. Assuming a prevalence of 69,300 AF patients aged 65–74 in Greece, the undiagnosed and untreated population is calculated as 69,300–59,714 = 9586 or 13.8% of the total AF population aged 65–74.*

**Table 1.**
*Baseline epidemiological and economic model parameters.*

modeled [9]. Treatment with OAC was assumed to reduce the risk of thromboembolic events [15]. Based on screening results, all patients with a true positive diagnosis of AF were assigned to treatment, while, on the other hand, patients with a true and false negative or false positive diagnosis were not assigned to treatment. Patients with an initial false negative diagnosis could be diagnosed after the initial screening by background screening. Patients with a true negative or false positive diagnosis were not subjected to stroke risk. Patients with a true positive were subject to the risk of bleeding events [16].

## 3. Data

### 3.1 Population

In Greece, AF prevalence among individuals aged 65–74 was reported at 5.73% (4.29 and 6.82% among men and women, respectively) [17] (**Table 1**). By multiplying this percentage by the total population in this age group, we estimated approximately 69,300 individuals aged 65–74 living with AF in Greece. Based on the calculation of market size for people in Greece diagnosed with and treated for AF (**Table 1**), 13.8% of them are estimated to be undiagnosed and untreated. It should be noted that in Greece, there is almost universal access to oral anticoagulation treatment for stroke prevention if AF is diagnosed, including access to prescription and reimbursement of pharmaceutical therapies by social insurance. Therefore, it can be safely estimated that the number of patients on anticoagulation prevention treatment equals the number of diagnosed AF patients in Greece. This model assumption is further tested by sensitivity analysis. Treated AF patients have a 75% lower stroke probability compared to untreated patients [15]. The 65–74-year age group was selected as candidates for screening due to the high probability of averting strokes among this age group as they age (study time horizon of 10 years) and before their mortality risk is affected by their age alone. Screening by electrocardiogram (ECG) in individuals aged >65 years during medical encounters is recommended by leading organizations such as the American Heart Association (AHA), the American Stroke Association (ASA), and the European Society of Cardiology (ESC) [15]. The risk of a bleeding event for patients on treatment was based on the ARISTOTLE trial [16].

### 3.2 Time horizon

Time horizon of the analysis was 10 years (2020–2030) to capture the intended benefits and harms of the intervention since stroke is a relatively rare event.

### 3.3 Scenarios

Two screening approaches are evaluated: a once-off screening with a 12-lead ECG (electrocardiograph) or a 48-hours Holter monitoring followed by a 12-lead ECG. We choose to examine an opportunistic screening with a long-term Holter since previous studies have shown that is a cost-effective strategy [9]. A current scenario was used to generate predictions regarding current AF management by 2030 (only random background diagnosis—current Scenario). Two additional scenarios were considered: a one-time screening model with a single 12-lead ECG (Scenario A) and an extended screening model with the use of a 48 hours-Holter device combined with a 12-lead

ECG (Scenario B). The clinical event of the study for all scenarios was ischemic stroke. Each scenario was assessed both in the total population aged 65–74 and those with baseline $CHA_2DS_2$-VASc score ≥ 3 or ≥ 4 (high-risk patients only).

### 3.4 Screening effectiveness

The model assumes the effectiveness of the current scenario (background diagnosis only) in terms of the prevalence of undiagnosed AF detected by screening as 1.00% or approximately 100 cases per annum. This was further tested in sensitivity analyses, as detailed below. According to Hindricks et al. [9], Scenario A would result in a 0.5% prevalence of undiagnosed AF detected by screening, whereas Scenario B [18] would result in a 13% prevalence (16% when high-risk population only, i.e., $CHA_2DS_2$-VASc score ≥ 3).

### 3.5 Costs

We estimated treatment, screening, and bleeding costs to be applied in the model (**Table 2**). Scenario A included screening cost for a 12-lead ECG. Scenario B included the screening cost for a Holter installation and removal and a 12-lead ECG. Both scenarios included the cost of treatment for those diagnosed, assuming market share and drug prices were constant across the model horizon. Current treatment market shares were derived from IQVIA data [19] and are assumed to be constant across the time horizon of the study. Current reimbursed prices (social insurance price—patient copayment) are derived from the Ministry of Health Drug Price Bulletin (2020) [20] and are used to calculate annual treatment costs, assuming compliance of 335 days a year for NOACs and 300 days for VKAs, based on current clinical practice. The model does not account for any discontinuations in treatment once treatment has commenced, other than the temporary discontinuation reflected in the compliance to treatment rates used for the calculation of the number of patients in **Table 1** and the permanent discontinuation after year 1 of treatment in the false-positive patients. According to the ESC AF Guidelines [9], bleeding risk should not withhold OAC treatment, and, in actual clinical practice in Greece, bleeding is usually addressed through temporary discontinuation. The cost of managing bleeding events that required hospitalization was retrieved from Kourlaba et al. [21].

| **Screening cost** | |
|---|---|
| ECG cost per individual (EOPYY Code 220000004) | 4.05€ |
| Holter Installation and Removal cost per individual (EOPYY Code 220000025) | 12.3€ |
| *Treatment cost market shares and (mean therapy costs per patient per annum, in €)* | |
| Eliquis® | 34.2% (285.17€) |
| Xarelto® | 32.6% (577.24€) |
| VKA | 18.9% (19.20€) |
| Pradaxa® | 14.3% (283.63€) |
| Per annum | 488.11€ |
| Bleeding cost | 1202.00 € |

**Table 2.**
*Screening and treatment cost.*

### 3.6 Analysis

For each scenario, 500 simulations (runs) were performed. Results were summarized using the median of all simulations. To include the appropriate uncertainty (stochastic variability), credible intervals (i.e., 2.5 and 97.5 percentiles of simulations) are also shown. Further increasing the number of runs had almost no impact on medians or credible intervals.

### 3.7 Sensitivity analysis

To examine the impact of different model assumptions, a series of univariate sensitivity analyses on the cumulative diagnoses of the screening intervention in the screening scenario in which we consider only individuals aged 65–74 with $CHA_2DS_2$-VASc score ≥ 4 was undertaken. These included the impact of a 25% increase/decrease in the prevalence of the undiagnosed AF population, 25% higher/lower efficacy of the 48 hours Holter +ECG intervention, and 50% reduction or 100% increase in background diagnosis.

## 4. Results

The model estimated that at the current scenario diagnosis rate (i.e., background diagnosis only), the projected number of AF detection and stroke events by 2030 among the total population aged 65–74 would be 840 (95% CrI: 775, 900) and 6585 (95% CrI:6390, 6785), respectively. Screening the same population according to Scenario A would result in 45 additional AF cases (95% CrI: −35, 144), a 5.3% increase from the current scenario. Applying screening according to Scenario B would result in an additional 1145 (95% CrI: 1015,1235) AF cases being detected, a 136.3% increase compared with background diagnosis only. Identification of additional AF patients and earlier treatment would lead to fewer ischemic strokes among cohorts screened. Ischemic strokes averted are estimated as follows: Scenario A, 15 (95% CrI: −100, 240) or a reduction of −0.23%, and Scenario B, 415 (95% CrI: 130, 650) or a reduction of −6.5%, compared to background diagnosis only (**Table 3**).

An alternative analysis considers only individuals in our age group with a $CHA_2DS_2$-VASc score ≥ 3, accounting for hypertension, diabetes mellitus, age, and sex as risk factors. These were the risk factors for which data were available in Greece from the EMENO study [13]. The model estimated that in 2020, there were 634,000 individuals with $CHA_2DS_2$-VASc score ≥ 3. In the current scenario, the projected number of AF detection and stroke events among those patients by 2030 would be 635 (95% CrI: 600, 676) and 5570 (95% CrI: 5435, 5680), respectively. Screening the same population according to Scenario A would result in 30 additional AF cases (95% CrI: −16, 80), a 4.7% increase from the current scenario. Applying screening according to Scenario B would result in an additional 925 (95% CrI: 846, 1010) AF cases being detected, a 145.0% increase, compared with background diagnosis only. Averted strokes are estimated at 20 (95% CrI: −160, 160), a – 0.36% reduction, and 350 (95% CrI: 130, 540), a – 6.7% reduction, respectively, compared to background diagnosis only (**Table 4**).

Should the analysis consider only individuals with a $CHA_2DS_2$-VASc score ≥ 4 (estimated to be 168,000, 95% Crl: 167,350–169,050, in 2020), the projected number of AF detection and stroke events among those patients by 2030 would be

| | Current scenario | Scenario A (ECG) | Scenario B (48 hours Holter) |
|---|---|---|---|
| Population in 65–74 group | 1,230,000 | 1,230,000 | 1,230,000 |
| Diagnosed population | 60,000 | 60,000 | 60,000 |
| Analysis population | 1,170,000 | 1,170,000 | 1,170,000 |
| Undiagnosed patients | 9586 (9365, 9815) | 9586 (9365, 9815) | 9586 (9365, 9815) |
| Number of AF detections | 840 (775, 900) | 885 (815, 967) | 1985 (1887, 2075) |
| Newly diagnosed population post-intervention | 8.76% | 9.23% | 20.7% |
| Number of ischemic strokes | 6585 (6390, 6785) | 6570 (6365, 6730) | 6170 (6010, 6390) |
| Additional AF diagnoses vs. current | NA | 45 (−35, 144) | 1145 (1015, 1235) |
| Relative difference in AF diagnoses vs. current (%) | NA | 5.3% (−1.5%, 13.2%) | 136.3% (121.4%, 151.1%) |
| Ischemic strokes averted vs. current | NA | 15 (−100, 240) | 415 (130, 650) |
| Relative difference in strokes vs. current scenario (%) | NA | −0.23% (−2.5%, +3.2%) | −6.5% (−3.5%, −8.4%) |

**Table 3.**
*Clinical outcomes, when total population aged 65–74 is screened. Ranges in brackets correspond to 95% credibility intervals.*

| | Current scenario | Scenario A (ECG) | Scenario B (48 hours Holter) |
|---|---|---|---|
| Analysis population | 634.000 | 634.000 | 634.000 |
| Number of AF detections | 635 (600, 676) | 665 (624, 705) | 1560 (1490, 1635) |
| Number of ischemic strokes | 5570 (5435, 5680) | 5550 (5428, 5670) | 5220 (5085, 5325) |
| Additional AF diagnoses vs. current | NA | 30 (−16, 80) | 925 (846, 1010) |
| Relative difference in AF diagnoses vs. current (%) | NA | 4.7% (−2.4%, 13.3%) | 145% (127.5%, 164.0%) |
| Ischemic strokes averted vs. current | NA | 20 (−160, 160) | 350 (130, 540) |
| Relative difference in strokes vs. current scenario (%) | NA | −0.36% (−2.9%, 2.8%) | −6.2% (−3.0%, −10.5%) |

**Table 4.**
*Clinical outcomes, when only individuals aged 65–74 with $CHA_2DS_2$-VASc score ≥ 3. Ranges in brackets correspond to 95% credibility intervals.*

315 (95% CrI: 280, 360) and 3475 (95% CrI: 3350, 3615), respectively. Screening the same population according to Scenario A would result in 10 additional AF cases (95% CrI: −50, 68), a 3.1% increase from the current scenario. Applying screening according to Scenario B would result in an additional 335 (95% CrI: 270, 450) AF cases being detected, a 106.3% increase, compared with background diagnosis only.

Averted strokes are estimated at 8 (95% CrI: −110, 200), a – 0.23% reduction, and 120 (95% CrI: 5, 250), a – 3.4% reduction, respectively, compared to background diagnosis only (**Table 5**).

Both screening strategies (Scenario A and B) led to increased costs, driven by screening costs and OAC treatment of newly detected AF cases. In the base case, incremental costs for a screening program compared with background diagnosis only were estimated at €4.93 million in Scenario A and €24.19 million in Scenario B. Cost per averted stroke was calculated at €322,882 in Scenario A and €52,013 in Scenario B, compared to background diagnosis only. If the target population for the screening intervention were limited to those with $CHA_2DS_2$-VASc score ≥ 3, corresponding incremental costs compared to background diagnosis only were calculated at €2.70 and €14.45 million for Scenario A and B, respectively. Cost per averted stroke was calculated at €128,739 in Scenario A and €35,021 in Scenario B, compared to background diagnosis only. If the target population for the screening intervention were limited to those with $CHA_2DS_2$-VASc score ≥ 4, corresponding incremental costs compared to background diagnosis only were calculated at €724,585 and €4.22 million for Scenario A and B, respectively. Cost per averted stroke was calculated at €84,300 in Scenario A and €28,952 in Scenario B, compared to background diagnosis only (**Table 6**).

Sensitivity analysis revealed that the variation in the undiagnosed AF population prevalence would substantially affect the expected cumulative diagnoses of the intervention (**Figure 2**). If a larger population were undiagnosed (25% increase), cumulative diagnoses among the $CHA_2DS_2$-VASc score ≥ 4 population would increase by 28.4%. If a smaller population were undiagnosed (25% decrease), diagnoses due to the intervention among the same population would decrease by 26.9%. Furthermore, fluctuations in the efficacy of the 48 hours Holter +ECG approach also affected model predictions. If efficacy were 25% lower than estimated, cumulative diagnoses among the $CHA_2DS_2$-VASc score ≥ 4 population would decrease by 25.4%, whereas if efficacy were 25% higher, cumulative incidence in this population would increase by 22.3%. Changes in the background diagnosis only had a marginal effect on estimated cumulative diagnoses (**Figure 2**).

| | **Current scenario** | **Scenario A (ECG)** | **Scenario B (48 hours Holter)** |
|---|---|---|---|
| Analysis population | 168.000 | 168.000 | 168.000 |
| Number of AF detections | 315 (280, 360) | 325 (285, 367) | 650 (600, 10) |
| Number of ischemic strokes | 3475 (3350, 3615) | 3467 (3355, 3612) | 3355 (3210, 3500) |
| Additional AF diagnoses vs. current | NA | 10 (−50, 68) | 335 (270, 420) |
| Relative difference in AF diagnoses vs. current (%) | NA | 3.1% (−11.0%, 17.1%) | 106.3% (84.3%, 127.4%) |
| Ischemic strokes averted vs. current | NA | 8 (−110, 200) | 120 (5, 250) |
| Relative difference in strokes vs. current scenario (%) | NA | −0.23% (−3.1%, +3.4%) | −3.4% (−0.4%, −9.6%) |

**Table 5.**
*Clinical outcomes, when only individuals aged 65–74 with $CHA_2DS_2$-VASc score ≥ 4. Ranges in brackets correspond to a 95% credibility interval.*

*DOI: http://dx.doi.org/10.5772/intechopen.1006642*

| | **Incremental screening cost (€)** | **Incremental OAC treatment costs (€)** | **Bleeding costs (€)[3]** | **Total cost (€)** | **Incremental averted strokes** | **Incremental cost per averted stroke (€)** | **Incremental cost per averted stroke (€), after allowing for stroke management cost*** |
|---|---|---|---|---|---|---|---|
| | | | | All individuals aged 65–74 | | | |
| Scenario A[1] | 4.73M | 197,685 | 1150 | 4.93 M | 15 | 329,155 | 322,882 |
| Scenario B[2] | 19.1M | 5.03 M | 29,315 | 24.19 M | 415 | 58,286 | 52,013 |
| | | | | Individuals aged 65–74 with $CHA_2DS_2$-VASc score ≥ 3 | | | |
| Scenario A[1] | 2.56 M | 131,790 | 768 | 2.70 M | 20 | 135,012 | 128,739 |
| Scenario B[2] | 10.36 M | 4.06 M | 23,680 | 14.45 M | 350 | 41,294 | 35,021 |
| | | | | Individuals aged 65–74 with $CHA_2DS_2$-VASc score ≥ 4 | | | |
| Scenario A[1] | 680,400 | 43,930 | 256 | 724,585 | 8 | 90,573 | 84,300 |
| Scenario B[2] | 2.74M | 1.47 M | 8576 | 4.22 M | 120 | 35,225 | 28,952 |

[1] *Scenario A cost calculations: Screening cost=Analysis population*ECG cost per individual, New OAC treatment costs=New diagnoses*mean drug cost*years, Total costs=Screening cost+New OAC treatment costs*
[2] *Scenario B cost calculations: Screening cost=Analysis population*(ECG cost per individual+Holter Installation and Removal cost per individual), New OAC treatment costs=New diagnoses*mean drug cost*years, Total costs=Screening cost+New OAC treatment costs*
[3] *Bleeding costs=Additional AF diagnoses*Probability of bleeding*Cost to Treat Bleeding*
**Stroke management cost estimated at € 6,273 by Vemmos et al. [6]*

**Table 6.**
*Economic analysis of screening scenarios versus current scenario.*

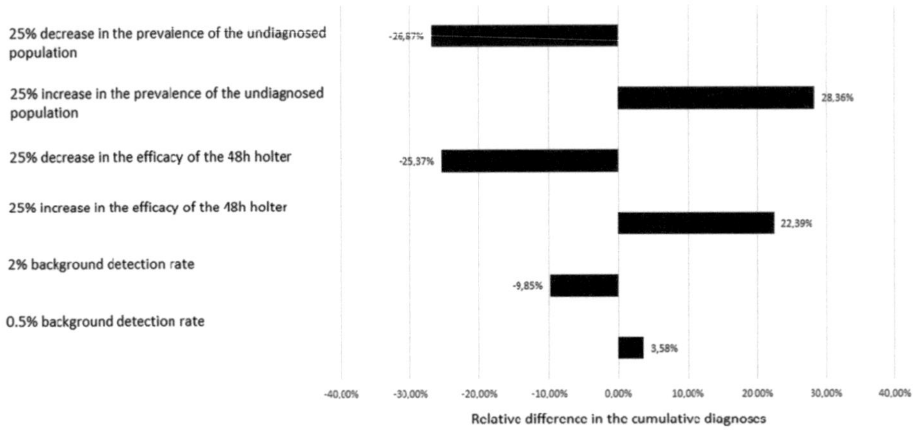


**Figure 2.**
*One-way sensitivity analysis: cumulative diagnoses vs. base parameter values (**Table 1**). Note: A value of zero describes no change from the projected cumulative incidence. A positive or a negative value means that the expected diagnoses are higher or lower, respectively, compared to that projected under the base scenario.*

## 5. Discussion

This study estimated the clinical impact and cost-effectiveness of one-time screening for AF of individuals upon reaching the age of 65 from the perspective of the Greek healthcare system. We analyzed 2 screening modalities: a one-time 12-lead ECG and a 48 hours continuous monitoring with a Holter followed by a 12-lead ECG. Both screening strategies led to better health outcomes (i.e., additional number of AF cases detected, and strokes avoided) compared with the current strategy of background diagnosis only, across all populations tested, i.e., total undiagnosed Greek population aged 65–74, individuals in the same age group with a $CHA_2DS_2$-VASc score $\geq 3$ and individuals in the same age group with a $CHA_2DS_2$-VASc score $\geq 4$. Results were more pronounced, in terms of improved health outcomes, when the 48 hours continuous monitoring with a Holter followed by a 12-lead ECG screening approach was applied to individuals in the 65–74 group with a $CHA_2DS_2$-VASc score $\geq 3$. On the contrary, lower incremental costs were estimated, when the 48 hours continuous monitoring with a Holter followed by a 12-lead ECG screening approach was applied to individuals in the 65–74 group with a $CHA_2DS_2$-VASc score $\geq 4$.

Our study adds to the existing evidence assessing the cost-effectiveness of systematic screening for AF. In the landmark SAFE study [22], which compared a control population over 65 years old with a population assigned to opportunistic or systematic screening for AF, both opportunistic and systematic screening was shown to lead to more cases of AF being detected, at an incremental cost that would be considered cost-effective. In a 2016 Cochrane Review on 'Systematic screening for the detection of atrial fibrillation' the SAFE trial was the only trial meeting the inclusion criteria and led to the Cochrane review concluding that both opportunistic pulse palpation and systematic screening will increase AF detection, a position endorsed by the European Heart Rhythm Association. European Heart Rhythm Association has also previously highlighted the potential benefit of targeting screening in high-risk populations and suggests systematic ECG screening can be considered in people aged 75 years or older, or those at high stroke risk [23].

In the STROKESTOP study by Svennberg et al. [2], mass screening for AF in a 75- to 76-year-old population identified a significant proportion of participants with untreated AF, whereas initiation of stroke prophylactic treatment was highly successful among individuals with newly diagnosed AF. The cost-effectiveness analysis of the study [24] estimated that screening 1000 individuals who matched the population of the STROKESTOP study resulted in 263 fewer patient years with undetected AF. This implied 8 fewer strokes, 11 more life-years, and 12 more quality-adjusted life years (QALYs) per 1000 screened individuals at an incremental cost of €50,012, or €4313 per QALY gained and €6583 per stroke averted.

A white paper by the AF-SCREEN International Collaboration [25] highlights how screen-detected AF found at a single timepoint or by intermittent ECG recordings over 2 weeks is not a benign condition and, with additional stroke factors, carries sufficient risk of stroke to justify consideration of anticoagulation. The paper also discusses the advantages of handheld ECG devices in providing a verifiable ECG trace that guidelines require for AF diagnosis, as well as the different settings for screening such as community and the clinic, which should be linked to a pathway for appropriate diagnosis and management if screening is to be effective.

Our age group was also found appropriate, as the review by Welton et al. [26] deemed a screening strategy with an initial screening age of 65 years and repeated screens every 5 years until age 80 years likely to be cost-effective if compliance with treatment does not decline with increasing age.

Another review by Fay et al. [27] confirmed that opportunistic screening via pulse palpation, with subsequent referral for 12-lead electrocardiogram testing, has been shown to cost-effectively identify individuals with asymptomatic AF. The review also focuses on those with an increased risk of AF, such as those aged ≥65 years or those diagnosed with or undergoing monitoring for hypertension.

Further, our selection of higher-risk populations $CHA_2DS_2$-VASc score of 3 or 4 is confirmed by previous screening studies. The REHEARSE-AF study recruited 1001 patients with a mean age of 72.6 years and $CHA_2DS_2$-VASc score of 3 and randomized them to twice-weekly home ECG screening using the AliveCor Kardia system or usual care. In the screening group, there were 19 new cases of AF detected over 1-year follow-up, compared to 5 in the usual care arm at a cost of $10,780 per AF diagnosis [28].

The ASSERT-II study used implantable subcutaneous ECG monitoring to detect AF over 16-month follow-up among 256 people with a mean age of 74 years and CHA2DS2VASc score of 4.1. The study found 34.4% of participants had at least one episode of AF lasting over 5 minutes. Short episodes of atrial arrhythmia were found in around one-third of all patients across studies where an implanted cardiac device or monitor was used for extended screening in high-risk individuals [29].

Our model scenario parameters are confirmed by a metanalysis of 25 unique (3 RCTs and 22 observational) studies (n = 88,786) from 14 countries, which revealed that systematic screening was more effective than opportunistic: 1.8% (95% CI 1.4 to 2.3%) vs. 1.1% (95% CI 0.6 to 1.6%), $p < 0.05$, GP-led screening was more effective than community-based: 1.9% (95% CI 1.4 to 2.4%) vs. 1.1% (95% CI 0.7 to 1.6%), $p < 0.05$, and repeated heart rhythm measurements were more effective than isolated assessments of rhythm: 2.1% (95% CI 1.5–2.8) vs. 1.2% (95% CI 0.8–1.6), $p < 0.05$ [30].

Our findings are also consistent with earlier studies assessing systematic screening in other settings [15]. The model by Oguz et al. [15] evaluated the clinical and economic impact of one-time screening for non-valvular AF (NVAF) with a single

12-lead ECG and a 14-day extended screening with a hand-held ECG device (Zenicor single-lead ECG, Z14) compared with no screening. It concluded that both screening strategies led to better health outcomes (ischemic strokes avoided: ECG 12-lead, 9.8 and Z14, 42.2; quality-adjusted life-years gained: ECG 12-lead, 31 and Z14, 131) and were cost-effective compared with no screening at a willingness-to-pay (WTP) threshold of $100,000 per QALY gained ($58,728/QALY with ECG 12-lead and $47,949/QALY with Z14 in 2016 US dollars).

To our knowledge, our study is the first to examine the cost efficiency of AF screening in Greece. In addition, our study is the first to examine the cost-effectiveness of both single time-point and extended 48-hour systematic screening in the country. Our study concluded that systematic screening for AF is associated with gains in health outcomes at an economically justifiable cost when assessed from a third-party payer perspective in Greece. Extended screening is estimated to detect more AF cases and have lower incremental cost per stroke averted than single time-point screening.

Our model projections are sensitive to the uncertainty of some of the underlying parameters. If the actual undiagnosed high-risk AF population is smaller than estimated, cumulative diagnoses are expected to substantially decrease. On the other hand, if the actual undiagnosed AF population is larger than estimated, cumulative diagnoses are expected to increase. Thus, the success of the screening campaign is strongly dependent on the size of the target population. The efficacy of the 48 hours Holter + ECG approach is an equally significant parameter that affects the model's projections; if the intervention has a higher efficacy than estimated, expected new diagnoses would be 22.4% higher compared to the status quo.

## 6. Limitations

As with all simulation studies, our findings are indicative and need to be confirmed with empirical evidence. Specific limitations arise from our choice of assumptions and limited data availability.

First, we assumed that all newly diagnosed individuals would commence treatment and stay on treatment without treatment discontinuation, for reasons presented in detail in previous sections and to avoid adding several assumptions for which data are unavailable in Greece to the model. This may overestimate treatment costs in both screening scenarios. As our primary objective was to model the public health impact of compared screening interventions in terms of new diagnoses and strokes averted, we deem this limitation to have only a limited impact on our findings.

Second, any false-positive individuals are assumed to remain under treatment for a year. After the year, the model assumes they will find out that they do not have AF and discontinue treatment. This would constitute wastage in resources dedicated to the treatment, which are nonetheless accounted for in the model and overestimate actual treatment cost, should detection of a false positive result be made earlier in time.

Third, all factors affecting stroke are assumed to be constant (e.g., no increase in hypertension) over the model period, except for the patient's age.

Fourth, market shares and prices for pharmaceutical therapies are assumed to be constant during the model time horizon. This may slightly overestimate treatment costs, provided pharmaceutical prices are expected to decrease over the study time frame.

Fifth, our study does not allow for the impact of diagnostic devices in watches and smartphones, which may increase both awareness of symptoms and number of patients seeking diagnosis and, therefore, reduce the population pool eligible for screening. This may impact on total intervention costs.

Finally, further evidence on the prevalence of undiagnosed AF—how it varies by age and how it can be modified by repeated screening—is required to ascertain whether repeated screening or screening at earlier ages would be effective.

## 7. Conclusions

Actively screening all individuals aged 65–74 with high risk for thromboembolic events, i.e., with a $CHA_2DS_2$-VASc score of $\geq 3$ or 4, would detect additional AF cases and prevent additional ischemic strokes compared to a current paradigm of background diagnosis only at a cost per averted stroke of €35,021 and €28,952, respectively. According to these results, implementing an AF screening and linkage to care program among high-risk adults aged 65–74 in Greece would constitute a critical strategy to avert strokes among this population in the next decade.

## Funding

This study was funded by Pfizer Hellas.

## Authors' contributions

Souliotis K: conception and design of the study, interpretation of the data, drafted the work, substantively revised it.

Golna C: conception and design of the study, interpretation of the data, drafted the work, substantively revised it.

Gountas I: design of the study, analysis of the data, drafted the work.

Trafalis D: design of the study, analysis of the data, interpretation of the data, drafted the work, substantively revised it.

Barmpouni M: design of the study, analysis of the data, interpretation of the data, substantively revised it.

Vemmos K: interpretation of the data, substantively revised it.

All authors have approved the submitted version and have agreed both to be personally accountable for their own contributions and to ensure that questions related to the accuracy or integrity of any part of the work, even ones in which the authors were not personally involved, are appropriately investigated, resolved, and the resolution documented in the literature.

## Conflict of interest

K Souliotis, I Gountas, and K Vemmos received consulting fees from Pfizer for the development of the public health impact analysis.

C Golna has no conflict of interest.

D Trafalis and M Barmpouni are Pfizer Hellas employees.

The authors have no other relevant affiliations or financial involvement with any organization or entity with a financial interest in or financial conflict with the subject matter or materials discussed in the manuscript apart from those disclosed.

## Notes/thanks/other declarations

The authors are willing to share the code used in this analysis with qualified external researchers. The requests are to be made to the corresponding author and will be appraised based on scientific merit.

## Author details

Kyriakos Souliotis[1,2*], Christina Golna[2], Ilias Gountas[1], Dimitrios Trafalis[3], Myrto Barmpouni[3] and Konstantinos Vemmos[4]

1 University of Peloponnese, Department of Social and Education Policy, Corinth, Greece

2 Health Policy Institute, Athens, Greece

3 Pfizer Hellas, Athens, Greece

4 Hellenic Stroke Organization, Athens, Greece

*Address all correspondence to: ksouliotis@uop.gr

## References

[1] Barbarossa A, Guerra F, Capucci A. Silent atrial fibrillation: A critical review. Journal of Atrial Fibrillation. 2014;**7**(3):1138. DOI: 10.4022/jafib.1138

[2] Svennberg E, Engdahl J, Al-Khalili F, Friberg L, Frykman V, Rosenqvist M. Mass screening for untreated atrial fibrillation: The STROKESTOP study. Circulation. 2015;**131**(25):2176-2184. DOI: 10.1161/circulationaha.114.014343

[3] Friberg L, Rosenqvist M, Lip GY. Evaluation of risk stratification schemes for ischaemic stroke and bleeding in 182 678 patients with atrial fibrillation: The Swedish atrial fibrillation cohort study. European Heart Journal. 2012;**33**(12):1500-1510. DOI: 10.1093/eurheartj/ehr488

[4] WilkinsE,WilsonL,WickramasingheK, Bhatnagar P, Leal J, Luengo-Fernandez R, et al. European cardiovascular disease statistics 2017. Brussels: European Heart Network; 2017

[5] Rienstra M, Lubitz SA, Mahida S, Magnani JW, Fontes JD, Sinner MF, et al. Symptoms and functional status of patients with atrial fibrillation: State of the art and future research opportunities. Circulation. 2012;**125**(23):2933-2943. DOI: 10.1161/circulationaha.111.069450

[6] Vemmos K, Boubouchairopoulou N, Stafylas P, Vitsou E, Giannakoulas G, Ntaios G, et al. Estimation of the economic burden of atrial fibrillation-related stroke in Greece. Expert Review of Pharmacoeconomics and Outcomes Research. 2022;**22**(3):429-435. DOI: 10.1080/14737167.2021.1979961

[7] Quinn FR, Gladstone D. Screening for undiagnosed atrial fibrillation in the community. Current Opinion in Cardiology. 2014;**29**(1):28-35. DOI: 10.1097/hco.0000000000000018

[8] Dobreanu D, Svendsen JH, Lewalter T, Hernández-Madrid A, Lip GY, Blomström-Lundqvist C. Current practice for diagnosis and management of silent atrial fibrillation: Results of the European heart rhythm association survey. Europace. 2013;**15**(8):1223-1225. DOI: 10.1093/europace/eut227

[9] Hindricks G, Potpara T, Dagres N, Arbelo E, Bax JJ, Blomström-Lundqvist C, et al. 2020 ESC guidelines for the diagnosis and management of atrial fibrillation developed in collaboration with the European Association for Cardio-Thoracic Surgery (EACTS): The task force for the diagnosis and management of atrial fibrillation of the European Society of Cardiology (ESC) developed with the special contribution of the European Heart Rhythm Association (EHRA) of the ESC. European Heart Journal. 2021;**42**(5): 373-498. DOI: 10.1093/eurheartj/ehaa612

[10] Wilson JMG, Jungner G. Principles and practice of screening for disease. Public health papers. Vol. 34. Geneva: World Health Organization; 1968

[11] Duncker D, Svennberg E. The catch in atrial fibrillation detection: don't forget to treat. The Lancet Healthy Longevity. 2021;**2**(8):e447-e448. DOI: 10.1016/s2666-7568(21)00176-8

[12] Hellenic Statistical Authority. Population and Housing Census. 2011. Available from: https://www.statistics.gr/en/2011-census-pop-hous

[13] Touloumi G, Karakosta A, Kalpourtzi N, Gavana M, Vantarakis A,

Kantzanou M, et al. High prevalence of cardiovascular risk factors in adults living in Greece: The EMENO National Health Examination Survey. BMC Public Health. 2020;**20**(1):1665. DOI: 10.1186/s12889-020-09757-4

[14] Eurohex. Life Tables Greece. 2021. Available from: http://www.eurohex.eu/IS/web/app.php/Ehleis/LifeGeographic?Typ=Life&SubTyp=None

[15] Oguz M, Lanitis T, Li X, Wygant G, Singer DE, Friend K, et al. Cost-effectiveness of extended and one-time screening versus no screening for non-valvular atrial fibrillation in the USA. Applied Health Economics and Health Policy. 2020;**18**(4):533-545. DOI: 10.1007/s40258-019-00542-y

[16] Dorian P, Kongnakorn T, Phatak H, Rublee DA, Kuznik A, Lanitis T, et al. Cost-effectiveness of apixaban vs. current standard of care for stroke prevention in patients with atrial fibrillation. European Heart Journal. 2014;**35**(28):1897-1906. DOI: 10.1093/eurheartj/ehu006

[17] Ntaios G, Manios E, Synetou M, Savvari P, Vemmou A, Koromboki E, et al. Prevalence of atrial fibrillation in Greece: The Arcadia rural study on atrial fibrillation. Acta Cardiologica. 2012;**67**(1):65-69. DOI: 10.1080/ac.67.1.2146567

[18] Diederichsen SZ, Haugan KJ, Kronborg C, Graff C, Højberg S, Køber L, et al. Comprehensive evaluation of rhythm monitoring strategies in screening for atrial fibrillation: Insights from patients at risk monitored long term with an implantable loop recorder. Circulation. 2020;**141**(19):1510-1522. DOI: 10.1161/circulationaha.119.044407

[19] IQVIA. MIDAS Data, Pfizer Hellas, DOTs Report, Atrial Fibrillation Indication. Athens, Greece: IQVIA; 2019

[20] Ministry of Health. Drug Price Bulletin. 2020

[21] Kourlaba G, Stefanou G, Tsalamandris S, Oikonomou E, Papageorgiou G, Nikas N, et al. Incidence and cost of bleeding events requiring hospitalization in patients with atrial fibrillation treated with acenocoumarol in Greece. Hellenic Journal of Cardiology. 2021;**62**(3):234-240. DOI: 10.1016/j.hjc.2020.06.013

[22] Hobbs FD, Fitzmaurice DA, Mant J, Murray E, Jowett S, Bryan S, et al. A randomised controlled trial and cost-effectiveness study of systematic screening (targeted and total population screening) versus routine practice for the detection of atrial fibrillation in people aged 65 and over. The SAFE study. Health Technology Assessment. 2005;**9**(40): iii-iv, ix-x, 1-74. DOI: 10.3310/hta9400

[23] Jones NR, Taylor CJ, Hobbs FDR, Bowman L, Casadei B. Screening for atrial fibrillation: A call for evidence. European Heart Journal. 2020;**41**(10):1075-1085. DOI: 10.1093/eurheartj/ehz834

[24] Aronsson M, Svennberg E, Rosenqvist M, Engdahl J, Al-Khalili F, Friberg L, et al. Cost-effectiveness of mass screening for untreated atrial fibrillation using intermittent ECG recording. Europace. 2015;**17**(7):1023-1029. DOI: 10.1093/europace/euv083

[25] Freedman B, Camm J, Calkins H, Healey JS, Rosenqvist M, Wang J, et al. Screening for atrial fibrillation: A report of the AF-SCREEN international collaboration. Circulation. 2017;**135**(19):1851-1867. DOI: 10.1161/circulationaha.116.026693

[26] Welton NJ, McAleenan A, Thom HH, Davies P, Hollingworth W, Higgins JP, et al. Screening strategies for atrial

fibrillation: A systematic review and cost-effectiveness analysis. Health Technology Assessment. 2017;**21**(29): 1-236. DOI: 10.3310/hta21290

[27] Fay MR, Fitzmaurice DA, Freedman B. Screening of older patients for atrial fibrillation in general practice: Current evidence and its implications for future practice. The European Journal of General Practice. 2017;**23**(1):246-253. DOI: 10.1080/13814788.2017.1374366

[28] Halcox JPJ, Wareham K, Cardew A, Gilmore M, Barry JP, Phillips C, et al. Assessment of remote heart rhythm sampling using the AliveCor heart monitor to screen for atrial fibrillation: The REHEARSE-AF study. Circulation. 2017;**136**(19):1784-1794. DOI: 10.1161/circulationaha.117.030583

[29] Healey JS, Alings M, Ha A, Leong-Sit P, Birnie DH, de Graaf JJ, et al. Subclinical atrial fibrillation in older patients. Circulation. 2017;**136**(14):1276-1283. DOI: 10.1161/circulationaha.117.028845

[30] Petryszyn P, Niewinski P, Staniak A, Piotrowski P, Well A, Well M, et al. Effectiveness of screening for atrial fibrillation and its determinants. A meta-analysis. PLoS One. 2019;**14**(3):e0213198. DOI: 10.1371/journal.pone.0213198

Chapter 4

# Atrial Fibrillation and Stroke Prevention

*Mohammad Montaser Atasi, Razan Dankar, Jamil Francis and Marwan M. Refaat*

## Abstract

Atrial fibrillation is the most common sustained arrhythmia encountered in adults and is associated with an increased morbidity and mortality due to both causing and contributing to an increase in the risk of stroke and heart failure. AF constitutes a significant public health concern. It is estimated that its management accounts for 1% of the National Health Service budget in the United Kingdom and between $6 and $26 billions of annual healthcare spending in the United States. This chapter includes the epidemiology and genetics of atrial fibrillation, with a special focus on the management of non-valvular atrial fibrillation, how and when to follow a rate control or rhythm control treatment strategy atrial fibrillation including catheter ablation. The chapter also includes assessment of a patient's risk of stroke in the setting of atrial fibrillation as well as the options for anticoagulation and left atrial appendage closure.

**Keywords:** atrial fibrillation, rate control, rhythm control, catheter ablation, appendage closure, anticoagulation, stroke

## 1. Introduction

Atrial fibrillation (AF) is the most common sustained arrhythmia found in adults, significantly increasing morbidity and mortality due to its role in elevating the risks of stroke and heart failure [1]. It is characterized by rapid and irregular beating of the atrial chambers of the heart, leading to a disorganized and ineffective atrial contraction. Triggers of AF can vary ranging from high sympathetic activity to any structural changes such as fibrosis, dilation, and hypertrophy, all of which alter the atrial architecture. Moreover, persistent AF can cause atrial fibrosis, which further disrupts the normal electrical conduction pathways. This arrhythmia can result in various complications, including stroke, heart failure, and other cardiovascular conditions, making it a significant public health concern. Symptoms of AF can vary, ranging from asymptomatic to palpitations, shortness of breath, chest pain, and fatigue. This chapter focuses on non-valvular atrial fibrillation and discusses the epidemiology and genetics of AF, outlining the strategies for implementing either rate control or rhythm control treatments, including catheter ablation. Additionally, the chapter addresses the assessment of stroke risk in AF patients and explores the options for anticoagulation and left atrial appendage closure. By providing a detailed understanding of these aspects, the chapter aims to equip healthcare professionals with the knowledge needed to effectively manage AF and mitigate its associated risks.

## 2. Epidemiology

Atrial fibrillation is the most prevalent cardiac arrhythmia with an estimated prevalence of 60 million cases around the globe [1]. It represents a significant global health challenge affecting individuals across diverse demographics and geographical regions and contributing to more than 8 million disability-adjusted life years [1].

The lifetime risk of developing AF is substantial, with estimates suggesting that approximately 33% of individuals will suffer from AF during their lifetime 1. It is estimated that between 6 and 12 million individuals are expected to suffer from AF in the United States by 2050, while approximately 17.9 million people in Europe are expected to be affected by the year 2060 [2]. In Asia, nearly 72 million individuals are estimated to experience AF by 2050 [3]. Data from the Framingham Heart Study (FHS) indicates that AF prevalence has increased by 3-folds over the past 50 years [4]. It is also important to note that nearly one-third of AF patients are asymptomatic, which might contribute to a decrease in the estimates of this arrhythmia's health burden [5].

In terms of incidence, AF commonly affects older adults, with the risk increasing significantly with age. However, it can also occur in younger individuals, particularly those with predisposing conditions or genetic predispositions. The incidence rates vary across different populations and regions, influenced by factors such as genetic predisposition, lifestyle habits, access to health care, and advancements in diagnostic technologies.

## 3. Risk factors

AF risk can vary considerably based on patient-level factors such as age, sex, race, and the burden of clinical risk factors. Modifiable risk factors play a pivotal role in shaping the lifetime risk of AF. Conditions like hypertension, type 2 diabetes mellitus, and physical inactivity independently increase the likelihood of developing AF, highlighting the importance of targeted interventions to mitigate these risk factors. Emerging research has identified novel risk factors for AF, including epigenetic markers of biological age and body composition [1]. These insights offer new avenues for understanding the pathophysiology of AF and developing innovative approaches to risk assessment and management.

There is growing evidence supporting the effectiveness of risk factor interventions in reducing the incidence of AF and preventing recurrent episodes. Lifestyle modifications, pharmacological interventions, and targeted therapies tailored to individual risk profiles hold promise in both primary and secondary prevention strategies for AF.

### 3.1 Non-modifiable risk factors

Advancing age is the single most important AF risk factor, with a dramatic increase after the age of 65 years [6]. Other non-modifiable risk factors include ethnicity, with lower incidence in Asians and Hispanics [7]. Underlying heart conditions and congenital heart disease also contribute to an increased AF risk.

### 3.2 Modifiable risk factors

Modifiable risk factors that contribute to AF include systemic or pulmonary hypertension, diabetes and endocrine disorders, smoking, alcohol consumption, obesity, and physical inactivity, as well as psychosocial factors [6, 7].

Future research endeavors should prioritize the comprehensive management of risk factors for AF, aiming for both primary prevention in at-risk populations and secondary prevention in individuals with established disease.

## 4. Genetics

Advancements in genetic research, particularly through genome-wide association studies (GWAS) conducted across diverse populations, have significantly expanded our understanding of the role of genetics in the development of AF [8]. Utilizing large-scale biobanks equipped with detailed phenotypic information has yielded valuable insights into the influence of both common and rare genetic variants on AF susceptibility and prognosis. Additionally, the development of polygenic risk scores has emerged as a valuable tool in refining individual risk stratification for AF and enhancing prognostic assessments, thereby facilitating more personalized approaches to patient care and management.

Nearly 140 AF loci and more than 150 functional candidate genes have been identified using GWAS studies [9, 10]. Several of the identified risk variants are

| Locus | Sentinel Variant | Nearest Gene(s) | Gene End Product | Function |
|---|---|---|---|---|
| 4q25 | rs2129977 | PITX2 | Pituitary Homeobox 2 | Transcription factor, role in cardiogenesis |
| 16q22.3 | rs2359171 | ZFHX3 | Zinc finger homeobox 3 | Transcription factor, role in cardiogenesis |
| 1q21.3 | rs11264280 | KCNN3 | KCa2.3 potassium channel | Atrial repolarization |
| 7q31.2 | rs11773845 | CAV1 | Caveolin-1 | Plasma membrane scaffolding protein |
| 10q25.1 | rs11598047 | NEURL | E3 ubiquitin ligase | PITX2 modulation |
| 12q24.21 | rs883079 | TBX5 | T-Box-5 | Transcription factor, role in cardiogenesis |
| 1q24.2 | rs72700114 | METTL11B, LINC01142 | Methyltransferase like 11B; Long intergenic non-protein coding RNA 1142 | Unknown |
| 1q24.2 | rs608930 | PRRX1 | Paired related homeobox 1 | Transcription factor, role in cardiogenesis |
| 9q22.33 | rs4385527 | C9orf3 | Aminopeptidase O | Angiotensin III cleavage to Angiotensin IV |
| 5q31.2 | rs34750263 | WNT8A | WNT8A Protein | Involved in embryo development |

**Table 1.**
*Main genetic variants involved in AF.*

positioned near genes linked to severe cardiac abnormalities in humans, such as GATA4, MYH6, NKX2–5, PITX2, and TBX5, where harmful mutations have been documented [10]. Additionally, these variants are located near genes critical for the function and structural integrity of striated muscles, including CFL2, MYH7, PKP2, RBM20, SGCG, and SSPN. Among the top 10 genetic loci identified, several sentinel variants have been determined and are highlighted in **Table 1** [9].

## 5. Non-invasive management and stroke prevention

There are three main goals in AF management. Firstly, restoring and preserving normal sinus rhythm, ensuring the stability of the heart's rhythm. Secondly, while AF may persist, controlling the heart rate to a normal or acceptable level is crucial for symptom management and preventing complications. The third main goal of management is the prevention of thromboembolic events through prophylactic measures, as AF predisposes individuals to thrombus formation, which can lead to serious adverse events including stroke.

### 5.1 Emergency electrical cardioversion

The most important consideration is the patient's stability. Unstable AF, like any other tachycardia, should be managed with emergency electrical cardioversion. Code should be activated, and crash cart, defibrillator, intubation equipment, and the relevant teams should be called. If the heart rate is above 150 beats per minute, immediate synchronized electrical cardioversion should be performed. Otherwise, it is appropriate for the clinician to look for another underlying etiology. If the clinician identified AF with rapid ventricular response or rapid atrial flutter, anticoagulation should be administered as soon as possible. Sedation although recommended should not be a reason to delay the lifesaving intervention. Midazolam, Etomidate, and Propofol are usually used with fentanyl for analgesia.

### 5.2 Non-emergent electrical cardioversion

In case of a stable patient with a first episode of non-valvular AF, electrical cardioversion is preferred in most cases even if the patient is asymptomatic. Especially if the patient is younger (<65 years). If the patient had AF episode before, then pharmacologic cardioversion could be followed by electrical cardioversion to restore sinus rhythm. The decision should take into consideration the strength and weaknesses of each approach and the patient preference.

Electrical cardioversion is beneficial in avoiding long-term drug side effects, like transient hypotension, QTc interval prolongation, and conversion of AF to atrial flutter. It reduces the need for prolonged telemetric monitoring and has superior efficacy when compared to pharmacologic cardioversion.

In preparation of the procedure, antiarrhythmic drugs could be administered to increase the likelihood of successful cardioversion, decrease cardioversion energy required as well as help in refractory patients. Ibutilide or verapamil may be useful in preventing early recurrences of AF after cardioversion, particularly if it is of recent onset [11, 12]. However, if the decision of long-term maintenance of sinus rhythm with antiarrhythmic drug therapy (such as amiodarone, flecainide, or propafenone) has been made, the same drug should be used prior to the electrical cardioversion.

The conversion of AF to sinus rhythm, whether it occurs spontaneously or intentionally, is linked to a significant temporary increase in the risk of thromboembolism, especially stroke. This is why it is important for patients with AF for more than 48 hours, uncertain duration, or high risk of thromboembolism to receive 4 consecutive weeks of therapeutic anticoagulation with warfarin (target INR > 2) or direct-acting oral anticoagulant (DOAC) before and after the electrical cardioversion. Alternatively, anticoagulation with heparin or a DOAC before, during, and after cardioversion along with precardioversion transesophageal echocardiography (TEE) could be done to rule out left atrial appendage thrombus in patients who have bleeding risk or were we do not want the cardioversion to be delayed.

On the day of the procedure, the patient should be fasting, oxygen saturation and electrolytes should be normalized, and anticoagulation status should be reviewed. The cardioversion shock should be synchronized to the QRS complex and should be delivered while the patient is under conscious sedation while having close vital monitoring and carbon dioxide monitored. Most cardioversions are well tolerated.

### 5.3 Pharmacological therapy

Medical management of AF holds many considerations and must be tailored to the patients need and to the clinical scenario that led to the development of the disease. The duration of AF, underlying cardiac disease, and other comorbidities are some of the factors that guide the clinician's decision.

For stable patients with AF, assess thromboembolic risk using the CHA2DS2-VASc score, and consider the initiation of anticoagulation. It is important to identify whom spontaneous restoration of normal sinus rhythm (conversion) is likely to happen, especially those short AF duration (<24 or < 48 hours versus longer duration), low episode number (first-detected AF versus recurrent AF or previous supraventricular arrhythmias), normal atrial size, and absence of underlying cause. Spontaneous conversion (SCV) rates range widely between 9 and 83% [13]. Moreover, risk factors for AF should be addressed. Hyperthyroidism, hypertension, heart failure, sleep apnea, and excess alcohol intake are modifiable precipitating factors that can be managed each with its own way.

When treating a patient with atrial fibrillation (AF), choosing between rhythm control and rate control is crucial. However, it is important to understand that this decision is complex, can change over time, and that these two strategies are not always mutually exclusive, depending on how they are defined.

#### *5.3.1 Rate control*

Rate control in the management of AF aims to regulate the heart rate to a normal or acceptable range to alleviate symptoms and prevent complications associated with rapid heart rates. Traditionally, the rate control strategy has been the primary approach for managing AF [14]. The AFFIRM trial, one of the largest clinical trials that included 4060 AF patients, demonstrated that the rhythm control strategy did not provide a survival advantage over rate control and was associated with a higher incidence of adverse drug effects [15]. The optimal heart rate for patients with atrial fibrillation was investigated in the RACE II trial which found no significant difference in mortality, hospitalizations for heart failure, arrhythmia-related symptoms, or thromboembolic complications when comparing heart rate control targets of below 80 beats per minute to those below 110 beats per minute [16]. Therefore, a lenient rate control of <100–110 is recommended by the European Society of Cardiology guidelines [14].

Several medications are commonly utilized for rate control in AF, primarily targeting the atrioventricular (AV) node to slow down the ventricular response to atrial fibrillation. The main drugs used in AF rate control are beta-blockers (BB), calcium channel blockers (CCB), amiodarone, and digoxin.

Beta-blockers (BB), such as metoprolol, atenolol, and carvedilol, work by blocking the beta-adrenergic receptors and are often first-line rate control agents [14]. They are particularly effective in patients with concomitant hypertension, coronary artery disease, or heart failure. BB are proven to effectively control the ventricular rate in AF and improve survival in patients with heart failure with reduced ejection fraction (HFrEF) [17].

Digoxin, a cardiac glycoside that increases vagal tone and reduces AV nodal conduction, is occasionally used for rate control, especially in patients with heart failure or those with reduced left ventricular function. It is typically used in patients who are not adequately controlled with BB and offers synergistic effects with BB. However, it should be used with caution to avoid its deleterious adverse events [18].

Non-dihydropyridine CCB, including diltiazem and verapamil, inhibits calcium influx into the cardiac cells, resulting in decreased AV nodal conduction. They are often used in patients with contraindications to BB and are a viable option in patients with heart failure with preserved ejection fraction (HFpEF). However, due to their negative inotropic effect, they may not be well tolerated at the doses needed for optimal ventricular rate control, potentially leading to increased mortality in patients with HFrEF [19].

Amiodarone is a class III antiarrhythmic agent that blocks multiple ion channels, thereby prolonging action potential duration and refractoriness. It is typically used in acute settings and as a last resort in patients who do not tolerate non-pharmacological rate control [14]. However, it can lead to thyroid, pulmonary, and hepatic toxicity.

### *5.3.2 Rhythm control*

In new onset AF (or flutter), rhythm control aims at the termination on the arrhythmic activity, restoration, and maintenance of sinus rhythm. This may lead to improvement in the symptoms and pretension of atrial remodeling. There are three types of cardioversions, namely pharmacologic cardioversion, planned electrical cardioversion, and interventional cardioversion. Those modalities are especially useful to prevent complications in patients with AF and rapid ventricular response and to improve outcomes for patients who have concomitant heart failure.

Because the AFFIRM trial-targeted patients over the age of 65 who were likely to have chronic and recurrent AF, this raised the question of whether implementing rhythm control early in the disease can improve long-term outcomes. Addressing this, the EAST-AFNET4 trial was conducted and included 22,635 patients within 12 months of their AF diagnosis [20]. The trial, which had a median follow-up period of five years, was stopped early because of the demonstrated efficacy of early rhythm control. Those in the early rhythm control group experienced significantly lower rates of cardiovascular mortality, stroke, heart failure hospitalization, and acute coronary syndrome-related hospitalizations. Other studies also showed similar findings, advocating for the adoption of early rhythm control strategies in the management of recently diagnosed AF [20–22]. **Table 2** summarizes the uses of rate vs. rhythm control.

| Aspect | Rate Control | Rhythm Control |
|---|---|---|
| Primary goal | Managing ventricular heart rate | Achieving and maintaining normal sinus rhythm |
| Treatment options | Beta blockers, calcium channel blockers, digoxin, and amiodarone | Flecainide, sotalol, amiodarone, dronedarone, dofetilide, disopyramide, dronedarone, flecainide, ibutilide, propofanone, ranolazine, quinidine, cardioversion, and ablation |
| Best suited for | Patients with multiple health issues, significant atrial enlargement, and long-standing AF | Younger patients, those with symptomatic AF, persistent heart failure despite rate control, and challenges in maintaining rate control |
| Advantages | Simple to start and often the first choice for new AF cases in hospital settings | Early rhythm control has been linked to reductions in overall mortality, cardiovascular mortality, strokes, and heart failure hospitalizations |
| Disadvantages | Long-term impacts are unclear, and patients might remain asymptomatic | Initiating antiarrhythmic drugs requires careful monitoring, and there are limited ablation facilities available. No clear benefit of maintaining sinus rhythm |

**Table 2.**
*Rate vs. rhythm control.*

To note, pharmacologic cardioversion can be done if AF onset is less than 48 hours and rate control is contraindicated or undesirable. Otherwise, proper anticoagulation for at least 3 weeks or ruling out thrombi through transesophageal echocardiography (TEE) before attempting rhythm control.

In long-term AF, we consider antiarrhythmic drugs to try to maintain the sinus rhythm or reduce the frequency and duration of AF episodes if the medications are generally tolerated, and it meets patient preference, young age, shorter history of AF, more symptoms, smaller LA, worse LV function, worse AV regurgitation, and generally difficult to control heart rate. Similar to rate control, they can control symptoms and improve quality of life. Even though quality of life improvement was higher in those receiving antiarrhythmics than those on rate controlling agents, the result is not clinically satisfactory [23].

Amiodarone, dofetilide, flecainide, propafenone, and sotalol are the commonly used antiarrhythmic drugs in AF. In the Canadian Trial of Atrial fibrillation, AFFIRM, and the SAFE-T randomized trials, amiodarone was more effective than the others, but held higher rate of discontinuation due to long-term adverse side effect [24, 25]. Echocardiogram and exercise or nuclear stress imaging test to screen for coronary heart disease should be done before starting any class Ic agent. Flecainide or propafenone are the first antiarrhythmic drug to be used in AF without structural heart disease or coronary artery disease. In contrast, Amiodarone, sotalol, and dofetilide are the most recommended first-line drugs in patients with structural heart disease and are acceptable in patients with coronary heart disease. Amiodarone and dofetilide are used in patients with AF and heart failure (HF) or those with a left ventricular ejection fraction less than 35 percent. However, amiodarone is the preferred option for patients with left ventricular hypertrophy.

Quinidine, procainamide, and especially disopyramide are strictly used in patients with vagally medicated AF. The long-lasting anticholinergic activity of disopyramide is helpful in controlling vagally induced AF especially in athletic young men with slow heart rates during rest or sleep, as long as the patient does not have prostatism or glaucoma. In contrast, adrenergically mediated AF that occur during exercise, beta blockers are used as first-line therapy, followed by sotalol and amiodarone.

### *5.3.3 Progression of atrial fibrillation*

AF commonly progress over time by becoming more sustained and with higher burden. Large non-randomized observational studies reported that AF progresses more frequently in patients treated with rate control, has HF, hypertension, history of stroke or transient ischemic attack and older age, when compared to those given rhythm control over 1 to 2 years period, although the absolute magnitude and difference have varied from one registry to another [26, 27]. The progression of AF is a complex process influenced not only by the choice between rhythm-control and rate-control strategies but also by factors such as age, comorbidities, structural problems, heart rate, and modifiable risk factors. Other non-randomized registries reported that rhythm control reduce the likelihood of development of dementia or worsening cardiac structural abnormalities.

### *5.3.4 Anticoagulation*

Patients with AF vary widely in their risk of developing a stroke and their tendency for bleeding. Many risk scores have been developed and validated throughout the years with a goal of accurately determine a patient's absolute risk of stroke, whether low (~ < 1%/y), intermediate (~1 to~2%/y), and high (~ > 2%/y). Even though including more predictors can improve the risk score, the absolute risk associated with a particular score level varies widely among different populations. The CHA 2 DS 2 -VASc score is considered the most validated score. However, the more recent ATRIA and GARFIELD-AF scores have better risk discrimination (c-index) compared with CHA 2 DS 2 -VASc, but their calibration and risk reclassification performance has not been as rigorously evaluated. For example, clinicians might find GARFIELD-AF better because it factors in the patient's smoking status, renal disease, and dementia [28, 29]. The decision of starting anticoagulation should be shared with the informed patient. The benefit should be weight against the risk of bleeding. The most studied bleeding risk scores (HAS-BLED, HEMORR 2 HAGES, and ATRIA) discriminate poorly between patients with and without bleeding. Therefore, clinicians use these scores to identify possible interventions to prevent bleeding on anticoagulation, like discontinuing antiplatelet medications or NSAIDs, or the use of left atrial appendage closure devices [30].

The ENGAGE AF-TIMI 48 trial concluded that AF burden might affect risk of thromboembolic events [31]. However, other randomized studies with level of certainty B recommend that the decision of initiating anticoagulation be based on the patient's risk of developing thromboembolic event (estimated annual risk ‡2%), regardless of the AF pattern [32].

For most patients with AF and an indication for anticoagulation, we recommend a direct oral anticoagulant (DOAC), rather than a vitamin K antagonist, for their safety, efficacy, and ease of use. DOACs include oral direct thrombin inhibitor dabigatran and direct factor Xa inhibitors (e.g., apixaban, edoxaban, and rivaroxaban) [33].

Long-term AF is a dynamic disease with changing risk for stroke. Disease progression, changing patient characteristics, and risk versus benefit prompt clinicians to reevaluate the need for and choice of stroke risk reduction therapy at periodic intervals. It is recommended to reassess stroke and bleeding risk, net clinical benefit, and proper dosing once a year [34].

### *5.3.5 Antithrombotic strategy after LAAC*

In patients who have history of major bleed, where long-term anticoagulation is contraindicated, clinicians may recommend a left atrial appendage closure (LAAC). There are variety of device options that will be mentioned in a later section. However, post implantation anticoagulation and antiplatelet therapy are worth mentioning because LAAC is done for patients who have a high risk of bleed in the first place.

In previous studies, after implanting a LAAC device, patients were given warfarin and aspirin for 45 days. If no device-related thrombosis (DRT) was found on a transesophageal echocardiogram (TEE) at the 45-day mark, warfarin was stopped. Patients then took aspirin and clopidogrel for 6 months, followed by aspirin alone indefinitely. This approach is the standard and recommended regimen after LAAC device implantation. Current guidelines suggest taking oral anticoagulants for 45 days and then switching to dual antiplatelet therapy (DAPT) for six months to manage DRT and reduce the risk of stroke. DOACs are thought to be more convenient than warfarin, and several observational studies have shown that they are non-inferior in terms of embolic events and bleeding risk; nevertheless, bigger RCTs are needed to confirm the findings [35].

## 6. Interventional management of atrial fibrillation

As previously discussed, depending on the strategy of treatment of the atrial fibrillation, one might opt for a rhythm control strategy [36].

In this section, we are going to review the interventional approach for treating atrial fibrillation to establish rhythm control, as well as some other catheter and interventions used in atrial fibrillation patients to decrease the rate of thromboembolic events.

### 6.1 Indications

The principal aim of AF ablation is to alleviate symptoms associated with atrial fibrillation (AF). According to prevailing guidelines in the United States and Europe, catheter ablation for AF holds a Class 1 designation (strongly recommended) for individuals with paroxysmal atrial fibrillation (PAF) who either cannot tolerate or do not respond to antiarrhythmic drug (AAD) therapy. It is classified as Class 2a (considered reasonable) as a primary treatment for individuals with PAF and for those with persistent AF who are either intolerant to or have failed AAD treatment. Additionally, it is considered Class 2b (may be considered) for patients with long-standing persistent AF [36].

Surgical ablation is deemed Class 1 for patients with all forms of AF who are undergoing open cardiac surgery, such as mitral valve (MV) replacement. Furthermore, it is classified as Class 1 for all forms of AF in patients undergoing closed cardiac surgery (e.g., aortic valve replacement or coronary artery bypass grafting) who are intolerant of or refractory to AAD [1], and as Class 2a for patients for whom AAD has not been attempted. Standalone surgical ablation is regarded as Class 2a for patients with persistent and longstanding persistent AF and as Class 2b for PAF, with catheter ablation being at least equally preferred in these patient subsets [36, 37].

In certain cohorts where pharmacological therapy is anticipated to have limited tolerability (e.g., in athletes or patients with tachy-brady syndrome lacking a pacemaker), AF ablation may be considered a viable first-line alternative [38]. Recent evidence suggests that first-line AF ablation may offer superior outcomes compared to AAD therapy in terms of AF recurrence in specific populations, irrespective of the patient's tolerance to pharmacological therapy [39]. Some patients with heart failure or hypertrophic cardiomyopathy may experience hemodynamic improvement with the maintenance of sinus rhythm (SR), thus making them suitable candidates for AF ablation [40]. The decision to proceed with AF ablation in any patient is personalized, considering factors such as the likelihood of efficacy, procedural risk, and patient preference for invasive procedures. Currently, discontinuation of anticoagulation is not a justification for AF ablation.

Anticoagulation for stroke and thromboembolism prevention should be continued based on clinical risk factors, such as the CHA2DS2-VASc score, although alternatives such as catheter left atrial appendage (LAA) occlusion may be offered to patients intolerant of long-term anticoagulation [41, 42].

In patients with moderate to severely reduced left ventricular (LV) function undergoing atrioventricular (AV) junction ablation for rate control of AF, the placement of a biventricular or His/left bundle branch area pacing lead is recommended [43].

Numerous trials have been conducted to assess the outcomes of ablation versus antiarrhythmic drug (AAD) therapy in patients unresponsive to at least one AAD. Trials involving patients with paroxysmal atrial fibrillation (PAF) exhibited success rates ranging from 59–89% at 12 months, while those with persistent AF demonstrated success rates of 59–80% at 6 or 12 months, in contrast to 5–23% and 9–58% for AAD, respectively [44].

A comprehensive meta-analysis of radiofrequency ablation (RFA) studies and AAD studies similarly concluded that RFA was more effective than AAD for AF control. Patients undergoing ablation tended to be younger, had longer AF duration, and had failed a greater number of AADs. Complication rates were 4.9% with ablation versus 30% with AAD; however, complications were generally less severe with AAD. Overall mortality was 0.7% with ablation versus 2.8% with AAD (0.6% sudden death and 0.5% treatment-related death) [45].

Trials investigating first-line pulmonary vein isolation (PVI) for PAF using either RFA (RAAFT, RAAFT-2) or cryoablation (STOP AF, EARLY-AF, and CRYO-FIRST) all demonstrated a reduction in AF recurrence (32% vs. 53%; relative risk, 0.62; 95% confidence interval [CI], 0.51–0.74; $p < 0.001$). Particularly, younger patients with PAF showed favorable outcomes with ablation [46, 47].

The efficacy of cryoballoon ablation appears comparable to RFA, as evidenced by the FIRE AND ICE trial. Phrenic nerve injury was more common with cryoablation but largely resolved within 6 months, resulting in a low permanent phrenic nerve injury rate. The CIRCA-DOSE study found no difference in the recurrence of PAF between groups using different PVI methods [48].

Though experience is limited, outcomes with laser balloon ablation demonstrate a high percentage of acute PVI that appears durable, with similar arrhythmia-free survival at 12 months compared with RFA PVI. However, the REAFFIRM study did not show added benefit to PVI with rotational activity or focal source mapping and ablation, necessitating further investigation of this technology [49].

The EAST-AFNET 4 trial provided evidence that early rhythm control in patients diagnosed with AF within a year was associated with a lower risk of adverse cardiac events (cardiovascular death, stroke, or heart failure hospitalization) when using class Ic agents or dronedarone combined with catheter ablation, when needed, in up to 20% of patients [50].

Trials of catheter ablation in patients with heart failure demonstrated improvement in cardiovascular outcomes, including mortality, compared with drug therapy alone; however, patients with more advanced heart failure may not benefit from catheter ablation compared with guideline-directed medical therapy [51, 52].

### *6.1.1 Outcomes and efficacy*

Numerous studies have been conducted to assess the comparative outcomes of ablation versus antiarrhythmic drug (AAD) therapy in patients resistant to at least one AAD. Trials involving patients with paroxysmal atrial fibrillation (PAF) revealed success rates ranging from 59–89% at 12 months, while those with persistent AF exhibited success rates of 59–80% at 6 or 12 months, in contrast to 5–23% and 9–58% for AAD, respectively [53–56].

A comprehensive meta-analysis of radiofrequency ablation (RFA) trials and AAD studies similarly indicated that RFA was more effective than AAD in managing AF. Patients undergoing ablation tended to be younger, with a longer AF duration, and had failed a greater number of AAD treatments. Complication rates were 4.9% with ablation versus 30% with AAD; however, AAD-related complications were generally less severe. The overall mortality rate was 0.7% with ablation versus 2.8% with AAD (0.6% sudden death and 0.5% treatment-related death) [57].

Trials focusing on pulmonary vein isolation (PVI) as a first-line treatment for PAF using either RFA or cryoablation consistently demonstrated a reduction in AF recurrence. Younger patients with PAF particularly benefited from ablation [58, 59] .

Cryoballoon ablation efficacy appears comparable to RFA, as evidenced by the FIRE AND ICE trial. Phrenic nerve injury was more frequent with cryoablation but often resolved within 6 months, resulting in a low permanent phrenic nerve injury rate. The CIRCA-DOSE study found no difference in PAF recurrence between PVI using contact force sensing RFA catheters and cryoballoon with varying dosing strategies [59, 60].

Although data on outcomes with laser balloon ablation are limited, there is a high percentage of acute PVI with apparent durability, comparable to RFA PVI at 12 months. However, studies like REAFFIRM have not shown added benefit to PVI with rotational activity or focal source mapping and ablation, necessitating further investigation of this technology [49].

The EAST-AFNET 4 trial demonstrated that early rhythm control in patients with recent AF diagnosis was associated with a lower risk of adverse cardiac events when utilizing antiarrhythmic medications combined with catheter ablation, if necessary [50].

### *6.1.2 Radiofrequency and cryoablation*

Unipolar radiofrequency ablation (RFA) stands as the prevailing method of ablation, where energy is administered from the catheter tip electrode, while an indifferent patch electrode on the patient's hip or thigh completes the circuit. Radiofrequency (RF) current, typically ranging from 450 to 500 KHz, induces resistive heating at or near the catheter tip-tissue interface, with thermal conduction extending lesion formation into deeper tissue. A tissue temperature of 50°C or above is necessary for irreversible cell death, with temperature feedback provided by a thermistor on the catheter tip to regulate power delivery and attain the preset temperature [61, 62].

To address potential coagulum formation from blood pool proteins hindering current delivery during ablation, catheter designs featuring irrigation are now favored.

With non-irrigated catheters, the maximal temperature is reached adjacent to the catheter's contact site, whereas irrigated catheters achieve maximal temperature deeper than the contact site due to the cooling and "rinsing" effect from irrigation. This allows for sustained higher power delivery without tip coagulum formation, facilitating the creation of larger lesions. Moreover, irrigated catheter designs are associated with a reduced likelihood of microembolism [63].

The cryoballoon emerged as an alternative to radiofrequency circumferential ablation for the pulmonary veins (PVs). Cryoablation employs a non-distensible multilayer balloon catheter (available in 28 mm and 23 mm diameter sizes) guided by a steerable sheath. Nitrous oxide refrigerant is introduced into the balloon through multiple jets, producing an equatorial band of freezing in the first-generation design and a nearly hemispheric freezing surface in the second-generation redesign, enhancing ablation contact. Typical freeze cycles last 300 seconds for first-generation balloons and 180–240 seconds for second-generation balloons, achieving temperatures of −50°C to −60°C. In a sizable randomized controlled trial, cryoballoon ablation demonstrated comparable efficacy and safety to RFA, albeit with a higher risk of acute phrenic nerve injury [64, 65].

### *6.1.3 Parameters and important factors*

During ablation procedures, the contact between the catheter and tissue plays a crucial role in lesion formation and can be continuously monitored using contact force sensing catheters [66]. These catheters employ high-precision optical or spring mechanism designs at the catheter tip to detect minor deflections or measure tip-tissue electrical coupling. When integrated with three-dimensional (3D) mapping systems, both the magnitude and direction of force can be accurately assessed [67, 68]. Notably, research has shown that surrogates for catheter contact, such as tactile feedback, fluoroscopic appearance, and electrogram amplitude, are less reliable indicators of lesion formation compared to contact force data [69].

The provision of contact force data has been shown to reduce both ablation and fluoroscopy times. Although the optimal contact force for catheter ablation has not been conclusively determined through prospective evaluation, expert consensus suggests a range of 5–10 grams as a minimum [69]. By combining contact force with other parameters such as ablation time, energy, and impedance change, a quantitative measurement of lesion delivery can be achieved. While contact force sensing catheter technology has been associated with improved first-pass pulmonary vein isolation (PVI) and medium-term outcomes in freedom from atrial fibrillation (AF), it may elevate the risk of collateral damage if the combination of power, contact force, and lesion duration exceeds safe thresholds [69, 70].

### *6.1.4 Imaging guidance*

Phased-array intracardiac echocardiogram (ICE) serves as a valuable tool in atrial fibrillation (AF) ablation procedures for real-time visualization of cardiac anatomy. It enables clinicians to visualize anatomy in real time, aiding in procedures such as trans-septal access and positioning of intracardiac catheters with visual confirmation of contact. Additionally, ICE allows for visual assessment of lesion formation during ablation procedures. It is also capable of early detection of thrombus formation on catheters or sheaths, as well as timely identification of pericardial effusions [71–73].

Furthermore, by integrating multiple two-dimensional ICE slices, 3D mapping systems can generate a comprehensive three-dimensional representation of cardiac anatomy. When used in conjunction with 3D mapping, ICE significantly reduces the reliance on fluoroscopy during AF ablation procedures, offering a safer and more efficient approach to treatment [74, 75].

#### *6.1.5 Three-dimensional mapping*

Modern electroanatomical mapping (EAM) systems offer high-resolution electrical data (voltage or activation time) overlaid onto an anatomical model, providing real-time visualization of catheter position. Bipolar voltage amplitude serves to identify areas of abnormal myocardium, with a consensus that voltage levels <0.4–0.5 mV indicate dense fibrosis or advanced disease in the atrium [76, 77].

Activation mapping demonstrates wavefront propagation either through isochronal topography or motion rendering, aiding in the visualization and analysis of re-entry circuits and focal tachycardia origins. Mapping systems allow for site tagging and display biophysical data in lesion tags, incorporating catheter position stability in millimeters, respiratory gating, radiofrequency application time in seconds, and contact force with predefined minimum thresholds in grams [78].

Integration with ultrasound and fluoroscopic imaging has been developed to harness the strengths of combined imaging modalities while reducing radiation exposure. Numerous mapping techniques and technologies are being investigated to identify critical substrate for ablation, particularly in patients with persistent AF, but none have demonstrated superiority over pulmonary vein isolation (PVI) alone [79, 80].

#### *6.1.6 New catheter technologies*

A promising technology is hot balloon ablation, which utilizes RF-superheated saline within a compliant balloon to create thermal lesions at the PV ostia through direct contact [81]. Additionally, multielectrode circular and mesh catheters positioned at the PV ostia aim to both record and selectively ablate sites of PV conduction [82, 83].

Irreversible electroporation or pulsed-field ablation (PFA) represents another highly promising approach, potentially offering improved efficacy with a wider safety margin. PFA is being extensively investigated across various catheter platforms. Initial safety and feasibility trials have shown promising results, with a high percentage of acute PV isolation rate and high durability, coupled with low one-year AF recurrence rates [84]. Ongoing prospective randomized trials comparing PFA to RF catheter ablation are currently underway, aiming to further evaluate its efficacy and safety profile.

#### *6.1.7 Trans-septal puncture*

Intracardiac echocardiography (ICE) serves as a valuable tool for visualizing cardiac landmarks and creating three-dimensional (3D) anatomical models. Key structures of interest include the fossa ovalis, membranous septum, left atrium (LA), pulmonary veins (PVs), and left atrial appendage (LAA). To initiate trans-septal access, a sheath with a dilator is introduced via a femoral vein and positioned over the membranous septum, with tenting directed toward the left PVs [85].

Under visualization with ICE or fluoroscopy, a trans-septal needle is advanced to puncture the membranous septum with controlled precision. Optionally, specific guidewires can aid in septal puncture to facilitate the advancement of the sheath across the membranous septum. Pressure waveforms can be monitored and recorded to confirm successful LA access [85].

### *6.1.8 General approach for ablation*

The fundamental strategy in ablation therapy for atrial fibrillation (AF) revolves around pulmonary vein isolation (PVI). Identification of trigger phenomena that initiate and sustain AF, along with evidence of AF triggers originating from the pulmonary veins (PVs), prompted the development of techniques focused on isolating the PVs. This approach became imperative as targeting specific PV trigger sites was often impractical, and ablating within a PV carried the risk of stenosis [86].

Early methods included segmental ablation, supported by mapping using multipolar circular electrode catheters positioned at the PV ostia, until electrical isolation of the PVs was achieved. Subsequent refinements led to PV ostial circumferential ablation, representing an evolution toward more comprehensive and effective PVI techniques [87].

Circumferential ablation of the antral left atrium (LA) surrounding the pulmonary veins (PVs), known as wide area circumferential ablation (WACA), has become widely accepted. The evolution toward the current WACA technique stemmed from accumulating evidence demonstrating reduced complications (such as decreased PV stenosis) and increased efficacy (including the elimination of antral triggers in addition to PV triggers) [88].

Achieving precise catheter positioning involves the utilization of supportive sheaths and controlled deflection to create continuous lesions along the intended ablation line. Establishing pulmonary vein isolation (PVI) is marked by the eradication of conduction both into (entry block) and out of (exit block) the PVs. Confirmation of exit block is often accomplished through pacing within the PVs, demonstrating capture of the PV muscle sleeve without altering the atrial rate [89].

Conduction to the PVs primarily occurs along the PV muscle sleeve extending directly from the adjacent atrium. However, conduction can also take place through epicardial pathways, including pathways from the superior vena cava (SVC) and posterior right atrium (RA) to right-sided PVs (septopulmonary bundles) [90], as well as through the vein of Marshall (VOM) to the left-sided PVs [91]. In cases where circumferential ablation fails, these alternative pathways of conduction must be identified and ablated, often at the carina between the PV ostia.

## 6.2 Ablation strategy

### *6.2.1 Left atrial posterior wall*

The posterior region of the left atrium (LA) can be targeted for isolation to reduce re-entry substrates, especially in cases of persistent atrial fibrillation (AF). After achieving pulmonary vein isolation (PVI) via wide area circumferential ablation (WACA), isolation of the posterior wall can be performed through linear ablation, forming continuous lesions that link the superior pulmonary veins (creating a "roof line") and the inferior pulmonary veins (forming a "floor line"). Successful isolation is confirmed by conduction block into and out of the posterior LA box, with any breakthrough indicating a gap that requires further ablation to establish a complete block [88, 92].

Similar to all linear ablation techniques, the primary challenge lies in ensuring lesion durability, as the recovery of one or more sites can create a substrate conducive to re-entrant tachycardia [93].

During ablation of the posterior left atrium (LA), it is crucial to determine the esophagus's location to prevent thermal injury, as the esophagus can be adjacent to any part of the posterior LA. Inserting a radiopaque esophageal temperature probe allows for fluoroscopic visualization of the esophageal position and monitoring of esophageal temperature during radiofrequency (RF) lesion delivery. An increase in temperature should lead to a reduction in energy delivery in that area. The temperature probe should be repositioned to remain as close as possible to the lesion delivery site as it changes [94].

PFA seems to be a safer option in avoiding esophageal injury when ablating the posterior wall [95].

Empirical posterior wall isolation (PWI) should not be combined with pulmonary vein isolation (PVI) during the initial ablation of persistent atrial fibrillation (AF). However, in specific patient groups—such as those with low voltage on the posterior wall, roof-dependent flutters, posterior wall triggers, or those undergoing redo ablation procedures with isolated pulmonary veins—there may be potential advantages.

In the POBI-AF (Comparison of Circumferential Pulmonary Vein Isolation Alone Versus Linear Ablation in Addition to Circumferential Pulmonary Vein Isolation for Catheter Ablation in Persistent Atrial Fibrillation) study, 217 patients with persistent atrial fibrillation (AF) were assigned randomly to either pulmonary vein isolation (PVI) alone or PVI combined with posterior wall box isolation (POBI). Following an average follow-up period of 16.2 months, the results showed no significant difference in freedom from AF between the two groups (50.5% for PVI alone compared to 55.9% for PVI plus POBI; $p = 0.5222$) [96].

Similar results were also found in a more recent RCT named the Catheter Ablation for Persistent Atrial Fibrillation (CAPLA) study, which involved 338 symptomatic persistent AF patients [80].

#### *6.2.2 Targeting the atrial flutter*

Typical atrial flutter, the most prevalent form of macro-reentry atrial flutter, involves the cavotricuspid isthmus (CTI) [97]. This condition frequently coexists with atrial fibrillation (AF), sharing a common pathological basis. Earlier research has demonstrated that pulmonary vein isolation (PVI) can markedly decrease the clinical recurrence of atrial arrhythmia in patients suffering from both AF and atrial flutter. However, more recent studies have shown that including CTI ablation in the treatment protocol significantly enhances clinical outcomes by further reducing the recurrence of atrial flutter [55, 98].

Ablation of the CTI is effectively accomplished by creating a continuous line of lesions from the inferior tricuspid valve annulus to the inferior vena cava, ensuring bidirectional block is achieved [99].

#### *6.2.3 How to test if the ablation is successful*

Confirmation of conduction block is essential for successful isolation of the pulmonary veins (PVs). Entrance block serves as an acceptable endpoint and can be verified using a circular or multisplined multielectrode mapping catheter positioned within each vein. If residual PV conduction is detected following circumferential ablation, the shortest left atrium to PV conduction pathways is targeted for additional ablation in the left atrium until all conduction into the vein is eliminated [89].

Differentiating pulmonary vein (PV) potentials from far-field potentials can be achieved through differential pacing maneuvers. Pacing from the far-field structure results in the advancement of far-field potentials and the delay of local PV potentials [89, 100].

### 6.3 Complications

Catheter ablation for AF is an advanced procedure. Its invasive nature necessitates vascular access, catheter navigation, and energy application within the left atrium (LA), which has a thin wall and is adjacent to organs that may be vulnerable to thermal injury. Consequently, AF ablation carries a significant complication rate. This is especially pertinent as the primary objective of the procedure in most cases is to alleviate symptoms [101].

The rate of complications following atrial fibrillation ablation is consistently documented in administrative databases, extensive registries, and randomized trials, ranging from 2.5–8% [102–105]. Whereas in-hospital death is extremely rare, ranging between 0.05 and 0.1% [106].

A recent meta-analysis of adjudicated safety outcomes from randomized controlled trials (RCTs) showed a notable reduction in the overall complication rate associated with atrial fibrillation (AF) catheter ablation in the more recent timeframe (2018–2022) compared to the prior five-year period (3.8% vs. 5.3%, respectively) [107].

The main complications of catheter ablation of AF are listed in the table below (adapted from 2024 European Heart Rhythm Association/Heart Rhythm Society/Asia Pacific Heart Rhythm Society/Latin American Heart Rhythm Society expert consensus statement on catheter and surgical ablation of atrial fibrillation) (**Table 3**) [101].

It is important to mention that the type of energy source for the ablation plays a role in the genre of complication but not in the rate of complications (RF vs. cryoballoon ablation) [48, 64].

Persistent phrenic nerve palsy following pulmonary vein isolation (PVI) is almost exclusively associated with cryoablation, whereas esophageal perforation is predominantly a complication of radiofrequency (RF) ablation [108].

The available data on pulsed-field ablation (PFA) are currently limited, yet the existing evidence suggests that its overall complication rate is comparable to those observed with the other two energy modalities. Due to the specific effect of electroporation on cardiomyocytes, adverse extracardiac effects such as esophageal damage are expected to be significantly limited, if not absent, after PFA [109–111].

Recent research indicates that the specific protocol used for RF ablation could influence the occurrence of asymptomatic cerebral emboli post-ablation. In a prospective, randomized study, it was found that high-power, short-duration (HPSD) RF ablation (70 W for 9–10 seconds) for pulmonary vein isolation (PVI) was linked to a significantly increased incidence of subclinical strokes detected by MRI, in comparison with conventional ablation guided by AI (25–40 W) [112].

Three primary forms of esophageal injury have been identified: atrioesophageal fistula (AEF), atrial-pericardial fistula, and esophageal hematoma. These complications arise due to thermal injury to the esophagus, which is situated near the posterior wall of the left atrium [113].

| Complication type | Complication rate, % |
|---|---|
| Periprocedural death | 0.05–0.1 |
| Atrioesophageal fistula | 0.02–0.1 |
| Periprocedural thromboembolic event | 0.15–0.5 |
| Cardiac tamponade | 0.4–1.3 |
| Severe pulmonary vein stenosis | 0–0.5 |
| Permanent phrenic nerve palsy | 0.08–0.1 |
| Vascular complications | 1–4[a] |
| Asymptomatic acute cerebral lesions | 5–30 |

[a]*Without ultrasound-guided vascular puncture.*

**Table 3.**
*Main complications of catheter ablation of atrial fibrillation.*

Esophageal perforation typically manifests through symptoms such as fever, chest pain or odynophagia, and neurological events (e.g., septic emboli). However, patients may also exhibit esophageal bleeding, hematemesis, systemic emboli, septic shock, or may succumb to the condition [108].

Another complication worth mentioning is the periprocedural thromboembolic events. These events predominantly present as strokes or transient ischemic attacks (TIA). In recent extensive studies, the occurrence of stroke or TIA following catheter ablation is reported to be between 0.15% and 0.5% [104, 106, 114].

Thromboembolic incidents generally happen within the first 24 hours post-ablation, with the elevated risk phase continuing throughout the initial two weeks after the procedure [115].

Possible causes of thromboembolic complications encompass thrombus formation on or within sheaths and ablation catheters inserted into the left atrium (LA), char formation at the ablation catheter tip, dislodgment of an existing LA thrombus, and the application of electrical cardioversion during the procedure. Consequently, it is advised to adhere to a rigorous anticoagulation protocol throughout the procedure. This includes the administration of heparin (prior to transseptal puncture), frequent measurement of activated clotting time (ACT), maintaining an ACT of at least 300 seconds, and paying close attention to sheath management [101].

A serious complication is cardiac tamponade. Cardiac tamponade continues to be the most common and potentially fatal complication associated with atrial fibrillation catheter ablation. According to recent extensive surveys, its occurrence has been reported to range between 0.4% and 1.3% [104, 106].

The markedly higher incidence of cardiac tamponade during atrial fibrillation (AF) ablation, in comparison with other cardiac electrophysiology procedures, can be ascribed to several procedural distinctions. These include the necessity for transseptal puncture, extensive manipulation and ablation within the heart, and the requirement for systemic anticoagulation during the procedure. The primary causes of cardiac perforation that result in cardiac tamponade during AF ablation are: (i) improperly directed transseptal puncture, where the puncture is performed too posteriorly, causing it to exit the right atrium (RA) into the pericardium before entering the left atrium (LA), or when the puncture is extended excessively, causing it to exit the LA through the roof, left atrial appendage (LAA), or the lateral LA wall; (ii) direct mechanical trauma to the LA during catheter manipulation and ablation; and (iii) overheating during the delivery of radiofrequency (RF) energy, which can occur with or without the formation of a steam pop. Additionally, excessive power, temperature, and force applied at the catheter tip can contribute to these complications [101].

Additionally, pulmonary vein (PV) stenosis is a known complication resulting from thermal damage during atrial fibrillation (AF) ablation procedures. The shift from ostial to antral ablation, along with the heightened awareness to avoid energy delivery within the PVs, has led to a substantial decrease in the occurrence of this issue. In recent extensive series of AF ablations, the incidence of severe PV stenosis has been reported to be between 0% and 0.5%, making it an exceedingly rare event [106, 116].

Managing pulmonary vein (PV) stenosis poses significant challenges. Interventional treatment becomes necessary when symptoms are present. For PV stenoses that are either asymptomatic or mildly symptomatic, a conservative approach with careful monitoring is recommended. Symptomatic relief has been noted even without treatment, as collateral vessel formation can occur following PV stenosis or occlusion [116].

Finally, a complication that is always concerning is the phrenic nerve palsy. Phrenic nerve palsy, a notable complication of atrial fibrillation (AF) ablation, arises from direct injury to the phrenic nerve (PN). The right PN is most frequently impacted due to its close proximity to ablation sites near the superior vena cava (SVC) and both right-sided pulmonary veins (PVs). It is situated slightly farther from the right inferior PV, making injury during ablation of this vein less frequent compared to the right superior PV (RSPV) ablation. The left PN can also be injured during ablation of the left atrial appendage (LAA) because it passes anterior to the LAA base. Although phrenic nerve palsy can occur with all forms of thermal AF ablation, the majority of cases are associated with cryoablation [48, 117, 118].

According to recent registries on pulsed field ablation (PFA), instances of phrenic nerve (PN) palsy are exceptionally uncommon when using the pentaspline, multi-electrode PFA catheter [109, 110].

Lastly, the most common complications in the ablation procedures are the vascular complications. Complications are usually groin hematoma, femoral artery pseudoaneurysm, arteriovenous fistula, and retroperitoneal bleeding are potential concerns. The current incidence rates for these complications are estimated to be between 1% and 4% [104, 106].

The majority of femoral hematomas are typically amenable to conservative management or intervention guided by ultrasound compression. Nonetheless, complications like femoral pseudoaneurysm, arteriovenous fistula, and retroperitoneal hemorrhage may necessitate blood transfusion and/or surgical or percutaneous intervention, resulting in elevated morbidity rates and prolonged hospitalization durations [119].

Moreover, a list of some complications that are very common but worth mentioning, with some description, found lately in the literature: air embolism, acute coronary artery stenosis and occlusion, mitral valve trauma and catheter entrapment, stiff left atrial syndrome, and gastric hypomotility [101].

## 7. Left atrial appendage

The left atrial appendage (LAA) is extensively recognized as the principal site for thrombus formation. This claim is well-supported by numerous prior studies, which have consistently shown a strong association between thrombus formation in the LAA and atrial fibrillation (AF) [120, 121]. The CHADS2 and CHA2DS2-VASc scoring systems are widely utilized to assess and predict stroke risk in patients with atrial fibrillation (AF) [122, 123].

Recently, left atrial appendage closure (LAAC) has gained prominence as an alternative therapeutic option for atrial fibrillation (AF) patients with elevated stroke risk. Although existing clinical outcome data for LAAC is limited, ongoing studies are anticipated to provide further insights, and advancements in LAAC device technology may enhance its efficacy.

The left atrial appendage (LAA) exhibits a distinct anatomy characterized by considerable variability in its size and shape. According to research by Ernst et al., the volume, length, width, and orifice diameter of the LAA were found to vary widely, measuring between 0.7 to 19.2 cc, 16 to 51 mm, 10 to 40 mm, and 5 to 27 mm, respectively [124]. The number of lobes can range from one to four [125].

Due to the anatomical diversity of the left atrial appendage (LAA), a customized procedural approach is necessary. Therefore, a preprocedural imaging assessment of the LAA's complexity and variability is crucial, especially for the percutaneous left atrial appendage closure (LAAC) procedure.

Whether via a TEE, CT or CMR, it is essential to measure the dimensions of the LAA to plan for the percutaneous LAA closure procedure or to document the absence of a thrombus intra-appendage.

Bleeding complications and non-adherence continue to pose significant challenges, particularly in elderly patients who are at an elevated risk for thromboembolic events related to atrial fibrillation (AF). Concerns about high bleeding risk led to approximately 40–50% of patients not receiving anticoagulation, despite its well-established benefits in preventing thromboembolic events [126, 127]. Consequently, mechanical preventive measures like surgical exclusion of the left atrial appendage (LAA) and percutaneous LAA closure (LAAC) have been implemented in clinical practice as a promising alternative to medical management for preventing thromboembolic events in patients with atrial fibrillation (AF).

It is noteworthy that the majority of LAAC trials do not specifically include AF patients who have had significant bleeding events following the use of non-vitamin K antagonist oral anticoagulants (NOACs).

### 7.1 LAA percutaneous closure

In recent years, various left atrial appendage closure (LAAC) devices have been designed and launched as alternatives to anticoagulant therapy for stroke prevention. The Percutaneous Left Atrial Appendage Transcatheter Occlusion (PLAATO) device, developed by eV3, Inc. in Plymouth, MA, USA, was the pioneering percutaneous device implanted in human subjects [128]. The device featured a self-expanding nitinol frame, covered with a non-thrombogenic polytetrafluoroethylene layer, and included anchors on three posts designed to secure it to the left atrial appendage (LAA). Prior studies have demonstrated that left atrial appendage closure (LAAC) using the PLAATO device is both safe and effective for patients with non-valvular atrial fibrillation (NVAF), and the device of the PLAATO trial is not available commercially anymore [129].

The Watchman device (Boston Scientific, Natick, Massachusetts) represents a specialized left atrial appendage closure (LAAC) device, following the PLAATO device. It received approval from the US Food and Drug Administration (FDA) subsequent to the completion of the pilot study in 2015 [130].

The Watchman device features a parachute-like shape and is self-expanding with a nitinol framework. It is encased in a polyethylene terephthalate fabric membrane that faces the left atrial body. This membrane serves to obstruct thrombus migration from the left atrial appendage (LAA) and encourages endothelialization. Available in five sizes, ranging from 21 to 33 mm, it is the most extensively researched device for left atrial appendage closure (LAAC).

The PROTECT-AF trial was a multicenter, randomized controlled study conducted across the USA and Europe from 2005 to 2012. A total of 707 patients with non-valvular atrial fibrillation (NVAF) and CHADS2 scores of ≥1 were randomly allocated in a 2:1 ratio to receive either left atrial appendage closure (LAAC) with the Watchman device or warfarin therapy. Warfarin treatment was maintained for 45 days post-device implantation, followed by clopidogrel for 6 months, with aspirin given indefinitely. The findings of this trial demonstrated that LAAC was comparable to warfarin alone in terms of preventing cardiovascular death, stroke, or systemic embolism in patients with NVAF [131].

A meta-analysis encompassing data from the PROTECT AF and PREVAIL trials over a 5-year period has shown that left atrial appendage closure (LAAC) using the Watchman device is effective in stroke prevention for non-valvular atrial fibrillation (NVAF), with outcomes comparable to those achieved with warfarin. Additionally, LAAC with Watchman provides further benefits, such as a reduction in major bleeding incidents, particularly hemorrhagic strokes, and a decrease in mortality rates [131].

The CAP Registry, involving 566 patients, indicated that Watchman implantation is a beneficial and safe alternative. It also demonstrated that the incidence of complications associated with Watchman implantation substantially declines as operator experience increases [132].

## Author details

Mohammad Montaser Atasi†, Razan Dankar†, Jamil Francis† and Marwan M. Refaat*†
Division of Cardiology, Department of Internal Medicine, American University of Beirut Faculty of Medicine and Medical Center (AUBMC), Beirut, Lebanon

*Address all correspondence to: mr48@aub.edu.lb

† All authors contributed equally.

## References

[1] Elliott AD et al. Epidemiology and modifiable risk factors for atrial fibrillation. Nature Reviews. Cardiology. 2023;**20**(6):404-417

[2] Lippi G, Sanchis-Gomar F, Cervellin G. Global epidemiology of atrial fibrillation: An increasing epidemic and public health challenge. International Journal of Stroke. 2021;**16**(2):217-221

[3] Chiang CE, Wang KL, Lip GY. Stroke prevention in atrial fibrillation: An Asian perspective. Thrombosis and Haemostasis. 2014;**111**(5):789-797

[4] Schnabel RB et al. 50 year trends in atrial fibrillation prevalence, incidence, risk factors, and mortality in the Framingham heart study: A cohort study. Lancet. 2015;**386**(9989):154-162

[5] Dilaveris PE, Kennedy HL. Silent atrial fibrillation: Epidemiology, diagnosis, and clinical impact. Clinical Cardiology. 2017;**40**(6):413-418

[6] Kornej J et al. Epidemiology of atrial fibrillation in the 21st century: Novel methods and new insights. Circulation Research. 2020;**127**(1):4-20

[7] Nesheiwat Z, Goyal A, Jagtap M. Atrial Fibrillation. In: StatPearls. Treasure Island (FL): StatPearls Publishing Copyright © 2024, StatPearls Publishing LLC; 2024

[8] Lee DSM, Damrauer SM, Levin MG. Genetics of atrial fibrillation. Current Opinion in Cardiology. 2023;**38**(3):162-168

[9] Kim JA, Chelu MG, Li N. Genetics of atrial fibrillation. Current Opinion in Cardiology. 2021;**36**(3):281-287

[10] Nielsen JB et al. Biobank-driven genomic discovery yields new insight into atrial fibrillation biology. Nature Genetics. 2018;**50**(9):1234-1239

[11] Tieleman RG et al. Verapamil reduces tachycardia-induced electrical remodeling of the atria. Circulation. 1997;**95**(7):1945-1953

[12] De Simone A et al. Pretreatment with verapamil in patients with persistent or chronic atrial fibrillation who underwent electrical cardioversion. Journal of the American College of Cardiology. 1999;**34**(3):810-814

[13] Pluymaekers N et al. Frequency and determinants of spontaneous conversion to sinus rhythm in patients presenting to the emergency department with recent-onset atrial fibrillation: A systematic review. Arrhythmia & Electrophysiology Review. 2020;**9**(4):195-201

[14] Hindricks G et al. 2020 ESC guidelines for the diagnosis and management of atrial fibrillation developed in collaboration with the European Association for Cardio-Thoracic Surgery (EACTS): The task force for the diagnosis and management of atrial fibrillation of the European Society of Cardiology (ESC) developed with the special contribution of the European heart rhythm association (EHRA) of the ESC. European Heart Journal. 2021;**42**(5):373-498

[15] Wyse DG et al. A comparison of rate control and rhythm control in patients with atrial fibrillation. The New England Journal of Medicine. 2002;**347**(23):1825-1833

[16] Van Gelder IC et al. Lenient versus strict rate control in patients with atrial

fibrillation. The New England Journal of Medicine. 2010;**362**(15):1363-1373

[17] Rienstra M et al. Beta-blockers and outcome in heart failure and atrial fibrillation: A meta-analysis. JACC Heart Fail. 2013;**1**(1):21-28

[18] Bavishi C, Khan AR, Ather S. Digoxin in patients with atrial fibrillation and heart failure: A meta-analysis. International Journal of Cardiology. 2015;**188**:99-101

[19] Montana PC et al. Safety and efficacy of Nondihydropyridine Calcium Channel blockers for acute rate control in atrial fibrillation with rapid ventricular response and comorbid heart failure with reduced ejection fraction. Cardiology in Review. 7 Aug 2023. DOI: 10.1097/CRD.0000000000000585 [Online ahead of print]

[20] Kim D et al. Comparative effectiveness of early rhythm control versus rate control for cardiovascular outcomes in patients with atrial fibrillation. Journal of the American Heart Association. 2021;**10**(24):e023055

[21] Waks JW, Zimetbaum P. Antiarrhythmic drug therapy for rhythm control in atrial fibrillation. Journal of Cardiovascular Pharmacology and Therapeutics. 2017;**22**(1):3-19

[22] Han S et al. Early rhythm control vs. rate control in atrial fibrillation: A systematic review and meta-analysis. Frontiers in Cardiovascular Medicine. 2023;**10**:978637

[23] Ha AC et al. Health-related quality of life in patients with atrial fibrillation treated with rhythm control versus rate control: Insights from a prospective international registry (registry on cardiac rhythm disorders assessing the control of atrial fibrillation: RECORD-AF). Circulation. Cardiovascular Quality and Outcomes. 2014;7(6):896-904

[24] Roy D et al. Amiodarone to prevent recurrence of atrial fibrillation. Canadian trial of atrial fibrillation investigators. The New England Journal of Medicine. 2000;**342**(13):913-920

[25] Singh BN et al. Amiodarone versus sotalol for atrial fibrillation. The New England Journal of Medicine. 2005;**352**(18):1861-1872

[26] Zhang YY et al. Predictors of progression of recently diagnosed atrial fibrillation in REgistry on cardiac rhythm DisORDers assessing the control of atrial fibrillation (RecordAF)-United States cohort. The American Journal of Cardiology. 2013;**112**(1):79-84

[27] De Vos CB et al. Progression of atrial fibrillation in the REgistry on cardiac rhythm disORDers assessing the control of atrial fibrillation cohort: Clinical correlates and the effect of rhythm-control therapy. American Heart Journal. 2012;**163**(5):887-893

[28] Singer DE et al. A new risk scheme to predict ischemic stroke and other thromboembolism in atrial fibrillation: The ATRIA study stroke risk score. Journal of the American Heart Association. 2013;**2**(3):e000250

[29] Fox KAA et al. Improved risk stratification of patients with atrial fibrillation: An integrated GARFIELD-AF tool for the prediction of mortality, stroke and bleed in patients with and without anticoagulation. BMJ Open. 2017;7(12):e017157

[30] Chao TF et al. Incident risk factors and major bleeding in patients with atrial fibrillation treated with Oral anticoagulants: A comparison of baseline, follow-up and Delta HAS-BLED scores with an approach

focused on modifiable bleeding risk factors. Thrombosis and Haemostasis. 2018;**118**(4):768-777

[31] Link MS et al. Stroke and mortality risk in patients with various patterns of atrial fibrillation: Results from the ENGAGE AF-TIMI 48 trial (effective anticoagulation with factor Xa next generation in atrial fibrillation-thrombolysis in myocardial infarction 48). Circulation: Arrhythmia and Electrophysiology. Jan 2017;**10**(1):e004267. DOI: 10.1161/CIRCEP.116.004267

[32] Steinberg BA et al. Higher risk of death and stroke in patients with persistent vs. paroxysmal atrial fibrillation: Results from the ROCKET-AF trial. European Heart Journal. 2015;**36**(5):288-296

[33] Ruff CT et al. Comparison of the efficacy and safety of new oral anticoagulants with warfarin in patients with atrial fibrillation: A meta-analysis of randomised trials. Lancet. 2014;**383**(9921):955-962

[34] Yoon M et al. Dynamic changes of CHA2DS2-VASc score and the risk of ischaemic stroke in Asian patients with atrial fibrillation: A Nationwide cohort study. Thrombosis and Haemostasis. 2018;**118**(7):1296-1304

[35] Magdi M et al. The WATCHMAN device and post-implantation anticoagulation management. A review of key studies and the risk of device-related thrombosis. American Journal of Cardiovascular Disease. 2021;**11**(6):714-722

[36] January CT et al. 2014 AHA/ACC/HRS guideline for the management of patients with atrial fibrillation: A report of the American College of Cardiology/American Heart Association task force on practice guidelines and the Heart Rhythm Society. Journal of the American College of Cardiology. 2014;**64**(21):e1-e76

[37] Calkins H et al. 2017 HRS/EHRA/ECAS/APHRS/SOLAECE expert consensus statement on catheter and surgical ablation of atrial fibrillation. Heart Rhythm. 2017;**14**(10):e275-e444

[38] Liu MB et al. Influence of endurance sports on atrial fibrillation ablation outcomes. Journal of Arrhythmia. 2022;**38**(5):694-709

[39] Cappato R et al. Updated worldwide survey on the methods, efficacy, and safety of catheter ablation for human atrial fibrillation. Circulation: Arrhythmia and Electrophysiology. 2010;**3**(1):32-38

[40] Almroth H et al. Haemodynamic changes after atrial fibrillation initiation in patients eligible for catheter ablation: A randomized controlled study. European Heart Journal Open. 2023;**3**(6):oead112

[41] Holmes DR et al. Prospective randomized evaluation of the watchman left atrial appendage closure device in patients with atrial fibrillation versus long-term warfarin therapy: The PREVAIL trial. Journal of the American College of Cardiology. 2014;**64**(1):1-12

[42] Holmes DR et al. Percutaneous closure of the left atrial appendage versus warfarin therapy for prevention of stroke in patients with atrial fibrillation: A randomised non-inferiority trial. Lancet (London, England). 2009;**374**(9689):534-542

[43] Huang W et al. Benefits of permanent his bundle pacing combined with atrioventricular Node ablation in atrial fibrillation patients with heart

failure with both preserved and reduced left ventricular ejection fraction. Journal of the American Heart Association. 2017;**6**(4):e005309

[44] Saglietto A et al. Catheter ablation vs. anti-arrhythmic drugs as first-line treatment in symptomatic paroxysmal atrial fibrillation: A systematic review and meta-analysis of randomized clinical trials. Frontiers in Cardiovascular Medicine. 2021;**8**:664647

[45] Elsayed M et al. Bayesian network meta-analysis comparing cryoablation, radiofrequency ablation, and antiarrhythmic drugs as initial therapies for atrial fibrillation. Journal of Cardiovascular Electrophysiology. 2022;**33**(2):197-208

[46] Kaba RA, Cannie D, Ahmed O. RAAFT-2: Radiofrequency ablation vs antiarrhythmic drugs as first-line treatment of paroxysmal atrial fibrillation. Global Cardiology Science & Practice. 2014;**2014**(2):53-55

[47] Morillo CA et al. Radiofrequency ablation vs antiarrhythmic drugs as first-line treatment of paroxysmal atrial fibrillation (RAAFT-2): A randomized trial. JAMA. 2014;**311**(7):692-700

[48] Kuck K-H et al. Cryoballoon or radiofrequency ablation for paroxysmal atrial fibrillation. New England Journal of Medicine. 2016;**374**(23):2235-2245

[49] Peigh G et al. Repeat pulmonary vein isolation with or without FIRM-guided ablation for recurrent atrial fibrillation with pulmonary vein reconnection. Journal of Cardiovascular Electrophysiology. 2020;**31**(5):1031-1037

[50] Kirchhof P et al. Early rhythm-control therapy in patients with atrial fibrillation. New England Journal of Medicine. 2020;**383**(14):1305-1316

[51] AlTurki A et al. Catheter ablation for atrial fibrillation in heart failure with reduced ejection fraction: A systematic review and meta-analysis of randomized controlled trials. BMC Cardiovascular Disorders. 2019;**19**:18

[52] Marrouche NF et al. Catheter ablation for atrial fibrillation with heart failure. The New England Journal of Medicine. 2018;**378**(5):417-427

[53] Pérez FJ et al. Long-term outcomes after catheter ablation of cavo-tricuspid isthmus dependent atrial flutter: A meta-analysis. Circulation. Arrhythmia and Electrophysiology. 2009;**2**(4):393-401

[54] Patel NJ et al. Contemporary utilization and safety outcomes of catheter ablation of atrial flutter in the United States: Analysis of 89,638 procedures. Heart Rhythm. 2016;**13**(6):1317-1325

[55] Wazni O et al. Randomized study comparing combined pulmonary vein-left atrial junction disconnection and cavotricuspid isthmus ablation versus pulmonary vein-left atrial junction disconnection alone in patients presenting with typical atrial flutter and atrial fibrillation. Circulation. 2003;**108**(20):2479-2483

[56] Natale A et al. Prospective randomized comparison of antiarrhythmic therapy versus first-line radiofrequency ablation in patients with atrial flutter. Journal of the American College of Cardiology. 2000;**35**(7):1898-1904

[57] Calkins H et al. Treatment of atrial fibrillation with antiarrhythmic drugs or radiofrequency ablation: Two systematic literature reviews and meta-analyses. Circulation: Arrhythmia and Electrophysiology. 2009;**2**(4):349-361

[58] Verma A et al. Approaches to catheter ablation for persistent atrial fibrillation. New England Journal of Medicine. 2015;**372**(19):1812-1822

[59] Hachem AH et al. Radiofrequency ablation versus Cryoablation in the treatment of paroxysmal atrial fibrillation: A meta-analysis. Cardiology Research and Practice. 2018;**2018**:6276241

[60] Andrade JG et al. The Cryoballoon vs irrigated radiofrequency catheter ablation (CIRCA-DOSE) study results in context. Arrhythmia & Electrophysiology Review. 2020;**9**(1):34-39

[61] Grubb NR, Furniss S. Radiofrequency ablation for atrial fibrillation. BMJ : British Medical Journal. 2001;**322**(7289):777-780

[62] Navaneethan U et al. Radiofrequency ablation devices. VideoGIE. 2017;**2**(10):252-259

[63] Müssigbrodt A et al. Irrigated tip catheters for radiofrequency ablation in ventricular tachycardia. BioMed Research International. 2015;**2015**:389294

[64] Shi L-B et al. Cryoballoon vs. radiofrequency catheter ablation: Insights from NOrwegian randomized study of PERSistent atrial fibrillation (NO-PERSAF study). Europace. 2021;**24**(2):226-233

[65] Straube F et al. Comparison of the first and second Cryoballoon. Circulation: Arrhythmia and Electrophysiology. 2014;**7**(2):293-299

[66] Kumar S et al. Predictive value of impedance changes for real-time contact force measurements during catheter ablation of atrial arrhythmias in humans. Heart Rhythm. 2013;**10**(7):962-969

[67] Gurevitz OT et al. Use of advanced mapping systems to guide ablation in complex cases: Experience with noncontact mapping and electroanatomic mapping systems. Pacing and Clinical Electrophysiology: PACE. 2005;**28**(4):316-323

[68] Kim YH et al. 2019 APHRS expert consensus statement on three-dimensional mapping systems for tachycardia developed in collaboration with HRS, EHRA, and LAHRS. Journal of Arrhythmia. 2020;**36**(2):215-270

[69] Ariyarathna N et al. Role of contact force sensing in catheter ablation of cardiac arrhythmias: Evolution or history repeating itself? JACC: Clinical Electrophysiology. 2018;**4**(6):707-723

[70] Okumura Y et al. A Systematical analysis of In vivo contact forces on virtual catheter tip/tissue surface contact during cardiac mapping and intervention. Journal of Cardiovascular Electrophysiology. 2008;**19**(6):632-640

[71] Wright M et al. Real-time lesion assessment using a novel combined ultrasound and radiofrequency ablation catheter. Heart Rhythm. 2011;**8**(2):304-312

[72] Sayseng V et al. Catheter ablation lesion visualization with intracardiac strain imaging in canines and humans. IEEE Transactions on Ultrasonics, Ferroelectrics, and Frequency Control. 2020;**67**(9):1800-1810

[73] Bunting E et al. Cardiac lesion mapping in vivo using Intracardiac myocardial Elastography. IEEE Transactions on Ultrasonics, Ferroelectrics, and Frequency Control. 2018;**65**(1):14-20

[74] Goyal SK, Stambler BS. Fluoroless catheter ablation of cardiac

arrhythmias. US Cardiology Review. 2018;**12**(2):107-109

[75] Zei PC et al. Safety and efficacy of minimal- versus zero-fluoroscopy radiofrequency catheter ablation for atrial fibrillation: A Multicenter, prospective study. The Journal of Innovations in Cardiac Rhythm Management. 2020;**11**(11):4281-4291

[76] Yamaguchi T, Fukui A, Node K. Bipolar voltage mapping for the evaluation of atrial substrate: Can we overcome the challenge of directionality? Journal of Atrial Fibrillation. 2019;**11**(5):2116

[77] Verma A et al. Pre-existent left atrial scarring in patients undergoing pulmonary vein antrum isolation: An independent predictor of procedural failure. Journal of the American College of Cardiology. 2005;**45**(2):285-292

[78] Quintanilla JG et al. Novel approaches to mechanism-based atrial fibrillation ablation. Cardiovascular Research. 2021;**117**(7):1662-1681

[79] Fink T et al. Stand-alone pulmonary vein isolation versus pulmonary vein isolation with additional substrate modification as index ablation procedures in patients with persistent and long-standing persistent atrial fibrillation: The randomized Alster-lost-AF trial (ablation at St. Georg Hospital for Long-Standing Persistent Atrial Fibrillation). Circulation. Arrhythmia and Electrophysiology. 2017;**10**(7):e005114

[80] Kistler PM et al. Effect of catheter ablation using pulmonary vein isolation with vs without posterior left Atrial Wall isolation on atrial arrhythmia recurrence in patients with persistent atrial fibrillation: The CAPLA randomized clinical trial. JAMA. 2023;**329**(2):127

[81] Satake S et al. Usefulness of a new radiofrequency thermal balloon catheter for pulmonary vein isolation: A new device for treatment of atrial fibrillation. Journal of Cardiovascular Electrophysiology. 2003;**14**(6):609-615

[82] Zylla MM et al. Implementation of the multielectrode radiofrequency-balloon in real-world clinical practice—Operator learning curve and procedural outcome at a high-volume center. Frontiers in Cardiovascular Medicine. 2023;**10**:1208250

[83] Wakamatsu Y et al. Hot balloon versus cryoballoon ablation for persistent atrial fibrillation: Lesion area, efficacy, and safety. Journal of Cardiovascular Electrophysiology. 2020;**31**(9):2310-2318

[84] Reddy VY et al. First-in-human clinical series of a novel conformable large-lattice pulsed field ablation catheter for pulmonary vein isolation. Europace: European Pacing, Arrhythmias, and Cardiac Electrophysiology: Journal of the Working Groups on Cardiac Pacing, Arrhythmias, and Cardiac Cellular Electrophysiology of the European Society of Cardiology. 2024;**26**(4):euae090

[85] Russo G, Taramasso M, Maisano F. Transseptal puncture: Procedural guidance, challenging situations and management of complications. EuroIntervention. 2021;**17**(9):720-727

[86] Nesapiragasan V et al. Catheter ablation approaches for the treatment of arrhythmia recurrence in patients with a durable pulmonary vein isolation. Balkan Medical Journal. 2023;**40**(6):386-394

[87] Yamada T. Pulmonary vein isolation with a multielectrode basket catheter. Indian Pacing and Electrophysiology Journal. 2007;7(2):97-109

[88] Proietti R et al. Comparative effectiveness of wide antral versus ostial pulmonary vein isolation: A systematic review and meta-analysis. Circulation. Arrhythmia and Electrophysiology. 2014;**7**(1):39-45

[89] Kircher S, Sommer P. Electro-physiological evaluation of pulmonary vein isolation. Journal of Atrial Fibrillation. 2013;**6**(3):934

[90] Barrio-Lopez MT et al. Epicardial connections involving pulmonary veins. Circulation: Arrhythmia and Electrophysiology. 2020;**13**(1):e007544

[91] Rodríguez-Mañero M, Schurmann P, Valderrábano M. Ligament and vein of Marshall. A therapeutic opportunity in atrial fibrillation. Heart Rhythm: The Official Journal of the Heart Rhythm Society. 2016;**13**(2):593-601

[92] Skeete J et al. Wide area circumferential ablation for pulmonary vein isolation using radiofrequency versus laser balloon ablation. Journal of Arrhythmia. 2022;**38**(3):336-345

[93] O'Neill L et al. Atrial tachycardia occurring after a prior atrial fibrillation ablation procedure: Does non-inducibility matter? Frontiers in Cardiovascular Medicine. 2022;**9**:1073239

[94] Ariyaratnam JP, Sanders P. Protecting the oesophagus during left atrial ablation: A surplus of options but an absence of evidence. Indian Pacing and Electrophysiology Journal. 2020;**20**(6):219-220

[95] Koruth JS et al. Pulsed field ablation versus radiofrequency ablation. Circulation. Arrhythmia and Electrophysiology. 2020;**13**(3):e008303

[96] Jm L et al. The electrical isolation of the left atrial posterior wall in catheter ablation of persistent atrial fibrillation. JACC: Clinical Electrophysiology. Nov 2019;**5**(11):1253-1261

[97] Calkins H et al. 2017 HRS/EHRA/ECAS/APHRS/SOLAECE expert consensus statement on catheter and surgical ablation of atrial fibrillation: Executive summary. Heart Rhythm. 2017;**14**(10):e445-e494

[98] Scharf C et al. Clinical significance of inducible atrial flutter during pulmonary vein isolation in patients with atrial fibrillation. Journal of the American College of Cardiology. 2004;**43**(11):2057-2062

[99] Jeong JH et al. Association of typical atrial flutter and cavotricuspid isthmus ablation on clinical recurrence after cryoballoon ablation for atrial fibrillation. Frontiers in Cardiovascular Medicine. 2023;**10**:1303635

[100] Ip JE et al. Method for differentiating left superior pulmonary vein exit conduction from pseudo-exit conduction. Pacing and Clinical Electrophysiology: PACE. 2013;**36**(3):299-308

[101] Tzeis S et al. European heart rhythm association/Heart Rhythm Society/Asia Pacific Heart Rhythm Society/Latin American Heart Rhythm Society expert consensus statement on catheter and surgical ablation of atrial fibrillation. Europace. 2024;**26**(4):euae043

[102] Dagres N et al. Complications of atrial fibrillation ablation in a high-volume center in 1,000 procedures: Still cause for concern? Journal of Cardiovascular Electrophysiology. 2009;**20**(9):1014-1019

[103] Deshmukh A et al. In-hospital complications associated with catheter ablation of atrial fibrillation in the United

States between 2000 and 2010: Analysis of 93 801 procedures. Circulation. 2013;**128**(19):2104-2112

[104] Wu L et al. Safety and complications of catheter ablation for atrial fibrillation: Predictors of complications from an updated analysis the National Inpatient Database. Journal of Cardiovascular Electrophysiology. 2021;**32**(4):1024-1034

[105] Packer DL et al. Effect of catheter ablation vs antiarrhythmic drug therapy on mortality, stroke, bleeding, and cardiac arrest among patients with atrial fibrillation: The CABANA randomized clinical trial. JAMA. 2019;**321**(13):1261-1274

[106] Arbelo E et al. Contemporary management of patients undergoing atrial fibrillation ablation: in-hospital and 1-year follow-up findings from the ESC-EHRA atrial fibrillation ablation long-term registry. European Heart Journal. 2017;**38**(17):1303-1316

[107] Benali K et al. Procedure-related complications of catheter ablation for atrial fibrillation. Journal of the American College of Cardiology. 2023;**81**(21):2089-2099

[108] Tilz RR et al. A worldwide survey on incidence, management, and prognosis of oesophageal fistula formation following atrial fibrillation catheter ablation: The POTTER-AF study. European Heart Journal. 2023;**44**(27):2458-2469

[109] Ekanem E et al. Multi-national survey on the methods, efficacy, and safety on the post-approval clinical use of pulsed field ablation (MANIFEST-PF). Europace: European Pacing, Arrhythmias, and Cardiac Electrophysiology: Journal of the Working Groups on Cardiac Pacing, Arrhythmias, and Cardiac Cellular Electrophysiology of the European Society of Cardiology. 2022;**24**(8):1256-1266

[110] Schmidt B et al. EUropean real-world outcomes with pulsed field ablatiOn in patients with symptomatic atRIAl fibrillation: Lessons from the multi-Centre EU-PORIA registry. Europace: European Pacing, Arrhythmias, and Cardiac Electrophysiology: Journal of the Working Groups on Cardiac Pacing, Arrhythmias, and Cardiac Cellular Electrophysiology of the European Society of Cardiology. 2023;**25**(7):euad185

[111] Reddy VY et al. Pulsed field ablation of paroxysmal atrial fibrillation: 1-year outcomes of IMPULSE, PEFCAT, and PEFCAT II. JACC. Clinical Electrophysiology. 2021;**7**(5):614-627

[112] Castrejón-Castrejón S et al. Multicenter prospective comparison of conventional and high-power short duration radiofrequency application for pulmonary vein isolation: The high-power short-duration radiofrequency application for faster and safer pulmonary vein ablation (POWER FAST III) trial. Journal of Interventional Cardiac Electrophysiology: An International Journal of Arrhythmias and Pacing. 2023;**66**(8):1889-1899

[113] Dagres N, Anastasiou-Nana M. Prevention of atrial-esophageal fistula after catheter ablation of atrial fibrillation. Current Opinion in Cardiology. 2011;**26**(1):1-5

[114] Hsu JC et al. Initial findings from the National Cardiovascular Data Registry of atrial fibrillation ablation procedures. Journal of the American College of Cardiology. 2023;**81**(9):867-878

[115] Kosiuk J et al. Early cerebral thromboembolic complications after radiofrequency catheter ablation of atrial

fibrillation: Incidence, characteristics, and risk factors. Heart Rhythm. 2014;**11**(11):1934-1940

[116] Hilbert S et al. Pulmonary vein collateral formation as a long-term result of post-interventional pulmonary vein stenosis. European Heart Journal. 2016;**37**(31):2474

[117] Andrade JG et al. Cryoablation or drug therapy for initial treatment of atrial fibrillation. The New England Journal of Medicine. 2021;**384**(4):305-315

[118] Mörtsell D et al. Cryoballoon vs. radiofrequency ablation for atrial fibrillation: A study of outcome and safety based on the ESC-EHRA atrial fibrillation ablation long-term registry and the Swedish catheter ablation registry. Europace: European Pacing, Arrhythmias, and Cardiac Electrophysiology: Journal of the Working Groups on Cardiac Pacing, Arrhythmias, and Cardiac Cellular Electrophysiology of the European Society of Cardiology. 2019;**21**(4):581-589

[119] Waigand J et al. Percutaneous treatment of pseudoaneurysms and arteriovenous fistulas after invasive vascular procedures. Catheterization and Cardiovascular Interventions: Official Journal of the Society for Cardiac Angiography & Interventions. 1999;**47**(2):157-164

[120] Stoddard MF et al. Left atrial appendage thrombus is not uncommon in patients with acute atrial fibrillation and a recent embolic event: A transesophageal echocardiographic study. Journal of the American College of Cardiology. 1995;**25**(2):452-459

[121] Blackshear JL, Odell JA. Appendage obliteration to reduce stroke in cardiac surgical patients with atrial fibrillation. The Annals of Thoracic Surgery. 1996;**61**(2):755-759

[122] Gage BF et al. Validation of clinical classification schemes for predicting stroke: Results from the National Registry of atrial fibrillation. JAMA. 2001;**285**(22):2864-2870

[123] Lip GYH et al. Refining clinical risk stratification for predicting stroke and thromboembolism in atrial fibrillation using a novel risk factor-based approach: The euro heart survey on atrial fibrillation. Chest. 2010;**137**(2):263-272

[124] Ernst G et al. Morphology of the left atrial appendage. The Anatomical Record. 1995;**242**(4):553-561

[125] Veinot JP et al. Anatomy of the normal left atrial appendage: A quantitative study of age-related changes in 500 autopsy hearts: Implications for echocardiographic examination. Circulation. 1997;**96**(9):3112-3115

[126] Birman-Deych E et al. Use and effectiveness of warfarin in Medicare beneficiaries with atrial fibrillation. Stroke. 2006;**37**(4):1070-1074

[127] Brass LM et al. Warfarin use among patients with atrial fibrillation. Stroke. 1997;**28**(12):2382-2389

[128] Sievert H et al. Percutaneous left atrial appendage transcatheter occlusion to prevent stroke in high-risk patients with atrial fibrillation: Early clinical experience. Circulation. 2002;**105**(16):1887-1889

[129] Block PC et al. Percutaneous left atrial appendage occlusion for patients in atrial fibrillation suboptimal for warfarin therapy: 5-year results of the PLAATO (percutaneous left atrial appendage Transcatheter occlusion) study.

JACC. Cardiovascular Interventions. 2009;**2**(7):594-600

[130] Sick PB et al. Initial worldwide experience with the WATCHMAN left atrial appendage system for stroke prevention in atrial fibrillation. Journal of the American College of Cardiology. 2007;**49**(13):1490-1495

[131] Reddy VY et al. 5-year outcomes after left atrial appendage closure: From the PREVAIL and PROTECT AF trials. Journal of the American College of Cardiology. 2017;**70**(24):2964-2975

[132] Reddy VY et al. Safety of percutaneous left atrial appendage closure: Results from the watchman left atrial appendage system for embolic protection in patients with AF (PROTECT AF) clinical trial and the continued access registry. Circulation. 2011;**123**(4):417-424

Chapter 5

# Current Evidence and Management in Left Atrial Appendage Exclusion

*Jakraphan Yu, Marc Leon, Manuel Quiroz-Flores and Chawannuch Ruaengsri*


## Abstract

Atrial fibrillation (AF) is the most common cardiac arrhythmia that is related to an increased risk of ischemic stroke and systemic embolism. While oral anticoagulation drugs remain the primary treatment for stroke prevention in AF patients, certain individuals face absolute or relative contraindications that preclude oral anticoagulants use. The left atrial appendage (LAA) has been found to be the main source of intracardiac thrombi in AF patients, which result in embolic stroke, a devastating morbidity. Over the past years, the LAA exclusion technique has emerged as an alternative and complimentary therapeutic strategy for stroke prevention In this chapter, the current evidence regarding LAA closure procedure from multiple guidelines, clinical trials, as well as the technique of LAA exclusion including both surgical and transcatheter approaches will be discussed. Moreover, we will demonstrate the essential factors to achieve optimal closure and translate to favorable clinical results and the ongoing trials and future trends in LAA exclusion procedures.


**Keywords:** left atrial appendage, occlusion, ligation, closure, atrial fibrillation

## 1. Introduction

Atrial fibrillation (AF) represents the most frequently observed cardiac arrhythmia, contributing significantly to increased morbidity, mortality, and healthcare costs [1–4]. Coumadin or oral vitamin K antagonist (VKA) has been demonstrated to decrease the risk of stroke by 60% compared with 20% stroke reduction rate by using antiplatelet agents [5]. In AF patients without valvular pathology, the CHA2DS2-VASc scoring system is used for therapeutic guidance strategies to prevent stroke [6–8]. For stroke prevention in non-valvular AF patients, excluding those with mechanical valve or moderate to severe mitral valve stenosis (MS), VKA and, more recently, direct oral anticoagulants have demonstrated substantial efficacy and are recommended for patients with CHA2DS2-VASc scores ≥1 (excluding sex-related factors) [9–12]. Nonetheless, certain patients cannot tolerate oral anticoagulation therapy due to relative or absolute contraindications. Therefore, the left atrial appendage (LAA) exclusion is considered as an alternative option, targeting the thrombogenic potential of the LAA, which is prone to thrombus formation due to hemodynamic stasis.



IntechOpen

The LAA is the sole structure within the LA that originates from the primitive atrium, with its development characterized by the formation of trabeculation and pectinate muscles, while other components originate from the pulmonary veins and possess a smooth endocardial surface. By the fourth week of gestation, the primitive atrium starts a rightward looping, positioning itself within developing heart. Around day 50 of embryonic development, the left atrium is completed with the addition of primordial pulmonary veins [13].

The LAA is close to vital structures (**Figure 1**) including the pulmonary artery (PA), the left circumflex artery (LCX), and the phrenic nerve. Its morphology varies widely, with common shapes categorized as "chicken wing" (48% prevalence), "cactus" (30%), "windsock" (19%), and "cauliflower" (3%) configurations. Each configuration exhibits distinct anatomical characteristics that may influence the success of LAA exclusion. The "cauliflower" morphology is associated with higher embolic risk due to its short length, wide and irregular neck, thicker muscle bundles, and variable lobes [13, 14].

The LAA functions as a contractile reservoir, which creates a suction effect during systole and acts as a conduit during diastole [13]. Additionally, the LAA contributes to the endocrine system by releasing about 30% of atrial natriuretic peptide in response to stretch. The studies in animal models also suggest the role of the LAA in thirst regulation under hypovolemic conditions [13, 15].

In AF patients, the LAA is responsible for approximately 90% of thrombus formation sources in non-valvular cases, as reduced blood flow velocity and stasis within the LAA increase thrombotic risk [16, 17]. The complex anatomy of the LAA, including trabeculations and morphology, contributes to stroke risk in AF. Imaging techniques, such as cardiac MRI, allow for detailed evaluation of LAA structure and flow to assess thrombotic potential. Conflicting data exists on the relationship between specific LAA morphologies and thromboembolic risk, but the condition of the LAA remains a significant predictor for stroke [13, 18].

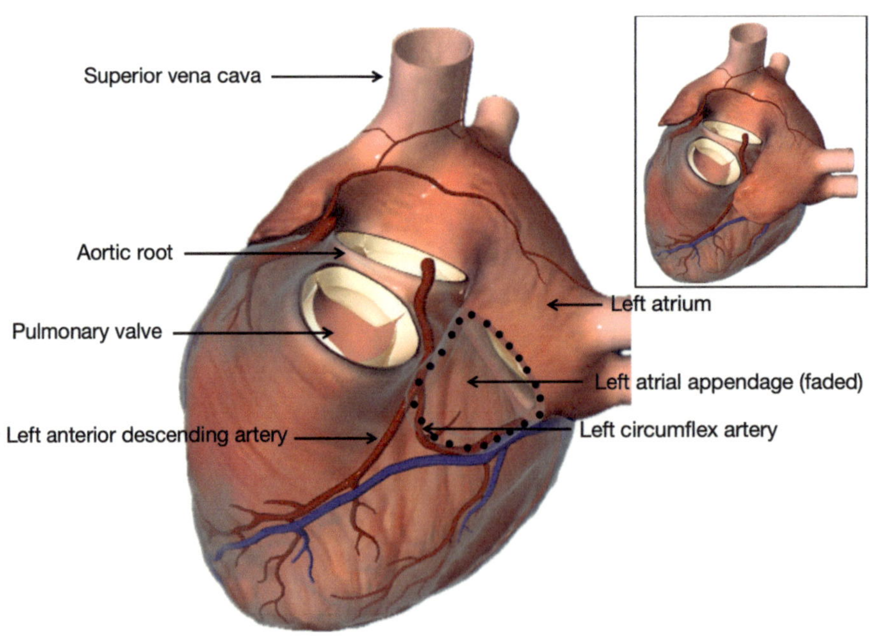


**Figure 1.**
*Left atrial appendage (LAA) with adjacent structures.*

Closure of the LAA has demonstrated advantages in numerous situations. Patients who undergo cardiac surgery usually receive surgery with Cox-maze IV procedure that includes LAA amputation/resection/ obliteration. Some non-randomized studies have indicated that LAA occlusion in patients who have had cardiac surgery can help reduce mortality, stroke, and thromboembolic events [19, 20]. A meta-analysis of five randomized controlled trials (RCTs) involving 5128 patients who underwent cardiac surgery with or without LAA occlusion demonstrated benefits in reducing thromboembolic events but did not show a reduction in all-cause mortality [21]. In contrast, for patients without a surgical indication, such as those with non-valvular atrial fibrillation, current guidelines recommend anticoagulants as the primary therapy to prevent thromboembolic events [22, 23]. A meta-analysis of three randomized controlled trials comparing percutaneous LAA closure to anticoagulation alone demonstrated that LAA closure provides advantages in reducing hemorrhagic stroke, cardiovascular mortality, and all-cause mortality, while maintaining a comparable stroke rate [24] According to current guidelines, percutaneous LAA closure may be considered for patients with contraindications to long-term anticoagulation therapy [22].

## 2. Therapeutic intervention

### 2.1 The transcatheter approach

The predominant percutaneous transcatheter approach involves delivering the device through femoral vein, traversing the inter-atrial septum, and anchoring it into the LAA ostium and neck in an antegrade fashion. Careful anatomical evaluation and selection can enable these percutaneous devices to be deployed safely and effectively. Conversely, inappropriate anatomical selection may lead to device malpositioning, which can result in prothrombotic foreign body exposure in the left atrium, device migration or embolization, or incomplete LAA neck closure, necessitating surgical correction [25–28]. Transesophageal echocardiogram (TEE) is very helpful for identifying the opening and the neck of the LAA, particularly if thrombus is present.

Growing expertise in percutaneous structural heart interventions has spurred the development of minimally invasive LAA exclusion technique via transcatheter methods [29]. Currently, multiple devices are specifically invented for transcatheter LAA occlusion, with the WATCHMAN and WATCHMAN FLX systems and the Amplatzer AMULET LAA Occluder being the most widely utilized in clinical practice. A thorough preoperative anatomy assessment is essential for all devices, involving the exclusion of intracardiac thrombus, confirmation of proper device placement, and evaluation of postoperative pericardial effusion, requiring skilled coordination of transesophageal echocardiogram (TEE) or intracardiac echocardiogram (ICE) and fluoroscopic imaging [30]. Computed tomography (CT scan) can assist in preprocedural planning by providing detailed information on the LAA dimension and shape [31]. Cardiac magnetic resonance imaging (C-MRI) provides further imaging benefits and aids in determining the device type and size [32, 33].

### 2.2 Watchman device

Among percutaneous LAA closure options, the Watchman device is currently the most widely used and only FDA-approved occluder for non-valvular AF patients eligible for long-term Coumadin treatment [13]. The Centers of Medicare and

Medicaid services recently approved reimbursement for this device implantation in non-valvular AF patients with CHA2DS2-VASC score ≥ 3, broadening its use for patients unable to undergo long-term Coumadin but able to tolerate short-term anticoagulation therapy [13]. The Watchman is the only one tested in randomized trials. The PROTECT-AF trial examined the Watchman left atrial appendage closure system for embolic protection in atrial fibrillation patients, with the primary endpoints including stroke, cardiovascular death, and systemic embolic events [34]. This device demonstrated non-inferiority to chronic warfarin use for stroke prevention and lower rates of cardiovascular death. However, high rates of periprocedural complications (pericardial effusion, procedure-related stroke events, device migration, and embolization) and excessive bleeding were noted. The impact of operator experience on procedural safety was further explored in the analysis involving patients from the PROTECT-AF trial and the subsequent non-randomized CAP registry (Continued Access to PROTECT-AF trial) [34]. Safety event rates decreased significantly between the initial and latter halves of both PROTECT-AF and CAP registry, with 10, 5.5, and 3.7% of patients experiencing device-related events in each respective phase ($P = 0.006$). The incidence of pericardial effusion dropped from 5% in PROTECT-AF trial to 2.2% in the CAP registry group ($P = 0.019$), while periprocedural stroke incidence declined from 0.9–0% respectively ($P = 0.039$) [34].

The PREVAIL Trial (Evaluation of the WATCHMAN LAA Closure Device in Patients with Atrial Fibrillation Versus Long Term Warfarin Therapy) is the second pivotal randomized trial that aimed to clarify early and late outcomes in stroke prevention [35]. Although the initial results showed reduced complication rates, longer follow-up indicated higher ischemic stroke incidence in the Watchman group, and the device did not show non-inferiority to warfarin therapy. Safety outcomes were encouraging, with major periprocedural complications reduced to 2.2% [35].

In a meta-analysis combining data from both trials (PROTECT-AF and PREVAIL registry) with findings from the CAP (Continued Access to PROTECT-AF) and CAP2 (Continued Access to PREVAIL), the Watchman device did not demonstrate a significant reduction in the efficacy endpoint compared to anticoagulation therapy (HR 0.79, $P = 0.22$) [36]. Nevertheless, individual components of the composite outcome revealed significant benefits from the Watchman device; reductions in hemorrhagic stroke, cardiovascular or unexplained death, and major bleeding were observed in patients implanted with the device compared to those on anticoagulation therapy. These advantages, however, were offset by an increased rate of ischemic stroke or systemic embolization in the device group (HR 1.95, $P = 0.05$), which could potentially be attributed to technical challenges, such as incomplete occlusion of the LAA, anatomical changes at the LAA ostium postprocedure leading to leakage, and clot formation on the device itself [36].

Both PROTECT-AF and PREVAIL trials, along with their CAP and CAP2 registries, shared similar inclusion criteria, requiring anticoagulation treatment for all individuals. However, data on the safety and efficacy on the Watchman device for individuals unable to tolerate oral anticoagulation therapy primarily was derived from case series and registries. The ASAP study, a prospective registry involving patients with a CHADS2 score > 1 who could not take oral anticoagulation, used dual antiplatelet therapy (Clopidogrel and Aspirin for 6 months followed by indefinite aspirin). This study achieved an annual ischemic stroke rate of 1.7%, a 77% reduction from the expect rate of 7.3% [37].

The EWOLUTION registry, a multicenter cohort study of 1025 Watchman recipients (73% of whom were unsuitable for oral anticoagulation therapy) reported an 84% reduction in ischemic stroke risk in 1 year compared with expected rates [38].

The ongoing ASAP-TOO trial seeks to evaluate the Watchman device's safety and effectiveness in patients ineligible for oral anticoagulation therapy, comparing it to single antiplatelet therapy or no therapy. Long-term data from this trial is expected to refine patient selection and clarity the use of the device in patients unable to use oral anticoagulation therapy [38].

The Watchman FLX, a next-generation device, features improvements such as 36 fixation anchors (the first Watchman generation has 10 fixation anchors) and broader size range, enhancing stability and safety. In a prospective trial of 400 patients, the Watchman FLX met primary effectiveness (≤ 0.5 cm peridevice leak at 1 year) and safety endpoints (0.5% complication rate) [39].

The CHAMPION-AF study is underway to compare the Watchman FLX to direct oral anticoagulants (DOAC) therapy in terms of stroke events, cardiovascular death, systemic embolism, and bleeding. Approved by CE Marked in 2019 and FDA in 2020, the Watchman FLX has largely superseded the original Watchman device in clinical practice due to its enhanced safety profile. Evolving evidence from randomized trials, observation studies, and registries supports the Watchman device as a viable option for stroke prevention in AF patients, particularly those at high risk of bleeding or contraindicated for long-term anticoagulation therapy. With the improved safety features of the Watchman FLX device, ongoing studies will further clarify its positioning relative to traditional anticoagulation therapy [40].

### 2.3 The Amplatzer device

The Amplatzer cardiac plug is a device designed for LAA occlusion made from a nitinol mesh with a polyester patch inspired by the Amplatzer septal occluders, featuring a self-expandable, fully retrievable, and repositionable device. Initial clinical trials at 10 European centers demonstrated a high operative success rate with 96.4% successfully implanted [41]. Despite this success, significant perioperative complications were reported in 7% of cases, including ischemic strokes (3 cases), device embolization (2 cases) but all successfully retrieved percutaneously, and pericardial effusions (5 cases). Data from the ACP European-market registry reflected similar outcomes. To reduce the risk of clot formation on the device, dual antiplatelet therapy (Aspirin + Clopidogrel) for one to 3 months postimplantation was advised [41].

The Amplatzer Amulet LAA occluder, a second-generation Amplatzer cardiac plug device, was developed with a wider lobe and additional stabilizing wires to enhance stability and accommodate larger LAA dimension. In the Amulet IDE study, 1878 patients with AF were randomized to receive either the Amulet or the first-generation Watchman device. The Amulet group achieved better occlusion rates but also had more instance of pericardial effusion. In a multicenter registry, the Amulet group achieved a 99% implantation success rate, with 98.2% effective LAA occlusion seen by follow-up transesophageal echocardiogram [42].

Rocca and colleagues published a meta-analysis of LAAO studies involving 4186 patients (3187 with the Amulet and 999 with the Watchman FLX). This analysis revealed that the Amulet group was associated with a higher rate of perioperative complications, mainly due to pericardial and major or intracranial bleeding, as well as a higher incidence of device-related leaks compared with the Watchman FLX group [43].

The PRAGUE-17 was a randomized study comparing LAA closure to direct oral anticoagulants (DOACs) with non-valvular AF, randomly assigning them to receive ether direct oral anticoagulants (primarily apixaban) or percutaneous LAA closure. Approximately 60% of the implanted devices were Amulet, with the remainder being the original Watchman or Watchman FLX devices. The primary outcome was a composite measure, including stroke, transient ischemic attack (TIA), cardiovascular death, bleeding, or complications related to the procedure or device. LAA closure was found to be noninferior to direct anticoagulants therapy for the primary endpoint. Non-procedural bleeding deviated between groups at about 6 months postoperatively, with more bleeding events occurring in the direct oral anticoagulants group compared to the LAA closure group [44].

The upcoming CATALYST trial, which aims to enroll over AF patients with a long-term oral anticoagulants indication, will further evaluate the safety and efficacy of LAA closure with the Amulet device compared to direct oral anticoagulants. Designed as a non-inferiority trial for stroke events, cardiovascular death, and systemic embolism, it will also assess superiority for non-procedural bleeding in the Amulet group relative to the direct oral anticoagulants group, providing a more robust evaluation of these therapies [40].

### 2.4 Percutaneous techniques

The Lariat device represents a percutaneous LAA exclusion method that combined both endocardial and epicardial approach. The procedure detail involves placing magnet-tipped wires on the endocardial and epicardial sites of the LAA, allowing the device to advance along this pathway to the LAA base. Here, a pre-tied suture is deployed to achieve complete blockage of LAA neck through ligation. In the United States large registry, the Lariat device showed a deployment success rate exceeding 95% with a perioperative complication rate of approximately 5%. The FDA has only approved the Lariat for soft tissue closure, making the use for LAA occlusion in the United States off-label. Due to its epicardial nature and minimal invasiveness without direct blood contact, this device may be particularly suitable for patients that do not tolerate antithrombotic therapy [45, 46].

### 2.5 Postimplantation antithrombotic therapy

Device-related thrombosis leads to ischemia and adverse cardiac events. The guideline for antithrombotic management following LAA occlusion remains unclear [47], and current practice often follows treatment protocols established in major trials. For patients with the Watchman device and a low bleeding risk, either Coumadin or direct anticoagulants are typically initiated alongside aspirin daily for 45 days or until adequate LAA closure is confirmed, after which the oral anticoagulant is discontinued and Clopidogrel is added to aspirin for 6 months. For Watchman patients with high bleeding risk, oral anticoagulant is avoided, with Clopidogrel combined with aspirin for 1 to 6 months based on LAA sealing, although this approach is currently off-label. This high bleeding risk protocol is also advised for patients with the Amplatzer cardiac plug/Amulet devices. For patients at extremely high bleeding risk, 2–4 weeks of single antiplatelet therapy (aspirin or Clopidogrel) may be considered based on expert opinion and limited non-randomized trial data. Patients who are unable to tolerate even this short antiplatelet therapy may be candidates for the Lariat device or an epicardial transcatheter approach or consider surgical approach of LAA exclusion [47].

A recent large multicenter study revealed that the type of antithrombotic used postoperatively was not a significant factor that contributed to device-related thrombosis. Given the flexibility in current guidelines, it is recommended that postoperative antithrombotic regimens be tailored individually, ideally in collaboration with a specialist managing the specific contraindications to oral anticoagulants [40].

## 3. Surgical approach

### 3.1 Epicardial LAA resection

LAA resection has been an integral part of the Cox Maze procedure and remains a cornerstone in surgical ablation [48]. This procedure is performed with cardiopulmonary bypass on an arrested heart, and LAA excision can be performed through an epicardial approach with subsequent oversewing or by inverting the LAA via the open left atrial incision site followed by endocardial excision and oversewing. LAA excision may be achieved by using a stapler device [49]. However, LAA stapling alone without excision has been associated with recanalization in the future [49]. When performing off-pump LAA excision, it is crucial to ensure that the device is applied to the neck/base of LAA without adjacent structures, minimizing bleeding risks [14].

The introduction of LAA clipping devices, particularly the FDA-approved AtriClip (AtriCure), has increased the adoption of LAA occlusion. This clip is straightforward to apply around the LAA epicardially and released to achieve complete occlusion. TEE is performed while the heart is beating to evaluate for any residual stump and ensure effectiveness of the device. Initial trials demonstrated approximately 95% success rate, and due to its safety, this clip device has largely supplanted the staplers [50]. The current advances in the delivery systems and design have enabled increased use of minimally invasive approaches. Preoperative imaging along with careful intraoperative evaluation of LAA anatomy is essential to achieve complete occlusion. Precision of device placement can be improved by dividing the Marshall ligament and gently dissecting the fat surrounding the pericardium to expose the neck and base of the LAA [14].

Recently, thoracoscopic appendage clip has gained popularity as a minimally invasive approach in patients without indication for cardiac surgery. This technique has demonstrated favorable long-term outcomes with no clip-related complication [51, 52]. Notably, a non-randomized study comparing thoracoscopic LAA clipping to the percutaneous occlusive device (Watchman) reported comparable outcomes over a follow-up period of 3–5 years [53]. The author emphasized the importance of a multidisciplinary heart-team approach, advocating that the choice between thoracoscopic clipping and percutaneous devices should be individualized based on the team's multidisciplinary evaluation. Another randomized study comparing these two methods found comparable efficacy, with significantly lower bleeding rates observed in the thoracoscopic clip group ($P = 0.002$) [54]. Consequently, thoracoscopic LAA occlusion with a clip may be preferable for patients with lone atrial fibrillation, a high stroke risk, and elevated bleeding risk, as percutaneous devices often require at least two antithrombotic agents postprocedure.

### 3.2 Endocardial LAA occlusion

Traditional methods of endocardial occlusion, such as purse-string closure of the ostium using Prolene suture in an interrupted pattern, have shown high rates of suture disruption leading to residual LAA flow up to 30% [49]. These techniques are typically performed with the patient on cardiopulmonary bypass, with the heart arrested through the left atrial incision to allow for controlled access while minimizing excessive retraction of the left atrium, there by reducing tissue tension, risking suture disruption later after weaning of cardiopulmonary bypass [14].

### 3.3 Literature reviews

Friedman et al. conducted a cohort analysis linking United States Medicare data with the STS database to evaluate the impact of LAA occlusion on thromboembolism readmission and mortality; the data revealed that LAA occlusion reduced thromboembolism risk, hemorrhagic stroke, and mortality. This extensive cohort study was the first to demonstrate a clear benefit for LAA occlusion in AF patients undergoing cardiac surgery [19]. Whitlock et al. published results from the LAAOS III trial and showed a significant benefit for LAA occlusion with a notable stroke reduction after 30 days [55]. These two significant literatures underscore the benefit of incorporating LAA occlusion in atrial fibrillation management for patients undergoing cardiac surgery, demonstrating reduced long-term stroke risk and improved survival [14]. Combining surgical ablation with LAA occlusion is likely to have a significant impact on long-term stroke and survival rates, and this approach should be considered if opportunities allowed [14].

Current evidence thus endorses LAA occlusion at a minimum. However, for atrial fibrillation patients requiring cardiac surgery, recent data suggests that goal-directed therapy should be based on individual factors. Factors influencing this decision may include advanced age, long-standing atrial fibrillation, a significant enlarged left atrium (more than 10 cm), calcified atrium, emergent surgery, and the surgeon's experience and proficiency with ablation techniques. When the aim is to restore normal sinus rhythm and maximize long-term survival, surgical atrial fibrillation ablation combined with LAA occlusion (ideally a bi-atrial Cox Maze procedure) is recommended. If stroke prevention alone is the goal, LAA alone may be sufficient [14].

## 4. Conclusion

In patients with atrial fibrillation (AF), LAA occlusion has demonstrated effectiveness in reducing stroke rates and thromboembolic complications through both surgical and percutaneous approaches. For those with non-valvular AF, LAA offers the potential advantage, as confirmed by transesophageal echocardiography (TEE), and following thorough discussions with the patient. Further research, including randomized controlled trials or large registry studies, is necessary to determine the most optimal treatment approach. Currently, we advocate for treatment decisions to be guided by a collaborative process involving both the heart team and the patient.

## Author details

Jakraphan Yu, Marc Leon, Manuel Quiroz-Flores and Chawannuch Ruaengsri*
Division of Cardiothoracic Surgery, Stanford University, Stanford, CA, USA

*Address all correspondence to: noot@stanford.edu

## References

[1] Khairallah F, Ezzedine R, Ganz LI, London B, Saba S. Epidemiology and determinants of outcome of admissions for atrial fibrillation in the United States from 1996 to 2001. The American Journal of Cardiology. 2004;**94**(4):500-504

[2] Lakshminarayan K, Solid CA, Collins AJ, Anderson DC, Herzog CA. Atrial fibrillation and stroke in the general medicare population: A 10-year perspective (1992 to 2002). Stroke. 2006;**37**(8):1969-1974

[3] Ott A, Breteler MM, de Bruyne MC, van Harskamp F, Grobbee DE, Hofman A. Atrial fibrillation and dementia in a population-based study. The Rotterdam Study. Stroke. 1997;**28**(2):316-321

[4] Benjamin EJ, Wolf PA, D'Agostino RB, Silbershatz H, Kannel WB, Levy D. Impact of atrial fibrillation on the risk of death: The Framingham Heart Study. Circulation. 1998;**98**(10):946-952

[5] Hart RG, Pearce LA, Aguilar MI. Meta-analysis: Antithrombotic therapy to prevent stroke in patients who have nonvalvular atrial fibrillation. Annals of Internal Medicine. 2007;**146**(12):857-867

[6] Beinart R, Heist EK, Newell JB, Holmvang G, Ruskin JN, Mansour M. Left atrial appendage dimensions predict the risk of stroke/TIA in patients with atrial fibrillation. Journal of Cardiovascular Electrophysiology. 2011;**22**(1):10-15

[7] John Camm A, Colombo A, Corbucci G, Padeletti L. Left atrial appendage closure: A new technique for clinical practice. Heart Rhythm. 2014;**11**(3):514-521

[8] Thambidorai SK, Murray RD, Parakh K, Shah TK, Black IW, Jasper SE, et al. Utility of transesophageal echocardiography in identification of thrombogenic milieu in patients with atrial fibrillation (an ACUTE ancillary study). The American Journal of Cardiology. 2005;**96**(7):935-941

[9] Gage BF, van Walraven C, Pearce L, Hart RG, Koudstaal PJ, Boode BS, et al. Selecting patients with atrial fibrillation for anticoagulation: Stroke risk stratification in patients taking aspirin. Circulation. 2004;**110**(16):2287-2292

[10] Gage BF, Waterman AD, Shannon W, Boechler M, Rich MW, Radford MJ. Validation of clinical classification schemes for predicting stroke: Results from the National Registry of Atrial Fibrillation. Journal of the American Medical Association. 2001;**285**(22):2864-2870

[11] Hindricks G, Potpara T, Dagres N, Arbelo E, Bax JJ, Blomstrom-Lundqvist C, et al. 2020 ESC Guidelines for the diagnosis and management of atrial fibrillation developed in collaboration with the European Association for Cardio-Thoracic Surgery (EACTS): The task force for the diagnosis and management of atrial fibrillation of the European Society of Cardiology (ESC) developed with the special contribution of the European Heart Rhythm Association (EHRA) of the ESC. European Heart Journal. 2021;**42**(5):373-498

[12] Steffel J, Heidbuchel H. 2021 European Heart Rhythm Association Practical Guide on the use of non-vitamin K antagonist oral anticoagulants in patients with atrial fibrillation: Comment-authors' reply. Europace. 2021;**23**(10):1685-1686

[13] Naksuk N, Padmanabhan D, Yogeswaran V, Asirvatham SJ. Left atrial appendage: Embryology, anatomy, physiology, arrhythmia and therapeutic intervention. JACC: Clinical Electrophysiology. 2016;**2**(4):403-412

[14] Badhwar V, Scott Rankin J, Lee R, McCarthy PM, Wei LM. Contemporary left atrial appendage management during adult cardiac surgery. The Journal of Thoracic and Cardiovascular Surgery. 2023;**165**(4):1398-1404

[15] Zimmerman MB, Blaine EH, Stricker EM. Water intake in hypovolemic sheep: Effects of crushing the left atrial appendage. Science. 1981;**211**(4481):489-491

[16] Mahilmaran A, Nayar PG, Sudarsana G, Abraham K. Relationship of left atrial appendage function to left ventricular function. Indian Heart Journal. 2004;**56**(4):293-298

[17] Blackshear JL, Odell JA. Appendage obliteration to reduce stroke in cardiac surgical patients with atrial fibrillation. The Annals of Thoracic Surgery. 1996;**61**(2):755-759

[18] Yamamoto M, Seo Y, Kawamatsu N, Sato K, Sugano A, Machino-Ohtsuka T, et al. Complex left atrial appendage morphology and left atrial appendage thrombus formation in patients with atrial fibrillation. Circulation: Cardiovascular Imaging. 2014;**7**(2):337-343

[19] Friedman DJ, Piccini JP, Wang T, Zheng J, Malaisrie SC, Holmes DR, et al. Association between left atrial appendage occlusion and readmission for thromboembolism among patients with atrial fibrillation undergoing concomitant cardiac surgery. Journal of the American Medical Association. 2018;**319**(4):365-374

[20] Zheng Y, Rao CF, Chen SP, He L, Hou JF, Zheng Z. Surgical left atrial appendage occlusion in patients with atrial fibrillation undergoing mechanical heart valve replacement. Chinese Medical Journal. 2020;**133**(16):1891-1899

[21] Mohamed MMG, Faisaluddin M, Kheiri B, Osman M. Meta-analysis of surgical left atrial appendage occlusion during cardiac surgery. The American Journal of Cardiology. 2021;**155**:150-151

[22] Van Gelder IC, Rienstra M, Bunting KV, Casado-Arroyo R, Caso V, Crijns H, et al. 2024 ESC Guidelines for the management of atrial fibrillation developed in collaboration with the European Association for Cardio-Thoracic Surgery (EACTS). European Heart Journal. 2024;**45**(36):3314-3414

[23] Joglar JA, Chung MK, Armbruster AL, Benjamin EJ, Chyou JY, Cronin EM, et al. 2023 ACC/AHA/ACCP/HRS guideline for the diagnosis and management of atrial fibrillation: A report of the American College of Cardiology/American Heart Association Joint Committee on Clinical Practice Guidelines. Circulation. 2024;**149**(1):e1-e156

[24] Turagam Mohit K, Osmancik P, Neuzil P, Dukkipati Srinivas R, Reddy VY. Left atrial appendage closure versus oral anticoagulants in atrial fibrillation. Journal of the American College of Cardiology. 2020;**76**(23):2795-2797

[25] Voskoboinik A, Lee RJ. Anatomic considerations for epicardial and endocardial left atrial appendage closure. Cardiac Electrophysiology Clinics. 2020;**12**(1):39-45

[26] Simard T, Jung RG, Lehenbauer K, Piayda K, Pracon R, Jackson GG, et al. Predictors of device-related

thrombus following percutaneous left atrial appendage occlusion. Journal of the American College of Cardiology. 2021;**78**(4):297-313

[27] Alkhouli M, Busu T, Shah K, Osman M, Alqahtani F, Raybuck B. Incidence and clinical impact of device-related thrombus following percutaneous left atrial appendage occlusion: A meta-analysis. JACC: Clinical Electrophysiology. 2018;**4**(12):1629-1637

[28] El-Gabry M, Shehada SE, Wendt D, Mourad F. Emergent surgical removal of a migrated left atrial appendage occluder. European Journal of Cardio-Thoracic Surgery. 2018;**54**(1):191-192

[29] Moss JD. Left atrial appendage exclusion for prevention of stroke in atrial fibrillation: Review of minimally invasive approaches. Current Cardiology Reports. 2014;**16**(2):448

[30] Urena M, Rodes-Cabau J, Freixa X, Saw J, Webb JG, Freeman M, et al. Percutaneous left atrial appendage closure with the AMPLATZER cardiac plug device in patients with nonvalvular atrial fibrillation and contraindications to anticoagulation therapy. Journal of the American College of Cardiology. 2013;**62**(2):96-102

[31] Holmes DR, Reddy VY, Turi ZG, Doshi SK, Sievert H, Buchbinder M, et al. Percutaneous closure of the left atrial appendage versus warfarin therapy for prevention of stroke in patients with atrial fibrillation: A randomised non-inferiority trial. Lancet. 2009;**374**(9689):534-542

[32] Hong SN, Rahimi A, Kissinger KV, Pedrosa I, Manning WJ, O'Halloran TD. Cardiac magnetic resonance imaging and the WATCHMAN device. Journal of the American College of Cardiology. 2010;**55**(24):2785

[33] Mohrs OK, Wunderlich N, Petersen SE, Pottmeyer A, Kauczor HU. Contrast-enhanced CMR in patients after percutaneous closure of the left atrial appendage: A pilot study. Journal of Cardiovascular Magnetic Resonance. 2011;**13**(1):33

[34] Reddy VY, Holmes D, Doshi SK, Neuzil P, Kar S. Safety of percutaneous left atrial appendage closure: Results from the Watchman Left Atrial Appendage System for Embolic Protection in Patients with AF (PROTECT AF) clinical trial and the Continued Access Registry. Circulation. 2011;**123**(4):417-424

[35] Holmes DR Jr, Kar S, Price MJ, Whisenant B, Sievert H, Doshi SK, et al. Prospective randomized evaluation of the Watchman Left Atrial Appendage Closure device in patients with atrial fibrillation versus long-term warfarin therapy: The PREVAIL trial. Journal of the American College of Cardiology. 2014;**64**(1):1-12

[36] Holmes DR Jr, Doshi SK, Kar S, Price MJ, Sanchez JM, Sievert H, et al. Left atrial appendage closure as an alternative to warfarin for stroke prevention in atrial fibrillation: A patient-level meta-analysis. Journal of the American College of Cardiology. 2015;**65**(24):2614-2623

[37] Reddy VY, Mobius-Winkler S, Miller MA, Neuzil P, Schuler G, Wiebe J, et al. Left atrial appendage closure with the Watchman device in patients with a contraindication for oral anticoagulation: The ASAP study (ASA Plavix Feasibility Study With Watchman Left Atrial Appendage Closure Technology). Journal of the American College of Cardiology. 2013;**61**(25):2551-2556

[38] Boersma LV, Ince H, Kische S, Pokushalov E, Schmitz T, Schmidt B,

et al. Efficacy and safety of left atrial appendage closure with WATCHMAN in patients with or without contraindication to oral anticoagulation: 1-year follow-up outcome data of the EWOLUTION trial. Heart Rhythm. 2017;**14**(9):1302-1308

[39] Kar S, Doshi SK, Sadhu A, Horton R, Osorio J, Ellis C, et al. Primary outcome evaluation of a next-generation left atrial appendage closure device: Results from the PINNACLE FLX trial. Circulation. 2021;**143**(18):1754-1762

[40] Rozen G, Margolis G, Marai I, Roguin A, Rahamim E, Planer D, et al. Left atrial appendage exclusion in atrial fibrillation. Frontiers in Cardiovascular Medicine. 2022;**9**:949732

[41] Park JW, Bethencourt A, Sievert H, Santoro G, Meier B, Walsh K, et al. Left atrial appendage closure with Amplatzer cardiac plug in atrial fibrillation: Initial European experience. Catheterization and Cardiovascular Interventions. 2011;**77**(5):700-706

[42] Lakkireddy D, Thaler D, Ellis CR, Swarup V, Sondergaard L, Carroll J, et al. Amplatzer Amulet left atrial appendage occluder versus Watchman device for stroke prophylaxis (Amulet IDE): A randomized, controlled trial. Circulation. 2021;**144**(19):1543-1552

[43] Della Rocca DG, Magnocavallo M, Gianni C, Mohanty S, Natale VN, Al-Ahmad A, et al. Procedural and short-term follow-up outcomes of Amplatzer Amulet occluder versus Watchman FLX device: A meta-analysis. Heart Rhythm. 2022;**19**(6):1017-1018

[44] Osmancik P, Herman D, Neuzil P, Hala P, Taborsky M, Kala P, et al. Left atrial appendage closure versus direct oral anticoagulants in high-risk patients with atrial fibrillation. Journal of the American College of Cardiology. 2020;**75**(25):3122-3135

[45] Miller MA, Gangireddy SR, Doshi SK, Aryana A, Koruth JS, Sennhauser S, et al. Multicenter study on acute and long-term safety and efficacy of percutaneous left atrial appendage closure using an epicardial suture snaring device. Heart Rhythm. 2014;**11**(11):1853-1859

[46] Moussa Pacha H, Al-Khadra Y, Soud M, Darmoch F, Moussa Pacha A, Alraies MC. Percutaneous devices for left atrial appendage occlusion: A contemporary review. World Journal of Cardiology. 2019;**11**(2):57-70

[47] Glikson M, Wolff R, Hindricks G, Mandrola J, Camm AJ, Lip GYH, et al. EHRA/EAPCI expert consensus statement on catheter-based left atrial appendage occlusion - An update. Europace. 2020;**22**(2):184

[48] Badhwar V, Rankin JS, Ad N, Grau-Sepulveda M, Damiano RJ, Gillinov AM, et al. Surgical ablation of atrial fibrillation in the United States: Trends and propensity matched outcomes. The Annals of Thoracic Surgery. 2017;**104**(2):493-500

[49] Lee R, Vassallo P, Kruse J, Malaisrie SC, Rigolin V, Andrei AC, et al. A randomized, prospective pilot comparison of 3 atrial appendage elimination techniques: Internal ligation, stapled excision, and surgical excision. The Journal of Thoracic and Cardiovascular Surgery. 2016;**152**(4):1075-1080

[50] Ailawadi G, Gerdisch MW, Harvey RL, Hooker RL, Damiano RJ Jr, Salamon T, et al. Exclusion of the left atrial appendage with a novel device: Early results of a multicenter trial. The Journal of Thoracic and Cardiovascular Surgery. 2011;**142**(5):1002-1009, 9 e1

[51] van Laar C, Verberkmoes NJ, van Es HW, Lewalter T, Dunnington G,

Stark S, et al. Thoracoscopic left atrial appendage clipping: A multicenter cohort analysis. JACC: Clinical Electrophysiology. 2018;**4**(7):893-901

[52] Kim JY, Jeong DS, Park SJ, Park KM, Kim JS, On YK. Long-term efficacy and anticoagulation strategy of left atrial appendage occlusion during total thoracoscopic ablation of atrial fibrillation to prevent ischemic stroke. Frontiers in Cardiovascular Medicine. 2022;**9**:853299

[53] Branzoli S, Guarracini F, Marini M, D'Onghia G, Penzo D, Piffer S, et al. Heart team for left atrial appendage occlusion: A patient-tailored approach. Journal of Clinical Medicine. 2021;**11**(1)

[54] Wang JL, Zhou K, Qin Z, Cheng WJ, Zhang LZ, Zhou YJ. Minimally invasive thoracoscopic left atrial appendage occlusion compared with transcatheter left atrial appendage closure for stroke prevention in recurrent nonvalvular atrial fibrillation patients after radiofrequency ablation: A prospective cohort study. Journal of Geriatric Cardiology. 2021;**18**(11):877-885

[55] Whitlock RP, Belley-Cote EP, Paparella D, Healey JS, Brady K, Sharma M, et al. Left atrial appendage occlusion during cardiac surgery to prevent stroke. The New England Journal of Medicine. 2021;**384**(22):2081-2091

Chapter 6

# Atrial Fibrillation in Heart Failure

*Ebru Sahin and Ali Oto*


## Abstract

Common risk factors, neurohormonal hyperactivation, development of fibrosis, and pathophysiological pathways such as electrophysiological remodeling result in frequent coexistence of atrial fibrillation and heart failure. Their coexistence results in an increase in mortality and morbidity compared to their isolated course. As the severity of the diseases increases, their potential to trigger and worsen each other also increases. Recent studies have introduced both pharmacologic and invasive treatment strategies to facilitate the management of these two comorbid conditions, resulting in a reduction in the clinical course, morbidity, and mortality. Slowing or reducing atrial and ventricular remodeling, modification of modifiable risk factors, prevention of stroke, restoration of early atrial fibrillation to physiologic sinus rhythm, and tight rate and rhythm control are important steps in improving the course of these two conditions. Compared to previous years, new pharmacotherapies in heart failure have come to the fore in terms of improving prognosis. Similarly, in the management of atrial fibrillation, catheter ablation techniques are becoming increasingly prominent in rhythm control. The aim of this chapter is to explain the pathophysiology underlying these two comorbid conditions according to the current literature and to review the current treatment modalities according to the latest guidelines.


**Keywords:** atrial fibrillation, atrial remodeling, heart failure, left ventricular dysfunction, stroke prevention, rate control, rhythm control, pharmacological strategy, catheter ablation

## 1. Introduction

The association of atrial fibrillation (AF) and heart failure (HF) is common due to the presence of common risk factors. The coexistence of these two major diseases worsens the prognosis compared to their independent course, resulting in increased mortality and morbidity. Age, obesity, sedentary lifestyle, hypertension, diabetes mellitus, chronic kidney disease, ischemic heart disease, and valvular heart disease are common risk factors and contribute to the development of atrial remodeling and diastolic dysfunction [1]. The prevalence of AF in HF patients varies between 10 and 57% depending on the severity of HF. As the New York Heart Association functional class (NYHA) increases from I to IV, the incidence of AF increases from 4 to 50% [2, 3]. In the Framingham cohort study, 37% of newly diagnosed AF patients had HF, whereas 57% of newly diagnosed HF patients had AF. The prevalence of AF increases in correlation with ejection fraction (EF) among HF subtypes. The prevalence of AF is higher in HF patients with preserved ejection fraction (HFpEF) than in HF



IntechOpen

patients with reduced ejection fraction (HFrEF). This prevalence is around 40–60% in HFpEF patients [4, 5].

Common risk factors, similarities in pathophysiology, and frequent coexistence create confusion as to whether these two conditions are the cause or consequence of each other. In recent years, there have been many advances in pharmacotherapy and interventional treatment of AF and HF, but the desired reduction in morbidity and mortality has still not been achieved. A better understanding of the pathophysiology of these two comorbid conditions and the relationship between them may lead to improved prognosis with strict follow-up and implementation of current treatment algorithms.

## 2. Pathophysiology

Although epidemiologic data show that AF and HF tend to coexist frequently, the causal relationships between these two conditions are not clearly established. AF maybe caused by a common triggering factor (such as diabetes, hypertension, obesity, sedentary lifestyle, sleep apnea, advanced age, smoking, coronary artery disease, renal insufficiency) or a substrate (a genetic or infectious factor) in individuals with HF. One of these two diseases may occur first and trigger the other, or both may become chronic and perpetuate each other in a vicious cycle [6]. A good understanding of the pathophysiology and clinical implications underpins the development of an appropriate treatment strategy for this challenging association.

### 2.1 AF as a cause

AF causes the abolition of atrial systole, ventricular chronotropic dysregulation, and irregular ventricular rhythm, resulting in poor hemodynamic outcomes.

Atrial systole contributes 25% to ventricular end-diastolic volume. Loss of atrial contribution may lead to worsening of HF. The prognosis may worsen in the presence of concomitant mitral stenosis, ischemic heart disease, and diastolic dysfunction [7].

Cardiac output depends on ventricular rate and stroke volume. In an uncontrolled AF, the ventricular rate also increases, and the duration of diastole shortens and becomes irregular, leading to suboptimal electromechanical function. Impaired ventricular filling results in a decrease in stroke volume. This worsens the prognosis, especially in HFpEF patients with diastolic dysfunction [6].

Decreased cardiac output and irregular ventricular rhythm observed in AF trigger neurohumoral mechanisms leading to worsening of HF. Increased levels of renin-angiotensin aldosterone system (RAAS), plasma norepinephrine, and endothelin have vasoconstrictive, proapoptotic, and adverse remodeling effects. Neurohumoral activation results in LV dysfunction and increased afterload [6, 8].

AF can also cause tachycardiomyopathy, a reversible left ventricular (LV) systolic dysfunction. Prolonged exposure to high heart rate results in morphologic and biochemical changes. The combination of extracellular matrix remodeling, decreased collagen content and cross-linking, significant changes in myocardial calcium processing and calcium-regulating proteins, myocardial mitochondrial damage, increased myocardial oxidative enzymes, and depletion of high-energy stores results in LV dilatation and impaired systolic function. With restoration of sinus rhythm, LV function can be restored within weeks [9, 10].

Patients with long-term symptomatic AF showed extensive LV fibrosis when evaluated by cardiac magnetic resonance (CMR). The degree of ventricular fibrosis was associated with AF burden, independent of advancing age and systolic dysfunction. Even patients with AF alone have been shown to have diffuse LV fibrosis in contrast to healthy controls [11]. The fibrosis-inducing and diastolic dysfunction effect of AF on the LV is an important risk factor for the development of HFpEF. In >50% of patients newly diagnosed with HFpEF, AF was previously or concurrently diagnosed [12]. However, AF is observed in approximately half of HF patients with LV systolic dysfunction and more than one-third of patients with AF have loss of LV systolic function [13, 14].

However, other causes of heart failure must be evaluated to manage the process correctly. Electrocardiography, echocardiography, cardiac magnetic resonance imaging, computed tomography, coronary angiography, and cardiac biopsy are evaluation tests used to differentiate structural diseases, valve diseases, pericardial and myocardial diseases, infiltrative and metabolic diseases, coronary artery diseases, pulmonary, and renal diseases in the etiology of heart failure.

### 2.2 AF as a consequence

The increase in LV filling pressure due to LV systolic and diastolic dysfunction observed in HF results in an increase in atrial filling pressure. Increased atrial wall stress causes atrial electrical and structural remodeling via renin-angiotensin system, calcium handling, profibrotic, and proinflammatory pathways.

Left ventricular dysfunction activates the renin-angiotensin pathway, mitogen-activated protein kinase (MAPK), the Janus kinase (JAK)/signal transducers and activators of transcription (STAT), transforming growth factor b1 (TGF-b1), angiotensin II activated platelet-derived growth factor A (PDGF-A), Rac1, and nuclear factor-kappa B (NF-kB) pathways and angiotensin II type 1 (AT-1) receptor-mediated myocyte hypertrophy, apoptosis, collagen deposition, and interstitial remodeling. This process resulting in atrial remodeling predisposes to AF development [7, 15].

As demonstrated in the sheep model, reduced L-type calcium-channel current causes an increase in intracellular calcium and consequent early and late after-depolarization. This automatic atrial activity triggers AF. In addition, the irregular ventricular rhythm observed in HF leads to decreased sarcoplasmic reticulum expression. Abnormal Ca handling leads to AF triggering [16].

Chronically reduced cardiac output leads to sustained adrenergic activation and increased levels of circulating noradrenaline and adrenaline. Beta-adrenergic stimulation initiates a cascade of proteins involved in calcium handling (ryanodine receptor 2 (RyR2), SERCA2a, and ICa-L), including protein kinase A mediated dephosphorylation. These proteins promote favorable conditions for delayed after-depolarizations. Direct effects upon Inward Rectifier (IK1) and Pacemaker (If) channels increase focal firing, whilst modulation of action potential duration (APD) via enhanced ICa-L (adrenergic) or IKAch (cholinergic) can promote phase 2 and phase 3 early after-depolarizations. The net effect is the promotion of conditions favorable to rapid firing and focal activity. In addition, b stimulation, via calcium activation of calmodulin and calcineurin, also activates transcription processes implicated in driving ultrastructural changes. Lastly, the effect of IKAch activity on APD abbreviation is thought to occur with significant regional variation, promoting conditions favorable for functional re-entry and pro-arrhythmia [17].

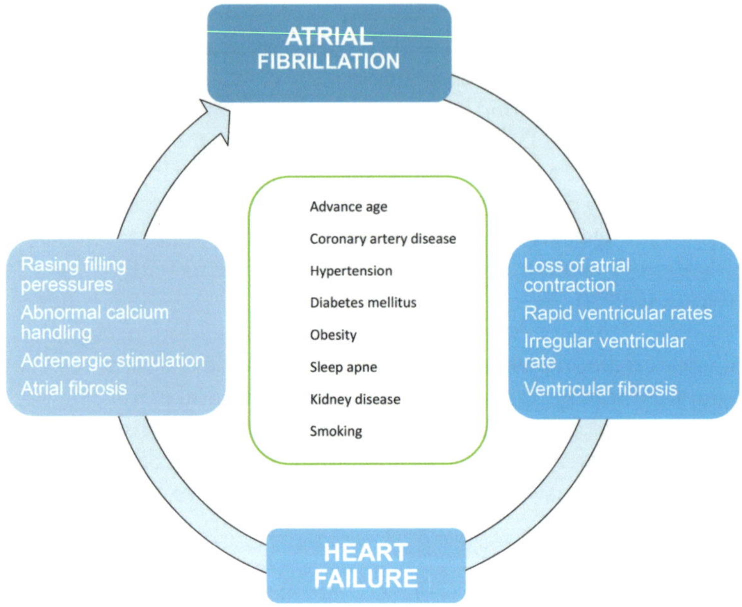


**Figure 1.**
*Pathophysiological interactions between AF and HF.*

In addition, functional mitral regurgitation resulting from systolic regurgitation and ventricular remodeling contributes to the development of AF. AF itself contributes to functional mitral regurgitation by causing atrial remodeling in addition to its contribution to ventricular dysfunction. This situation once again reveals the confusion of whether AF is cause or effect (**Figure 1**) [18].

## 3. Management of AF in HF

Managing the association of HF and AF requires a multifactorial approach. The patient's history, physical examination, clinical presentation, and comorbidities should be well evaluated. As in all AF patients, a holistic approach including stroke prevention, controlling symptoms with rate or rhythm control, managing cardiovascular risk factors, lifestyle modification, and increasing compliance with treatment is recommended in AF patients with HF [19].

### 3.1 Risk factor modification and HF medical therapy

Lifestyle modification and modification of common risk factors are often missed steps in this management process. A Mediterranean diet with a low intake of salt and fat benefits HF and AF patients [20]. Regular exercise has a positive impact, assisting in weight loss [21]. Alcohol reduction and smoking cessation could also eliminate HF decompensation and control AF in a better way [22, 23].

Although treatment for HFpEF is not as clear as for HFrEF, Angiotensin-neprilysin inhibitor (ARNI), angiotensin-converting enzyme inhibitors (ACEIs), and angiotensin receptor blockers (ARBs) are recommended in HF patients, The use of beta-blockers, mineralocorticoid antagonists (MRAs), and sodium-glucose cotransporter 2 (SGLT2) at the maximum tolerated dose contributes to mortality and morbidity. In addition, with optimal maximal medical therapy, the incidence of AF in HF patients is reduced [1, 4, 19, 24]. ACEIs, ARBs, and MRA reduce the incidence of AF in patients with HFrEF, possibly as a result of reverse remodeling because this AF protective effect is not seen in patients with a normal EF and no cardiomyopathy [25]. Sacubitril-valsartan has incremental efficacy over ACE inhibitors/ARBs and is the treatment of choice when available for patients with symptomatic HFrEF (up to an approximate EF <50%), with no interaction by baseline AF status [26]. SGLT2 inhibitors have beneficial effects in HFrEF regardless of AF status, improving symptoms, HF hospitalization risk, and mortality [27]. Statins also prevent new-onset AF. Cardiac resynchronization therapy (CRT) provides AV, interventricular, and intraventricular conduction and complements HF medical therapy to maintain sinus rhythm [19, 28].

### 3.2 Stroke prevention

As shown in the Framingham Heart Study, AF is associated with a fivefold increase in stroke risk. In the absence of other risk factors for stroke, this risk decreases, but the risk increases exponentially with the addition of HF and other risk factors [29]. Although there are many risk scores, the CHADS2-VASc is one of the most commonly used when deciding to start anticoagulation for the prevention of stroke, a devastating consequence of AF. "C" in the score defines congestive HF. HF in the score is independent of EF. Each HF patient receives one point on the score. If the CHA2DS2-VASc Score is ≥1 in men and ≥2 in women, class IIA is recommended, and if the CHA2DS2-VASc Score is ≥2 in men and ≥3 in women, class IA and recommendation level anticoagulation is recommended [19].

The etiology of AF and comorbid conditions should also be considered when choosing anticoagulant therapy. VKAs (vitamin K antagonists) are recommended as the gold standard in the presence of mechanical valves, moderate to severe mitral stenosis, and antiphospholipid syndrome. In patients with non-valvular AF, Non-Vitamin K Oral Anticoagulants (NOACs) are recommended to be preferred as anticoagulant agents due to similar or better efficacy levels with VKAs and less bleeding risk [1, 3, 19].

Left atrial appendage (LAA) closure is recommended in patients with contraindications to anticoagulant therapy or high thrombotic and hemorrhagic risk [1, 19].

### 3.3 Rate control

Control of ventricular rate is an important step in the holistic approach to AF in terms of symptom control. The choice of medical therapy for AF patients with HF should be based on ventricular systolic function. Uncertainties remain as to what the optimal rate should be. Current ESC guidelines recommend a heart rate below 100–110 bpm. However, it is not recommended to decrease the rate below 70 bpm because it increases the need for a pacemaker [30].

Beta-blockers are the first-line treatment option for rate control in patients with HFrEF. Beta blockers also contribute to prognosis by reducing mortality in HFrEF patients in sinus rhythm. However, this effect on prognosis is not observed when AF is added [31]. Again, in a meta-analysis including 11 randomized clinical trials by Kotecha et al., no contribution to mortality was observed with beta-blockers [32]. However, beta-blockers are preferred as the first choice in the HFrEF-AF patient group because of their good symptom control and favorable effects on LV function. In cases where rate control cannot be achieved, digoxin should be the second choice in addition to treatment. They can be used as the first choice in decompensated HF. They reduce hospitalization without contributing to survival. They may also be the sole treatment option when beta blockers are contraindicated [33].

Non-dihydropyridine calcium-channel blockers, like verapamil and diltiazem, have a negative inotropic effect on LV contractility, leading to a decrease in EF and impaired pump function. Their use is not recommended in HFrEF and decompensated HF [1, 19]. Non-dihydropyridine calcium-channel blockers are a treatment option for the HFpEF-AF patient group. There is no evidence that they increase morbidity and adversely affect prognosis in this patient group [3]. Amiodarone is a treatment option for rate control in new-onset HF or when dual therapy is not sufficient to achieve rate control. In the current ESC guidelines, amiodarone is included as class IIB for rate control [19].

In patients who cannot achieve rate control despite pharmacotherapy and ablation, atrioventricular (AV) node ablation and permanent pacemaker implantation are options to achieve rate and symptom control. In addition to this, in patients with AF-HF coexistence, AV node ablation is mandatory if cardiac resynchronization therapy (CRT) is to be performed [34, 35]. The APAF-CRT study was planned in patients with narrow QRS who had persistent AF, were severely symptomatic, had been hospitalized for HF at least once in the last year, were unsuitable for AF ablation, or had failed AF ablation. Study results showed that AV node ablation + CRT treatment was superior to pharmacological rate control treatment, regardless of EF, in patients with severe symptomatic, persistent AF and narrow QRS who were hospitalized for HF at least once in the last year [35].

### 3.4 Rhythm control

Rhythm control and ventricular rate control are recommended treatment strategies in atrial fibrillation. Recent clinical trials have demonstrated the prognostic benefit of early rhythm control strategies and AF catheter ablation. The current ESC guideline recommends a rhythm control strategy with a class I recommendation level for symptom control and improvement of quality of life in all symptomatic patients [19]. Rhythm control can be achieved by pharmacologic agents or ablation and restoration of sinus rhythm by electrical or medical cardioversion.

Cardioversion is used in acute rhythm control. While electrical cardioversion is mostly preferred in patients with hemodynamic instability due to AF, pharmacologic or electrical cardioversion are effective treatment methods that can be preferred in hemodynamically stable AF patients [1]. Electrical cardioversion is more effective than pharmacologic cardioversion alone [36]. Thromboembolic risk is present in both methods, and the patient should be evaluated for anticoagulation.

Antiarrhythmic agents that can be used in pharmacologic rhythm control include amiodarone, dofetilide, dronaderone, flecainide, propafenone, and sotalol. When using these agents, care should be taken in terms of their proarrthymic effects as well as their antiarrhythmic effects. The choice of which antiarrhythmic agent for which patient depends on ventricular function, presence or absence of structural heart disease, and comorbid conditions. IC antiarrhythmic agents are commonly used in patients with AF, but when HF is added, this group of antiarrhythmic agents leads to increased mortality. Their use in HF-AF coexistence is contraindicated [37]. Dronaderone is similar to amiodarone in chemical structure, but its use is not recommended in HFrEF because of recurrent hospitalization and increased mortality [38]. In HFrEF, current guidelines recommend the use of amiodarone and dofetilide with class IIa recommendation level. Sotalol is at the IIb recommendation level, while the use of Flecainide and propafenone is not recommended due to poor prognostic results [1]. Amiodarone is a Class III antiarrhythmic agent with a natural effect on survival that is frequently preferred in patients with HFrEF and has beta-blockade, negative inotropic, and vasodilator effects. Caution should be exercised in terms of side effect profile when used for long-term rhythm control [39]. Dofetilide is a Class III antiarrhythmic agent and is effective in restoring sinus rhythm and preventing recurrence. However, torsades de pointes are frequent side effects and should be used with caution and the patient should be hospitalized for up to 3 days [3]. Amiodarone dronaderone, flecainide, propafenone, and dofetilide can be used as antiarrhythmic agents with a class IIa recommendation level in patients with normal LV function, no structural heart disease, no NYHA class III–IV or no decompensated period in the last 4 weeks [1].

The other strategy for rhythm control is catheter ablation and the main goal is pulmonary vein isolation with various techniques. Radiofrequency ablation after mapping, cryoablation, ultra-low temperature cryoablation, pulsed-field ablation are some ablation techniques used [24].

Another method that can be preferred before atrioventricular nodal ablation and permanent pacemaker implantation in symptomatic patients resistant to medical treatment and catheter ablation is the Cox Maze procedure (CMP), which is a surgical ablation method. In the Cox Maze III procedure, incisions are made and stitched to create a conduction block in both atria to prevent AF. In the Cox Maze IV procedure, bipolar radiofrequency or cryoballoon is used. The newer Cox Maze IV procedure has lower morbidity and mortality rates than procedure III. CMP was found to be equally effective in patients with paroxysmal and nonparoxysmal AF. It is the recommended method before AV node ablation to restore sinus rhythm alone or simultaneously with cardiac surgery in patients resistant to Group I–III antiarrhythmic therapy and catheter-based therapy. A consensus has not yet been reached on surgical ablation in the presence of HF and AF due to the lack of randomized studies on this procedure. However, ablation with a surgical procedure can be considered as a rhythm control strategy to be applied before AV node ablation and pacing in patients resistant to other rhythm control methods, with high efficiency, low mortality and morbidity, and in patients whose diagnosis of tachycardiomyopathy is confirmed by imaging studies and other differential diagnostic tests [40].

In many randomized trials and meta-analyses in HF patients, AF ablation as a rhythm control strategy has been found to be safer and more effective than antiarrhythmic drugs in terms of achieving and maintaining sinus rhythm, reducing AF burden, symptom control, and improving quality of life. Recent randomized controlled trials have also shown positive effects of ablation as a rhythm control strategy on LVEF, mortality, and hospitalizations [41–45].

### 3.5 Rate control vs. rhythm control

Although AF is more common in the HFpEF group, the treatment and management algorithm in the HFrEF group is better defined.

The Atrial Fibrillation and Congestive Heart Failure (AF-CHF), Atrial Fibrillation Follow-up Investigation of Rhythm Management (AFFIRM), and Rate Control Versus Electrical Cardioversion (RACE) trials using pharmacological methods for rhythm control based on pre-catheter ablation showed no difference or superiority in all-cause mortality and cardiovascular death. In the AF-CHF study in which 1376 patients with HFrEF (EF < 35%) and AF were randomized to antiarrhythmic therapy (82% amiodarone) and rate control groups, no difference in mortality, stroke, symptoms, or quality of life was found in rhythm control compared to rate control, but an increase in hospitalization, bradycardia, and need for cardioversion was observed. However, these studies were performed in the pre-ablation period and difficulties in adjusting the optimal dose of antiarrhythmic agents, side effect profile, and difficulties in monitoring and managing these agents contributed to these results [46–48].

The AATAC trial included patients with persistent AF, dual-chamber implanted cardioverter-defibrillator (ICD), or cardiac resynchronization (CRT) defibrillator, HF with NYHA class II–III, and LVEF ≤40% who were randomized to catheter ablation or amiodarone. Catheter ablation resulted in not only a significant improvement of LVEF and 6-minutes-walking distance but also a relative risk reduction in hospitalization and all-cause mortality of 45 and 56%, respectively [49].

The CASTLE- AF study including patients with HFrEF and AF showed that catheter ablation for AF in patients with HF was associated with a significantly lower rate of the composite end point of death from any cause or hospitalization for worsening HF than medical therapy with an absolute risk reduction of 16.1%. There was an increase in EF with ablation. However, the distribution of outcomes differed between patient groups. NYHA I-II, nonischemic cardiomyopathy patients benefited more, while patients with EF > 25 or NYHA III and above did not benefit [41].

The CAMERA-MRI trial compared catheter ablation and medical rate control in patients with idiopathic cardiomyopathy and suspected tachycardia mediated with LVEF ≤45% regarding the primary endpoint of LVEF change. EF, BNP, and NYHA functional classes were improved with catheter ablation [38].

A sub-analysis of the CABANA trial for patients with concomitant AF and HF showed a reduction of the primary composite endpoint of death, disabling stroke, serious bleeding, or cardiac arrest, and all-cause mortality by AF ablation compared to drug therapy including rate or rhythm control drugs [42].

The EAST-AFNET 4 trial randomized patients with early AF (diagnosed ≤1 year before enrollment) and cardiovascular risk factors to early rhythm control (with anti-arrhythmic drug (AAD) or catheter ablation) or usual care. 19.4% of patients received AF catheter ablation. The study was terminated early after the primary endpoint of CV death, stroke, heart failure, or hospitalization with acute coronary syndrome showed significant efficacy of the rhythm control strategy [50].

The CASTLE-HTx study investigated the efficacy and safety of AF ablation in end-stage HF patients with symptomatic AF referred for heart transplantation or left ventricular assist device. As a result, when AF ablation was performed in end-stage HF patients with AF, there was a significant reduction in the sum of clinical events consisting of death, left ventricular assist device implantation, or emergency heart transplantation [51].

As a result of all these studies, the ESC-AF guideline recommends class I for patients with tachycardia-induced cardiomyopathy and catheter ablation in selected HFrEF patients with a class IIa recommendation level in the management of AF in HF [19]. The AHA AF guideline recommends catheter ablation as an AF management strategy in patients with AF-mediated cardiomyopathy suspected, early-stage AF, no significant ventricular scar on CMR, paroxysmal and early-stage permanent AF, and younger patients without significant other comorbidities, with a recommendation level of class I if accompanied by HFrEF and class IIa if accompanied by HFpEF [1, 24].

*DOI: http://dx.doi.org/10.5772/intechopen.1006110*

## 4. Conclusion

AF and HF are two diseases that frequently occur together and have common risk factors. Although the pathophysiology of the relationship has been largely elucidated, the chicken-egg relationship and the cause-effect relationship remain partially unclear. Effective drug treatments and interventional procedures applied separately for HF and AF have begun to reduce the burden of AF-HF association. Although management algorithms have been developed in the light of current studies, more randomized studies are needed on this subject, especially in the HFpEF group.

## Author details

Ebru Sahin* and Ali Oto
Memorial Ankara Hospital, Department of Cardiology, Ankara, Turkey

*Address all correspondence to: ebru_sahin@ymail.com

## References

[1] Joglar JA, Chung MK, Armbruster AL, Benjamin EJ, Chyou JY, Cronin EM, et al. 2023 ACC/AHA/ACCP/HRS guideline for the diagnosis and management of atrial fibrillation: A report of the American college of cardiology/American heart association Joint Committee on Clinical Practice Guidelines. Circulation. 2024;**149**(1):E1-E156. DOI: 10.1161/CIR.0000000000001193

[2] De Ferrari GM, Klersy C, Ferrero P, Fantoni C, Salerno-Uriarte D, Manca L, et al. Atrial fibrillation in heart failure patients: Prevalence in daily practice and effect on the severity of symptoms. Data from the ALPHA study registry. European Journal of Heart Failure. 2007;**9**:502-509. DOI: 10.1016/j.ejheart.2006.10.021

[3] Tsigkas G, Apostolos A, Despotopoulos S, Vasilagkos G, Kallergis E, Leventopoulos G, et al. Heart failure and atrial fibrillation: New concepts in pathophysiology, management, and future directions. Heart Failure Reviews. 2022;**27**(4):1201-1210. DOI: 10.1007/s10741-021-10133-6

[4] Fauchier L, Bisson A, Bodin A. Heart failure with preserved ejection fraction and atrial fibrillation: Recent advances and open questions. BMC Medicine. 2023;**21**:1. DOI: 10.1186/s12916-023-02764-3

[5] Zafrir B, Lund LH, Laroche C, Ruschitzka F, Crespo-Leiro MG, Coats AJS, et al. Prognostic implications of atrial fibrillation in heart failure with reduced, mid-range, and preserved ejection fraction: A report from 14 964 patients in the European society of cardiology heart failure long-term registry. European Heart Journal. 2018;**39**(48):4277-4284. DOI: 10.1093/eurheartj/ehy626

[6] Ling LH, Kistler PM, Kalman JM, Schilling RJ, Hunter RJ. Esc of atrial fibrillation and heart failure. Nature Reviews. Cardiology. 2016;**13**(3):131-147. DOI: 10.1038/nrcardio.2015.191

[7] Luong C, Barnes ME, Tsang TSM. Atrial fibrillation and heart failure: Cause or effect? Current Heart Failure Reports. 2014;**11**(4):463-470. DOI: 10.1007/s11897-014-0229-1

[8] Bergau L, Bengel P, Sciacca V, Fink T, Sohns C, Sommer P. Atrial fibrillation and heart failure. Journal of Clinical Medicine. 29 Apr 2022;**11**(9):2510. DOI: 10.3390/jcm11092510

[9] Patel HJ, Pilla JJ, Polidori DJ, Pusca SV, Plappert TA, Sutton MSJ, et al. Ten weeks of rapid ventricular pacing creates a long-term model of left ventricular dysfunction. The Journal of Thoracic and Cardiovascular Surgery. 2000;**119**(4 I):834-841. DOI: 10.1016/S0022-5223(00)70021-3

[10] Gopinathannair R, Etheridge SP, Marchlinski FE, Spinale FG, Lakkireddy D, Olshansky B. Arrhythmia-induced cardiomyopathies: Mechanisms, recognition, and management. Journal of the American College of Cardiology. 2015;**66**(15):1714-1728. DOI: 10.1016/j.jacc.2015.08.038

[11] Ling LH, Kistler PM, Ellims AH, Iles LM, Lee G, Hughes GL, et al. Diffuse ventricular fibrosis in atrial fibrillation: Noninvasive evaluation and relationships with aging and systolic dysfunction. Journal of the American College of Cardiology. 2012;**60**(23):2402-2408. DOI: 10.1016/j.jacc.2012.07.065

[12] Zakeri R, Chamberlain AM, Roger VL, Redfield MM. Temporal

relationship and prognostic significance of atrial fibrillation in heart failure patients with preserved ejection fraction: A community-based study. Circulation. 2013;**128**(10):1085-1093. DOI: 10.1161/CIRCULATIONAHA.113.001475

[13] Santhanakrishnan R, Wang N, Larson MG, Magnani JW, McManus DD, Lubitz SA, et al. Atrial fibrillation begets heart failure and vice versa: Temporal associations and differences in preserved versus reduced ejection fraction. Circulation. 2016;**133**(5):484-492. DOI: 10.1161/CIRCULATIONAHA.115.018614

[14] Pabel S, Sossalla S. Atrial fibrillation and heart failure: Novel insights into the chicken and egg dilemma. European Heart Journal. 2022;**43**(36):3376-3378. DOI: 10.1093/eurheartj/ehac257

[15] Okada M, Yamawaki H, Hara Y. Angiotensin II enhances interleukin-1 beta-induced MMP-9 secretion in adult rat cardiac fibroblasts. The Journal of Veterinary Medical Science. 2010;**72**(6):735-739. DOI: 10.1292/jvms.09-0582

[16] Clarke JD, Caldwell JL, Horn MA, Bode EF, Richards MA, Hall MCS, et al. Perturbed atrial calcium handling in an ovine model of heart failure: Potential roles for reductions in the L-type calcium current. Journal of Molecular and Cellular Cardiology. 2015;**79**:169. DOI: 10.1016/j.yjmcc.2014.11.017

[17] Chen PS, Chen LS, Fishbein MC, Lin SF, Nattel S. Role of the autonomic nervous system in atrial fibrillation: Pathophysiology and therapy. Circulation Research. 2014;**114**(9):1500. DOI: 10.1161/CIRCRESAHA.114.303772

[18] Gertz ZM, Raina A, Saghy L, Zado ES, Callans DJ, Marchlinski FE, et al. Evidence of atrial functional mitral regurgitation due to atrial fibrillation: Reversal with arrhythmia control. Journal of the American College of Cardiology. 2011;**58**(14):1474-1481. DOI: 10.1016/j.jacc.2011.06.032

[19] Hindricks G, Potpara T, Dagres N, Arbelo E, Bax JJ, et al. 2020 2019 guidelines for the diagnosis and management of atrial fibrillation developed in collaboration with the European association for cardio-thoracic surgery (EACTS): The task force for the diagnosis and management of atrial fibrillation of the European society of cardiology (ESC) developed with the special contribution of the European Heart Rhythm Association (EHRA) of the ESC. European Heart Journal. 2021;**42**(5):373-498. DOI: 10.1093/eurheartj/ehaa612

[20] Barrio-Lopez MT, Ruiz-Canela M, Ramos P, Tercedor L, Ibañez Criado JL, Ortiz M, et al. PREvention of recurrent arrhythmias with mediterranean diet (PREDIMAR) study in patients with atrial fibrillation: Rationale, design and methods. American Heart Journal. 2020;**220**:127-136. DOI: 10.1016/j.ahj.2019.10.009

[21] Lavie CJ, Pandey A, Lau DH, Alpert MA, Sanders P. Obesity and atrial fibrillation prevalence, pathogenesis, and prognosis: Effects of weight loss and exercise. Journal of the American College of Cardiology. 2017;**70**(16):2022-2035. DOI: 10.1016/j.jacc.2017.09.002

[22] Voskoboinik A, Prabhu S, Han LL, Kalman JM, Kistler PM. Alcohol and atrial fibrillation: A sobering review. Journal of the American College of Cardiology. 2016;**68**(23):2567-2576. DOI: 10.1016/j.jacc.2016.08.074

[23] Zhu W, Guo L, Hong K. Relationship between smoking and adverse outcomes in patients with atrial fibrillation:

A meta-analysis and systematic review. International Journal of Cardiology. 2016;**222**:289-294. DOI: 10.1016/j.ijcard.2016.07.220

[24] Maddox TM, Januzzi JL, Allen LA, Breathett K, Brouse S, Butler J, et al. 2024 ACC expert consensus decision pathway for treatment of heart failure with reduced ejection fraction: A report of the American college of cardiology solution set oversight committee. Journal of the American College of Cardiology. 2024;**83**(15):1444-1488. DOI: 10.1016/j.jacc.2023.12.024

[25] Vermes E, Tardif JC, Bourassa MG, Racine N, Levesque S, White M, et al. Enalapril decreases the incidence of atrial fibrillation in patients with left ventricular dysfunction. Circulation. 2003;**107**(23):2926-2931. DOI: 10.1161/01.CIR.0000072793.81076.D4

[26] McMurray JJV, Packer M, Desai AS, Gong J, Lefkowitz MP, Rizkala AR, et al. Angiotensin-neprilysin inhibition versus enalapril in heart failure. The New England Journal of Medicine. 2014;**371**(11):132-133. DOI: 10.1056/NEJMoa1409077

[27] Packer M, Anker SD, Butler J, Filippatos G, Pocock SJ, Carson P, et al. Cardiovascular and renal outcomes with empagliflozin in heart failure. The New England Journal of Medicine. 2020;**383**(15):1413-1424. DOI: 10.1056/NEJMoa2022190

[28] Padeletti L, Musilli N, Porciani MC, Colella A, Di Biase L, Ricciardi G, et al. Atrial fibrillation and cardiac resynchronization therapy: The MASCOT study. Europace. 2003;**5**(s1):S49-S54. DOI: 10.1016/j.eupc.2004.07.007

[29] Kannel WB, Wolf PA, Benjamin EJ, Levy D. Prevalence, incidence, prognosis, and predisposing conditions for atrial fibrillation: Population-based estimates. The American Journal of Cardiology. 1998;**82**(8A):2N-9N. DOI: 10.1016/s0002-9149(98)00583-9

[30] Mareev Y, Cleland JGF. Should β-blockers be used in patients with heart failure and atrial fibrillation? Clinical Therapeutics. 2015;**37**(10):2215-2224. DOI: 10.1016/j.clinthera.2015.08.017

[31] Kotecha D, Holmes J, Krum H, Altman DG, Manzano L, Cleland JGF, et al. Efficacy of β blockers in patients with heart failure plus atrial fibrillation: An individual-patient data meta-analysis. Lancet. 2014;**384**(9961):2235-2243. DOI: 10.1016/S0140-6736(14)61373-8

[32] Kotecha D, Flather MD, Altman DG, Holmes J, Rosano G, Wikstrand J, et al. Heart rate and rhythm and the benefit of beta-blockers in patients with heart failure. Journal of the American College of Cardiology. 2017;**69**(24):2885-2896. DOI: 10.1016/j.jacc.2017.04.001

[33] Kotecha D, Bunting KV, Gill SK, Mehta S, Stanbury M, Jones JC, et al. Effect of digoxin vs bisoprolol for heart rate control in atrial fibrillation on patient-reported quality of life: The RATE-AF randomized clinical trial. Journal of the American Medical Association. 2020;**324**(24):2497. DOI: 10.1001/jama.2020.23138

[34] Gasparini M, Leclercq C, Lunati M, Landolina M, Auricchio A, Santini M, et al. Cardiac resynchronization therapy in patients with atrial fibrillation: The CERTIFY study (cardiac resynchronization therapy in atrial fibrillation patients multinational registry). JACC Heart Failure. 2013;**1**(6):500-507. DOI: 10.1016/j.jchf.2013.06.003

[35] Brignole M, Pokushalov E, Pentimalli F, Palmisano P, Chieffo E,

Occhetta E, et al. A randomized controlled trial of atrioventricular junction ablation and cardiac resynchronization therapy in patients with permanent atrial fibrillation and narrow QRS. European Heart Journal. 2018;**39**(45):3999-4008. DOI: 10.1093/eurheartj/ehy555

[36] Crijns HJGM, Weijs B, Fairley AM, Lewalter T, Maggioni AP, Martín A, et al. Contemporary real life cardioversion of atrial fibrillation: Results from the multinational RHYTHM-AF study. International Journal of Cardiology. 2014;**172**(3):588-594. DOI: 10.1016/j.ijcard.2014.01.099

[37] Noseworthy PA, Van Houten HK, Gersh BJ, Packer DL, Friedman PA, Shah ND, et al. Generalizability of the CASTLE-AF trial: Catheter ablation for patients with atrial fibrillation and heart failure in routine practice. Hear Rhythm. 2020;**17**(7):1057-1065. DOI: 10.1016/j.hrthm.2020.02.030

[38] Prabhu S, Taylor AJ, Costello BT, Kaye DM, McLellan AJA, Voskoboinik A, et al. Catheter ablation versus medical rate control in atrial fibrillation and systolic dysfunction: The CAMERA-MRI study. Journal of the American College of Cardiology. 2017;**70**(16):1949-1961. DOI: 10.1016/j.jacc.2017.08.041

[39] Reddy YNV, Borlaug BA, Gersh BJ. Management of atrial fibrillation across the spectrum of heart failure with preserved and reduced ejection fraction. Circulation. 2022;**146**(4):339-357. DOI: 10.1161/CIRCULATIONAHA.122.057444

[40] Khiabani AJ, Schuessler RB, Damiano RJ Jr. Surgical ablation of atrial fibrillation in patients with heart failure. The Journal of Thoracic and Cardiovascular Surgery. 2021;**162**(4):1100-1105. DOI: 10.1016/j.jtcvs.2020.05.125

[41] Marrouche NF, Brachmann J, Andresen D, Siebels J, Boersma L, Jordaens L, et al. Catheter ablation for atrial fibrillation with heart failure. The New England Journal of Medicine. 2018;**378**(5):417-427. DOI: 10.1056/NEJMoa1707855

[42] Rettmann ME, Holmes DR, Monahan KH, Breen JF, Bahnson TD, Mark DB, et al. Treatment-related changes in left atrial structure in atrial fibrillation: Findings from the CABANA imaging substudy. Circulation: Arrhythmia and Electrophysiology. 2021;**14**(5):E008540. DOI: 10.1161/CIRCEP.120.008540

[43] Chen S, Pürerfellner H, Meyer C, Acou WJ, Schratter A, Ling Z, et al. Rhythm control for patients with atrial fibrillation complicated with heart failure in the contemporary era of catheter ablation: A stratified pooled analysis of randomized data. European Heart Journal. 2020;**41**(30):2863-2873. DOI: 10.1093/eurheartj/ehz443

[44] Pan KL, Wu YL, Lee M, Ovbiagele B. Catheter ablation compared with medical therapy for atrial fibrillation with heart failure: A systematic review and meta-analysis of randomized controlled trials. International Journal of Medical Sciences. 2021;**18**(6):1325. DOI: 10.7150/ijms.52257

[45] Turagam MK, Garg J, Whang W, Sartori S, Koruth JS, Miller MA, et al. Catheter ablation of atrial fibrillation in patients with heart failure: A meta-analysis of randomized controlled trials. Annals of Internal Medicine. 2019;**170**(1):41-50. DOI: 10.7326/M18-0992

[46] Roy D, Talajic M, Nattel S, George Wyse D, Dorian P, Lee KL, et al. Rhythm control versus rate control for atrial fibrillation and heart failure.

The New England Journal of Medicine. 2008;**358**(25):2667-2677. DOI: 10.1056/NEJMoa0708789

[47] Freudenberger RS, Wilson AC, Kostis JB. Comparison of rate versus rhythm control for atrial fibrillation in patients with left ventricular dysfunction (from the AFFIRM study). The American Journal of Cardiology. 2007;**100**(2):247-252. DOI: 10.1016/j.amjcard.2007.02.101

[48] Hagens VE, Crijns HJGM, Van Veldhuisen DJ, Van Den Berg MP, Rienstra M, Ranchor AV, et al. Rate control versus rhythm control for patients with persistent atrial fibrillation with mild to moderate heart failure: Results from the rate control versus electrical cardioversion (RACE) study. American Heart Journal. 2005;**149**(6):1106-1111. DOI: 10.3390/medicina58060743

[49] Di Biase L, Mohanty P, Mohanty S, Santangeli P, Trivedi C, Lakkireddy D, et al. Ablation versus amiodarone for treatment of persistent atrial fibrillation in patients with congestive heart failure and an implanted device. Circulation. 2016;**133**(17):1637-1644. DOI: 10.1161/CIRCULATIONAHA.115.019406

[50] Kirchhof P, Camm AJ, Goette A, Brandes A, Eckardt L, Elvan A, et al. Early rhythm-control therapy in patients with atrial fibrillation. The New England Journal of Medicine. 2020;**383**(14):1305-1316. DOI: 10.1056/NEJMoa2019422

[51] Sohns C, Fox H, Marrouche NF, Crijns HJGM, Costard-Jaeckle A, Bergau L, et al. Catheter ablation in end-stage heart failure with atrial fibrillation. The New England Journal of Medicine. 2023;**389**(15):1380-1389. DOI: 10.1056/NEJMoa2306037

Chapter 7

# Interaction between Atrial Fibrillation and Heart Failure: Recent Advances

*Jovany Castro-Lara, Sandra Sánchez-Cassio and Manuel Alejandro Vera-Fuentes*

## Abstract

A continuous relationship exists between atrial fibrillation and heart failure, where each condition can cause or exacerbate the other. Determining which condition occurs first can pose a significant challenge, as they share various risk factors and intrinsically related pathophysiology. Such is their correlation that a prevalence nearing 60% of atrial fibrillation in de novo heart failure patients and a 37% prevalence of heart failure in newly occurring atrial fibrillation patients have been reported. These conditions have a negative synergistic effect on quality of life, exercise capacity, and hospital readmission. Significant advances have been made in recent years in the diagnosis and treatment of atrial fibrillation and heart failure, with recent guidelines from the American Heart Association (AHA) guidelines, all aimed at establishing comprehensive treatment leading to beneficial cardiovascular outcomes.

**Keywords:** atrial fibrillation, heart failure, recent advances, diagnosis, treatment

## 1. Introduction

Atrial fibrillation (AF) is the most common cardiac arrhythmia worldwide, affecting 1% of the population and is associated with high cardiovascular morbidity and mortality. It is now understood that heart failure is the most common complication and cause of death in AF patients, with a much greater risk of death from heart failure compared to stroke [1, 2].

Among heart failure (HF) patients, over half suffer from AF; the two are entities that relate to each other, with one facilitating the occurrence of the other and vice versa. AF is associated with dysfunction and pathological remodeling of the myocardium, an alteration termed atrial myopathy [1, 3]. The prevalence of each is increasing globally, with this trend expected to continue due to population aging [2, 4].

There are multiple studies in the literature evaluating the optimal therapy for managing patients with atrial fibrillation and heart failure, with two strategies (rhythm control and rate control) not mutually exclusive, and their outcomes are dependent on multiple factors, including clinical characteristics, associated comorbidities, timing of onset, and cardiac anatomical alterations. In this chapter, we summarize recent advances and a body of evidence on the comprehensive treatment of AF in heart failure.

## 2. Epidemiology

In the United States, AF prevalence is projected to increase to 12.1 million by 2030, a similar trend in Europe, where prevalence was 8.8 million in 2010, estimated to rise to 17.9 million by 2060. Similarly, a substantial increase in HF prevalence is expected due to population aging. Although guideline-directed medical therapy (GDMT) is associated with a 25% reduction in all-cause mortality at 24 months in HF patients, mortality remains high [4].

An analysis of Framingham Heart Study participants demonstrated that 32% of patients diagnosed with HF had a history of AF, with an additional 30% diagnosed with AF subsequently. AF prevalence differs depending on left ventricular ejection fraction (LVEF), with a Swedish analysis showing higher prevalence in patients with preserved LVEF (LVEF <40%: 53%; LVEF 40–49%: 60%, and LVEF ≥50%: 65%) [4].

The onset of AF in patients with heart failure with reduced ejection fraction (HFrEF) increases as their functional class worsens, averaging 4% in NYHA class I to 50% in NYHA class IV heart failure, reflecting the progression of underlying myocardial disease and predicting a worse prognosis upon presentation [1].

Multiple risk factors are associated with the onset of atrial fibrillation, which are also shared for heart failure development. Obesity has been linked to increased incidence, decreased activity levels, and sedentary lifestyle associated with symptom worsening, and alcohol consumption is related to AF recurrence (**Table 1**) [1, 4].

## 3. Pathophysiology of atrial fibrillation and heart failure

There are multiple mechanisms through which HF can lead to the development of AF and vice versa. Pulmonary congestion in HF patients depends on the left atrial pressure due to its direct connection with the pulmonary veins. The elevation of left ventricular (LV) diastolic pressure influences congestion through its effects on the left atrium (LA). Left atrial pressure is determined by the pressure-volume relationship during filling, such that left atrial mean pressure depends on myocardial properties, atrioventricular coupling, and its anatomical relationship with the pericardium [1].

| |
|---|
| Advanced age |
| Smoking |
| Obesity |
| Hypertension |
| Coronary and peripheral artery disease |
| Diabetes |
| Chronic kidney disease |
| Metabolic syndrome |
| Sleep apnea |
| Alcohol consumption |

**Table 1.**
*Risk factors present in patients with heart failure for the development of atrial fibrillation.*

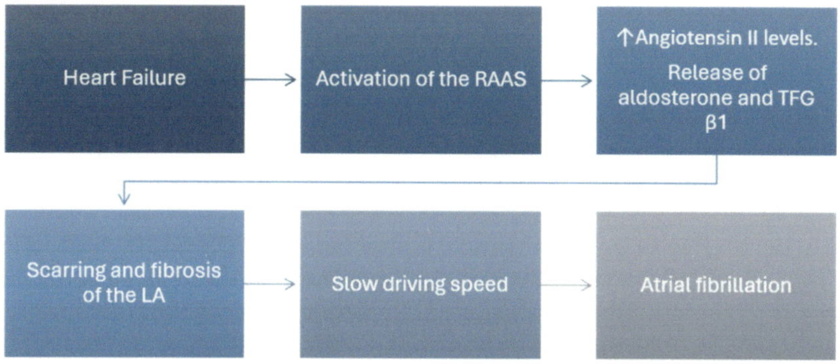


**Figure 1.**
*Pathophysiology in the generation of atrial fibrillation in heart failure. RAAS: renin-angiotensin-aldosterone system; TGF-β1: transforming growth factor beta 1; LA: left atrium.*

Once elevated, atrial pressure leads to fibrosis and scarring, resulting in slower conduction velocity with a shorter action potential duration, thereby promoting the initiation and perpetuation of AF (**Figure 1**) [4].

Chronic AF induces intracellular oxidative stress, leading to calcium overload and activation of the inflammatory cascade. These processes contribute to the perpetuation of the arrhythmia and remodeling of the LA, resulting in fibrosis, thereby influencing the success of rhythm control strategies [3].

In patients with AF, LV filling is affected by a loss of effective atrial contractility and shorter diastolic filling times due to increased heart rate and irregular rhythm. Both factors lead to decreased cardiac output and elevated cardiac pressures. LA dilation can result in functional mitral regurgitation, associated with a high symptom burden and poor quality of life [4].

The impairment of ventricular function is such that the positive effect of beta-blockers on mortality in HF patients disappears when the patient has AF instead of sinus rhythm, despite maintaining controlled heart rate (**Figure 2**) [1, 3].

Studies utilizing cardiac magnetic resonance imaging (CMRI) have shown that patients with AF scheduled for pulmonary vein isolation (PVI), regardless of whether they have preserved or impaired LV function, exhibited significantly prolonged T1 relaxation times (an early marker of fibrosis) compared to a healthy control group. After catheter ablation (3–6 months) and restoration to a stable sinus rhythm, T1 times significantly decreased to normal values [3].

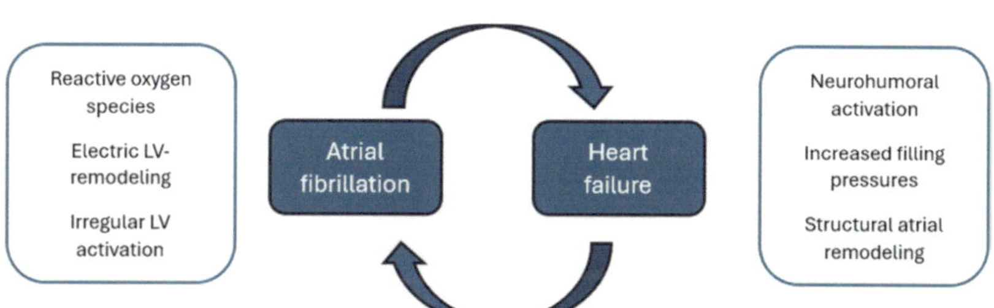


**Figure 2.**
*Synergistic effect between atrial fibrillation and heart failure. LV: left ventricle.*

While the definitive diagnosis of atrial myopathy is histological, clinically the degree of atrial remodeling can be inferred from the extent of atrial dilation, dysfunction assessed via strain, and fibrosis detected through CMRI [1].

## 4. Diagnosis of heart failure in patients with atrial fibrillation

Due to the overlap of symptoms and findings between AF and HF, there is an underdiagnosis of HF, particularly in cases where the left ventricular ejection fraction is preserved. Therefore, the Heart Failure Association (HFA)/European Society of Cardiology (ESC) consensus [5] recommends suspect the diagnosing heart failure with preserved ejection fraction (HFpEF) in AF patients using the following criteria:

- N-terminal pro-brain natriuretic peptide (NT-proBNP) levels:

  o Major criterion: >660 picograms (pg/ml)

  o Minor criterion: 375–660 pg/ml

- Brain natriuretic peptide (BNP) levels:

  o Major criterion: >240 pg/ml

  o Minor criterion: 105–240 pg/ml

- Echocardiographic criteria:

  o Major criterion: left atrial volume index >40 $ml/m^2$

  o Minor criterion: left atrial volume index 34–40 $ml/m^2$

## 5. Treatment of atrial fibrillation in patients with heart failure

The American Heart Association (AHA) recommends a comprehensive treatment strategy that includes targeted therapy for both AF and HF, along with aggressive lifestyle modifications to reduce cardiovascular risk factors [6, 7].

### 5.1 Rhythm control vs. rate control

Currently, two therapeutic strategies are accepted for AF patients: rhythm control aims to restore sinus rhythm, while rate control targets reducing ventricular rate without stopping AF. In the past 5 years, several significant studies have been published investigating the optimal therapeutic strategy (**Table 2**) [3].

There is substantial evidence supporting the use of catheter ablation for AF in patients with HF. However, rhythm control with drugs also appears beneficial. In the EAST-AFNET 4 (Early Rhythm-Control Therapy in Patients with Atrial Fibrillation) trial [15], patients with signs and symptoms of HF assigned to early rhythm control (with AF diagnosed ≤1 year) had a significantly lower risk of cardiovascular deaths, strokes, HF hospitalization, or acute coronary syndrome (antiarrhythmic therapy: 31 amiodarone, 33 flecainide, 10 dronedarone, and less than 10% ablation).

| Trial | Objective | Type of trial | Population type sample size (n) | Primary endpoint | Results |
|---|---|---|---|---|---|
| AFFIRM Trial (2000) [8] | Comparison of rate control and rhythm control in patients with AF. | Multicenter, randomized | Patients with AF and high risk of stroke or death<br>n = 4060 patients. | 5-year mortality | 23.8% in the rhythm control group and 21.3% in the rate control group (HR 1.15; 95% CI 0.99–1.34; p = 0.08) |
| AATAC Trial (2016) [9] | Catheter ablation vs. amiodarone for the treatment of persistent AF in patients with congestive heart failure and an implanted device. | Multicenter, randomized | Patients with persistent AF, with a dual-chamber ICD or CRT-D, CHF (NYHA II to III), and LVEF <40%<br>n = 203 patients | Recurrence of AF | Amiodarone therapy had a significantly higher likelihood of AF recurrence (HR 2.5; 95% CI 1.5–4.3; p < 0.001) |
| CAMERA-MRI Trial (2017) [10] | Catheter ablation vs. medical rate control in atrial fibrillation and systolic dysfunction. | Multicenter, randomized | Patients with persistent AF and idiopathic cardiomyopathy (LVEF ≤45%)<br>n = 66 patients. | Change in LVEF assessed by CMRI at 6 months | Absolute LVEF improved by 18 ± 13% in the ablation group compared with 4.4 ± 13% in the rate control group (p < 0.0001). |
| CASTLE-AF Trial (2018) [11] | Effect of catheter ablation for atrial fibrillation with heart failure. | Multicenter, randomized | Patients with symptomatic paroxysmal or persistent AF not responsive to antiarrhythmic drugs vs. medical therapy (rate or rhythm control).<br>n = 363 patients. | Combination of all-cause mortality or hospitalization for worsening HF | Primary endpoint occurred in 28.5% in the ablation group vs. 44.6% in the medical therapy group (HR 0.62; 95% CI 0.43–0.87; p = 0.007). NNT = 6. |
| CABANAA Trial (2019) [12] | Effect of catheter ablation vs. antiarrhythmic drug therapy in AF. | Multicenter, randomized | Patients with symptomatic AF with one or more risk factors for stroke<br>n = 2204 patients. | Combination of death, disabling stroke, serious bleeding, or cardiac arrest | Primary endpoint occurred in 8% in the ablation group vs. 9.2% in the drug therapy group (HR 0.86; 95% CI 0.65–1.15; p = 0.30) |
| APAF-CRT trial (2021) [13] | AV junction ablation and cardiac resynchronization therapy for patients with permanent AF and narrow QRS vs. medical rate control. | Multicenter, randomized | Patients with severe symptomatic permanent AF >6 months with narrow QRS and at least one hospitalization for HF<br>n = 133 patients. | Time to all-cause mortality | Primary endpoint occurred in 11% in the ablation + CRT group vs. 29% in the medical control group (HR 0.26; 95% CI 0.10–0.65; p = 0.004) |

| Trial | Objective | Type of trial | Population type sample size (n) | Primary endpoint | Results |
|---|---|---|---|---|---|
| CASTLE-Htx Trial (2023) [14] | Catheter ablation in end-stage heart failure with AF vs. medical therapy alone. | Single-center. | Patients with symptomatic AF and end-stage heart failure referred for heart transplant evaluation. n = 194 patients. | Combination of all-cause mortality, ventricular assist device implantation, or urgent heart transplant | Primary endpoint occurred in 8% in the ablation group vs. 30% in the medical therapy group (HR 0.24; 95% CI 0.11–0.52; $p < 0.001$). NNT = 5. |

*AF: atrial fibrillation; ICD: implantable cardioverter defibrillator; CRT: cardiac resynchronization therapy; HF: heart failure; LVEF: left ventricular ejection fraction; CMRI: cardiac magnetic resonance imaging; AV: atrioventricular; NNT: number needed to treat; HR: hazard ratio.*

**Table 2.**
*Clinical trials evaluating rhythm control vs. rate control strategies in atrial fibrillation.*

Both therapeutic strategies have been cornerstones of atrial fibrillation treatment, making it crucial to determine which is superior in improving clinical outcomes. A recently published meta-analysis evaluated the efficacy of rhythm control (Class IA, IC, or III antiarrhythmic drugs, catheter ablation, and electrical cardioversion) and rate control (beta blockers, digitalis, or calcium antagonists) in patients with non-valvular AF. The primary outcome was cardiovascular (CV) death, with secondary outcomes including all-cause death, stroke, and HF hospitalization. With a sample of 17,536 patients from 18 analyzed studies and an average follow-up of 28.5 months, the rhythm control strategy reduced CV death (HR 0.78; 95% CI, 0.62–0.96), stroke (HR 0.80; 95% CI, 0.64–0.99) and HF hospitalization (HR 0.80; 95% CI, 0.69–0.94), but not all-cause death (HR 0.86; 95% CI, 0.73–1.02) compared to a rate control strategy (15). In the subgroup of patients with HF, rhythm control reduced CV mortality by 41% (HR 0.59; 95% CI, 0.36–0.97), all-cause mortality (HR 0.83; 95% CI, 0.70–0.98), stroke risk (HR 0.619; 95% CI, 0.385–0.996), and HF hospitalizations (HR 0.81; 95% CI, 0.68–0.97). The type of AF (paroxysmal/persistent) did not show differences in CV death [16].

## 5.2 The role of ablation in rhythm control

In recent decades, ablation has become an effective and safe treatment for the management of AF. The decision regarding patient eligibility should be made on an individualized basis, considering factors such as age, duration of AF, comorbidities, atrial dilation, and the presence of fibrosis [17].

### *5.2.1 Catheter ablation in patients with AF and HF*

Clinical trials have demonstrated the benefits of catheter ablation in patients with AF and left ventricular systolic dysfunction; findings have confirmed the importance of the cardiac substrate in achieving the reversal and maintenance of sinus rhythm, with an inversely proportional relationship between the response and the degree of myocardial dysfunction.

Determining which condition presents first becomes relevant when evaluating the efficacy of catheter ablation; patients who develop HF first have a worse prognosis, a lower likelihood of presenting AF-mediated cardiomyopathy, and a worse prognosis after ablation [17].

Therefore, it is important to have objective tools to determine which patients are more likely to respond to ablation. The ANTWERP score has been developed to predict response in patients with HF and reduced ejection fraction, with an area under the curve of 0.86 (95% CI 0.82–0.89; $p < 0.001$). For total scores of 0, 1, 2, 3, 4, and 5–6, the response rates are 94, 92, 82, 51, 40, and 17%, respectively (**Table 3**) [17, 18].

| Parameter | Score |
|---|---|
| QRS complex width >120 milliseconds | 2 points |
| Known etiology | 2 points |
| Paroxysmal atrial fibrillation | 1 point |
| Severe atrial dilation | 1 point |
| *Total score ≤2 points: benefit of early referral for catheter ablation.* | |

**Table 3.**
*ANTWERP score.*

It has been demonstrated that catheter ablation in patients with AF and heart failure with reduced ejection fraction has benefits beyond rhythm control, significantly reducing arrhythmia recurrences and the risk of cardiovascular events compared to pharmacological therapy, even in heart failure with preserved ejection fraction [17].

### *5.2.2 Surgical ablation in patients with AF and HF*

The Cox-MAZE procedure is the most effective curative surgical intervention for patients with AF who do not respond to medical therapies. Developed by Dr. James Cox in the 1980s, it consists of complex sequential atriotomy incisions in a labyrinth-shaped pattern with scar tissue formation that prevents the spread of abnormal impulses. It was initially applied in patients with isolated AF; however, with the passage of time and emerging evidence, its use was expanded to patients undergoing concomitant cardiac surgical procedures [19–21].

The procedure has improved its effectiveness and reduction in operating time, currently the Cox-MAZE III version is considered the standard surgical treatment, as a safe and effective technique when performed concomitantly with other cardiac surgical procedures (mitral valve, aortic, tricuspid, congenital heart disease, and coronary revascularization) [21].

Today, the use of cryothermy and radiofrequency energy to create auricular lesions (Cox-MAZE III/IV procedure) has replaced the scalpel incision technique. Its effectiveness has been demonstrated by freedom of atrial tachyarrhythmia in up to 92% at 1 year and 84% at 5 years (with or without the use of antiarrhythmic drugs). It is important that patients who maintain sinus rhythm at 10 years have a better survival rate compared to those who have one or more episodes of atrial tachyarrhythmia (84 vs. 77%, p = 0.03) (**Table 4**) [21, 27].

| Authors | Quiruric plan | Findings |
|---|---|---|
| Churyla et al. [22] | AVR + CSA | N = 15,596 (5167 ablation, 2983 LAA closure)<br>No differences in mortality or stroke incidence<br>Increased incidence in PPM implantation in ablation group |
| Mehaffey et al. [23] | MVS + CSA | N = 1675 (1044 CSA)<br>Decreased utility of CSA from 2011 to 2018 |
| Guo et al. [24] | AVR + CSA | N = 108 (58 CSA)<br>Decrease in mid-term recurrence of AF with CSA<br>Improvement in all-cause mortality at 12 months (100% in CSA vs. 89% in isolated AVR) |
| Cheng et al. [25] | CABG + CSA<br>Valve + CSA<br>AS + CSA | N = 11,459<br>CSA associated with lower risk of all-cause mortality and ischemic stroke<br>Superior long-term survival after CABG or AVRMVR +CSA<br>No increase in postoperative complication rates |
| Kim et al. [26] | MVS + CSA | N = 9501 (5508 CSA)<br>Reduced risk of composite event (mortality, CVA, and major bleeding) |

*AF: atrial fibrillation; AS: aortic surgery; AVR: aortic valve replacement/repair; CABG: coronary artery bypass grafting; CMP-IV: Cox-Maze procedure- IV; CSA: concomitant surgical ablation; CVA: cerebrovascular accident; LAA: left atrial appendage; MVS: mitral valve surgery; PPM: permanent pacemaker.*

**Table 4.**
*Clinical trials evaluating the safety and effectiveness of concomitant surgical ablation.*

Therefore, the Society of Thoracic Surgeons (STS) proposes that CSA should be performed in all patients undergoing first-time non-emergent cardiac surgery for aortic or mitral valve (Class I recommendation) and for coronary revascularization (Class II recommendation). This recommendation is supported by recently proposed guidelines from the American College of Cardiology/American Heart Association/American College of Chest Physicians/Heart Rhythm Society with a Class IIa recommendation [7].

Although guidelines support its widespread use, outcomes will depend on proper patient selection, surgeon experience, and clinical context, emphasizing the importance of the heart team decision-making with an individualized approach (**Table 5**) [28].

Recent technological advancements have led to the development of novel techniques such as hybrid ablation, which combines minimally invasive surgical ablation with percutaneous catheter ablation to create endocardial and epicardial lesions. This technique should be used in selected patients with persistent or long-standing persistent atrial fibrillation, especially when antiarrhythmic drugs and catheter ablation have been unsuccessful. It is essential to perform hybrid ablation in experienced centers with collaboration between cardiac electrophysiology and cardiac surgery teams [29].

### 5.3 Role of guideline-directed medical therapy (GDMT)

Guideline-directed medical therapy (GDMT) has changed the prognosis of patients with HF. However, once AF is present, it influences the effectiveness of some drugs for HF [4].

#### *5.3.1 Angiotensin-converting enzyme inhibitors (ACEI) and angiotensin receptor blockers (ARB)*

Several mechanisms by which angiotensin II mediates AF include its binding to its receptor, resulting in the production of transforming growth factor-beta 1 (TGF-β1), which promotes fibroblast proliferation. Another mechanism is increased systemic vascular resistance, sympathetic activity, and myocardial fibrosis, leading to increased left atrial pressure affecting atrial myocyte action potential [4].

There exists numerous Trials Providing Evidence for ACEI/ARB benefit on AF:

- SOLVD Trial [30] (effect of enalapril on survival in patients with reduced left ventricular ejection fraction and congestive heart failure): in a sub-analysis

| | **Paroxysmal AF** | **Persistent AF** |
|---|---|---|
| LAVI < 34 ml/m$^2$ | PVI + LAAO | PVI + box + LAAO<br>LA open → + mitral isthmus line |
| LAVI > 34 ml/m$^2$ | PVI + box + LAAO | PVI + box + LAAO<br>LA open → + mitral isthmus line |
| LAVI > 70 ml/m$^2$ | PVI + box + LAAO | No ablation |

*AF: atrial fibrillation; LAVI: left atrial volume index; PVI: pulmonary vein isolation; LAAO: left atrial appendage occlusion; box: left atrial posterior wall.*

**Table 5.**
*Concomitant surgical ablation options for AF.*

of 374 patients without a history of AF at a single center, patients assigned to enalapril were less likely to develop AF.

- Trandolapril in patients with left ventricular systolic dysfunction after a myocardial infarction was associated with a reduction in AF incidence [31].

- Val-HeFT Trial [32] (a randomized trial of the angiotensin-receptor blocker valsartan in chronic heart failure): among 4395 patients in sinus rhythm, 5.12% in the valsartan group developed AF compared to 7.95% of patients assigned to placebo (HR 0.63; 95% CI: 0.49–0.81; p = 0.0003).

- CHARM Trial [33] (mortality and morbidity reduction with candesartan in patients with chronic heart failure and left ventricular systolic dysfunction): patients assigned to candesartan were less likely to develop AF during follow-up across the spectrum of left ventricular ejection fraction.

#### *5.3.2 Angiotensin-neprilysin inhibitors*

Currently, sacubitril/valsartan has been shown to be superior to ACE inhibitors in reducing morbidity and mortality in patients with HFrEF. Although the data are inconclusive, some studies suggest it may promote reverse atrial remodeling among patients with AF [4, 34].

#### *5.3.3 Beta blockers (BB)*

Beta blockers are first-line drugs for rate control in AF, reducing mortality, hospitalizations, and symptom burden in HFrEF. They prevent adverse remodeling and promote positive remodeling, resulting in reduced left atrial pressure, preventing atrial ischemia and fibrosis [4].

The benefits of beta blockers in HFrEF may be attenuated by the presence of AF. A meta-analysis including patients from COPERNICUS, MERIT-HF, CIBIS-II, and SENIORS showed that BB did not reduce HF hospitalizations or mortality in patients with AF. Another meta-analysis with >18,000 patients associated BB with a significant reduction in mortality in HFrEF patients in sinus rhythm but not in those with AF (HR 0.97; 95% CI: 0.83–1.14; p = 0.73) [4].

Several considerations should be made regarding these results. In the second meta-analysis, AF status was determined at randomization, without characterizing AF as paroxysmal or permanent. About 4.7% of patients in sinus rhythm developed AF during follow-up, and this risk was reduced by 33% with beta blockers. Patients with AF likely had permanent AF, so the apparent reduction in BB efficacy applies predominantly to patients with permanent AF and not those with paroxysmal AF. Finally, the trials included patients with controlled heart rates [1].

These points are important as beta blockers have shown better outcomes with higher doses (carvedilol 25 mg twice daily, metoprolol succinate 200 mg/day, and bisoprolol 10 mg/day). Thus, the meta-analysis results suggest that patients with intrinsically slower permanent AF due to conduction system disease may not benefit from aggressive BB optimization. It is reasonable to consider that low doses are equally effective as higher doses in permanent AF with controlled heart rate in HFrEF, and optimizing dosing in patients with paroxysmal AF will improve survival and reduce incident AF episodes [1].

#### *5.3.4 Mineralocorticoid receptor antagonists*

Patients with chronic kidney disease and type 2 diabetes have a higher risk of developing AF, associated with increased morbidity and mortality. This was addressed in a post hoc analysis of the FIDELIO-DKD [35] (effect of finerenone on chronic kidney disease outcomes in type 2 diabetes), where finerenone reduced the risk of AF onset by 29% (HR 0.71; 95% CI: 0.53–0.94; $p = 0.0164$) [36]. Similarly, a secondary analysis of EMPHASIS-HF found that eplerenone significantly reduced the incidence of AF compared to placebo [37].

#### *5.3.5 Sodium-glucose cotransporter 2 inhibitors (SGLT-2i)*

The precise mechanism by which SGLT-2i reduces HF hospitalizations and cardiovascular mortality is unknown. They have a significant natriuretic effect, reducing intravascular volume and blood pressure, decreasing preload and afterload, and reducing sympathetic hyperactivity. Although different studies (DAPA-HF [38], EMPEROR-Preserved [39], and DELIVER [40]) did not demonstrate a reduction in AF incidence, the benefits of SGLT-2i were consistent among patients with and without AF, improving symptoms, reducing the risk of HF hospitalization, and mortality [4, 41].

#### *5.3.6 Digoxin*

Digoxin is useful for heart rate control in patients with AF due to its vagomimetic effects, slowing sinoatrial and atrioventricular conduction without negative inotropic effects. An analysis of the Swedish HF Registry found that digoxin was associated with reduced HF hospitalizations and mortality among patients with HF and AF, contrary to patients with HF without AF history, where a higher risk of hospitalization and mortality was observed [42].

In the RATE-AF trial [43] (Effect of Digoxin vs. Bisoprolol for Heart Rate Control in Atrial Fibrillation on Quality of Life), among patients with HFrEF and permanent AF, symptom endpoints favored digoxin. Therefore, its use should be at the lowest effective dose, avoiding levels ≥1.2 ng/ml associated with higher mortality [1].

### 5.4 Anticoagulation in patients with AF and HF

One of the therapeutic goals in managing atrial fibrillation (AF) is the prevention of stroke and improvement of symptoms. Anticoagulation therapy reduces the risk of stroke by nearly two-thirds, although it carries an increased risk of bleeding. Patients with HFrEF and AF have a higher risk of embolic events originating in the LA and an increased risk of thrombi in the left ventricle [1, 44].

The American Heart Association (AHA) recommends using the CHA2DS2-VASc score to guide anticoagulant therapy in patients with AF and HFrEF to prevent stroke. Direct oral anticoagulants (DOACs) are recommended as the first-line treatment, with warfarin as an alternative. For patients with a long-term contraindication to oral anticoagulation, left atrial appendage closure should be considered [6].

DOACs are preferred over warfarin due to a lower risk of bleeding, greater convenience, and potentially greater reduction in stroke incidence. The combination of antiplatelet agents with anticoagulants increases the risk of bleeding and mortality without reducing ischemic events. Therefore, patients with non-ischemic cardiomyopathy, AF, and HFrEF should be treated with anticoagulation alone [1].

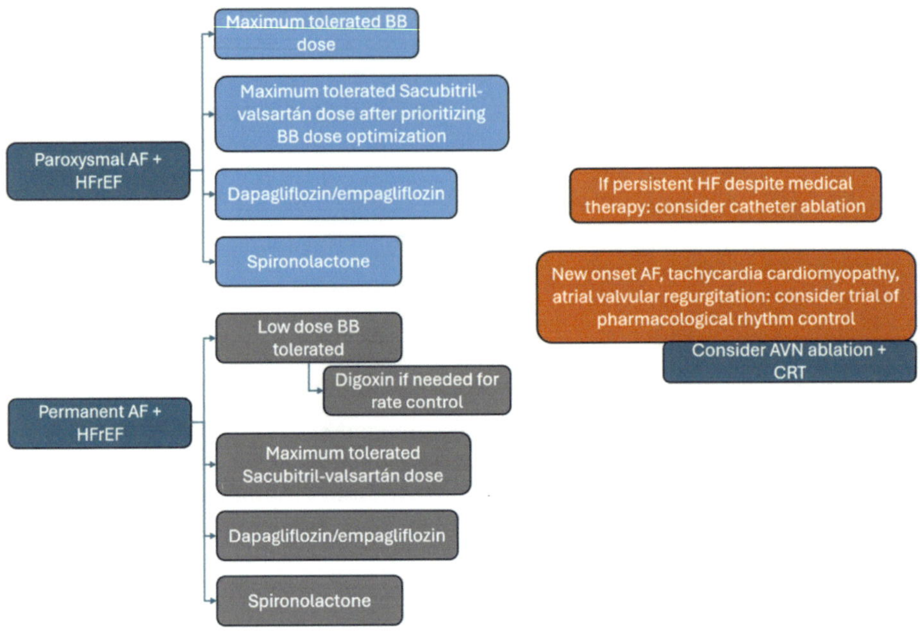


**Figure 3.**
*Approach to medical treatment and rhythm control in HFrEF based on the status of AF. AF: atrial fibrillation. HFrEF: heart failure with reduced ejection fraction. BB: beta blocker. HF: heart failure. AVN: atrioventricular node. CRT: cardiac resynchronization therapy.*

The treatment of AF in the context of heart failure is complex, but recent advances in catheter-based strategies have shown potential in improving clinical outcomes. Restoring sinus rhythm, preferably through catheter ablation, should be the primary goal in patients with heart failure. If restoration of sinus rhythm is unattainable and AF is deemed permanent, timely discussion with the patient regarding the potential benefits of atrioventricular node ablation and cardiac resynchronization therapy (CRT) implantation is warranted (**Figure 3**) [3, 7].

## 6. AF-induced cardiomyopathy (AF-CM)

Atrial fibrillation-induced cardiomyopathy (AF-CM) is part of a group of myocardial disorders known as arrhythmia-induced cardiomyopathies (AiCM), which are characterized by left ventricular dysfunction that may potentially be reversible. The likelihood of developing this cardiomyopathy increases when a patient exhibits a mean heart rate >100 beats per minute, atrial fibrillation, and/or a burden of premature ventricular contractions ≥10%, with no other identifiable cause of left ventricular dysfunction [45].

AF-CM is defined as systolic dysfunction of the left ventricle in patients with paroxysmal or persistent atrial fibrillation despite adequate heart rate control. Ambulatory Holter monitoring is crucial for detecting AF-CM, as it helps exclude inadequate heart rate control [45, 46].

The risk of developing ventricular dysfunction not only depends on the type of arrhythmia but also on its duration and frequency. Persistent tachycardia leads to structural changes that result in systolic dysfunction and dilation of the left ventricle (LV), and in some cases, this dilation can affect both ventricles with thinning, with or without hypertrophy of the cardiac mass. The progression of these changes includes a decrease in systemic arterial pressure with an increase in LV and pulmonary artery pressure, leading to a decline in cardiac output, ejection fraction, and cardiac volumes [45, 47].

Due to the reversible nature of AF-CM once the tachyarrhythmia is eliminated, timely and targeted treatment plays an essential role. Following elimination, most patients typically experience improved left ventricular function within 4–12 weeks, along with symptom improvement in at least one functional class of heart failure [45, 46].

Among rhythm control therapies, ablation has achieved sinus rhythm restoration in 50–88% of patients with paroxysmal and persistent AF-CM. In contrast, antiarrhythmic drugs have a success rate ranging from 30 to 50%, often interrupted due to frequent side effects [45].

## 7. Advances in the prognosis of atrial fibrillation on heart failure

Patients with HF who subsequently receive a diagnosis of AF are associated with a greater burden of symptoms and hospitalizations regardless of their left ventricular ejection fraction (LVEF). An analysis of patients from the ENGAGE AF-TIMI 48 study found that patients with AF and HF with reduced ejection fraction (HFrEF) had a higher rate of mortality and hospitalizations compared to those with preserved LVEF [4, 48].

The prognosis in cardiovascular outcomes is not only affected when a patient with HF receives a de novo diagnosis of AF, but also when AF is preexisting. This was addressed in a recent issue of the Journal of the American College of Cardiology, where Prasada et al. evaluated the perioperative risk of AF; in a sample of 8,635,758 patients who underwent non-cardiac surgical interventions (16.4% with preexisting AF), AF was associated with a higher risk of mortality (OR 1.31; 95% CI: 1.30–1.32), heart failure (OR 1.31; 95% CI: 1.30–1.33), and stroke (OR: 1.40; 95% CI: 1.37–1.43) [2].

## 8. Conclusions

Atrial fibrillation and heart failure are two entities that coexist in a prevalent manner, therefore it is always worth investigating this scenario and using therapeutic tools to control both according to the GDMT.

The evidence in recent years suggests that early rhythm control, primarily through ablation, may delay the perpetuation and progression of AF, leading to better clinical outcomes in patients with non-permanent AF, with the timing of intervention being a determinant factor of success.

## Conflict of interest

The authors declare no conflict of interest.

## Author details

Jovany Castro-Lara[1*], Sandra Sánchez-Cassio[2] and Manuel Alejandro Vera-Fuentes[3]

1 Department of Internal Medicine, Zone General Hospital No. 1 "Dr. Abraham Azar Farah" IMSS, San Francisco de Campeche, Campeche, Mexico

2 Department of Cardiology, Regional General Hospital No. 1 "Ignacio García Téllez" IMSS, Mérida, Yucatán, Mexico

3 Department of Cardiology, High Specialty Medical Unit, National Medical Center "Ignacio García Téllez" IMSS, Mérida, Yucatán, Mexico

*Address all correspondence to: castrolarajovany@gmail.com

IntechOpen

## References

[1] Reddy YNV, Borlaug BA, Gersh BJ. Management of atrial fibrillation across the spectrum of heart failure with preserved and reduced ejection fraction. Circulation. 2022;**146**(4):339-357

[2] Prasada S, Desai MY, Saad M, Smilowitz NR, Faulx M, Menon V, et al. Preoperative atrial fibrillation and cardiovascular outcomes after noncardiac surgery. Journal of the American College of Cardiology. 2022;**79**(25):2471-2485

[3] Bergau L, Bengel P, Sciacca V, Fink T, Sohns C, Sommer P. Atrial fibrillation and heart failure. JCM. 2022;**11**(9):2510

[4] Newman JD, O'Meara E, Böhm M, Savarese G, Kelly PR, Vardeny O, et al. Implications of atrial fibrillation for guideline-directed therapy in patients with heart failure. Journal of the American College of Cardiology. 2024;**83**(9):932-950

[5] Pieske B, Tschöpe C, De Boer RA, Fraser AG, Anker SD, Donal E, et al. How to diagnose heart failure with preserved ejection fraction: The HFA–PEFF diagnostic algorithm: A consensus recommendation from the Heart Failure Association (HFA) of the European society of cardiology (ESC). European Heart Journal. 2019;**40**(40):3297-3317

[6] Gopinathannair R, Chen LY, Chung MK, Cornwell WK, Furie KL, Lakkireddy DR, et al. Managing atrial fibrillation in patients with heart failure and reduced ejection fraction: A scientific statement from the American heart association. Circulation: Arrhythmia and Electrophysiology. 2021;**14**(7):688-705

[7] Joglar JA, Chung MK, Armbruster AL, Benjamin EJ, Chyou JY, Cronin EM, et al. ACC/AHA/ACCP/HRS Guideline for the Diagnosis and management of atrial fibrillation: A Report of the American college of cardiology/American heart association Joint Committee on Clinical Practice Guidelines. Circulation. 2024;**149**(1):1-156

[8] Wyse DG, Waldo AL, DiMarco JP, Domanski MJ, RosenbergY, Schron EB, et al. A comparison of rate control and rhythm control in patients with atrial fibrillation. The New England Journal of Medicine. 2002;**347**(23):1825-1833

[9] Di Biase L, Mohanty P, Mohanty S, Santangeli P, Trivedi C, Lakkireddy D, et al. Ablation versus amiodarone for treatment of persistent atrial fibrillation in patients with congestive heart failure and an implanted device: Results from the AATAC multicenter randomized trial. Circulation. 2016;**133**(17):1637-1644

[10] Prabhu S, Taylor AJ, Costello BT, Kaye DM, McLellan AJA, Voskoboinik A, et al. Catheter ablation versus medical rate control in atrial fibrillation and systolic dysfunction. Journal of the American College of Cardiology. 2017;**70**(16):1949-1961

[11] Marrouche NF, Brachmann J, Andresen D, Siebels J, Boersma L, Jordaens L, et al. Catheter ablation for atrial fibrillation with heart failure. The New England Journal of Medicine. 2018;**378**(5):417-427

[12] Packer DL, Mark DB, Robb RA, Monahan KH, Bahnson TD, Poole JE, et al. Effect of catheter ablation vs antiarrhythmic drug therapy on mortality, stroke, bleeding, and cardiac arrest among patients with atrial fibrillation. JAMA. 2019;**321**(13):1261-1274

[13] Brignole M, Pentimalli F, Palmisano P, Landolina M, Quartieri F, Occhetta E, et al. AV junction ablation and cardiac resynchronization for patients with permanent atrial fibrillation and narrow QRS: The APAF-CRT mortality trial. European Heart Journal. 2021;**42**:4731-4739

[14] Sohns C, Fox H, Marrouche NF, Crijns HJGM, Costard-Jaeckle A, Bergau L, et al. Catheter ablation in end-stage heart failure with atrial fibrillation. The New England Journal of Medicine. 2023;**389**(15):1380-1389

[15] Kirchhof P, Camm AJ, Goette A, Brandes A, Eckardt L, Elvan A, et al. Early rhythm-control therapy in patients with atrial fibrillation. The New England Journal of Medicine. 2020;**383**(14):1305-1316

[16] Zafeiropoulos S, Doundoulakis I, Bekiaridou A, Farmakis IT, Papadopoulos GE, Coleman KM, et al. Rhythm vs rate control strategy for atrial fibrillation. JACC: Clinical Electrophysiology. 2024;**10**(7):S24055 00X24001877

[17] Tzeis S, Gerstenfeld EP, Kalman J, Saad EB, Shamloo AS, Andrade JG, et al. European Heart Rhythm Association/ heart rhythm society/Asia pacific heart rhythm society/Latin American heart rhythm society expert consensus statement on catheter and surgical ablation of atrial fibrillation. Heart Rhythm. 2024;**26**:1-107

[18] Novel Score Predicts Heart Failure Improvement after Atrial Fibrillation Ablation. Available from: https://www.escardio.org/The-ESC/Press-Office/Press-releases/novel-score-predicts-heart-failure-improvement-after-atrial-fibrillation-ablatio

[19] Schuessler RB, Damiano RJ. Patient-specific surgical strategy for atrial fibrillation: Promises and challenges. Heart Rhythm. 2007;**4**(9):1222-1224

[20] Cox JL, Schuessler RB, D'Agostino HJ, Stone CM, Chang BC, Cain ME, et al. The surgical treatment of atrial fibrillation. III. Development of a definitive surgical procedure. The Journal of Thoracic and Cardiovascular Surgery. 1991;**101**(4):569-583

[21] Medical Policy & Technology Assessment Committee (MPTAC). CG-SURG-05 Maze Procedure. Clinical UM Guideline. 2024. Available from: https://www.anthem.com/dam/medpolicies/abc/active/guidelines/gl_pw_a051146.html

[22] Churyla A, Andrei AC, Kruse J, Cox JL, Kislitsina ON, Liu M, et al. Safety of atrial fibrillation ablation with isolated surgical aortic valve replacement. The Annals of Thoracic Surgery. 2021;**111**(3):809-817

[23] Mehaffey JH, Krebs E, Hawkins RB, Charles EJ, Tsutsui S, Kron IL, et al. Variability and utilization of concomitant atrial fibrillation ablation during mitral valve surgery. The Annals of Thoracic Surgery. 2021;**111**(1):29-34

[24] Guo R, Fan C, Sun Z, Zhang H, Sun Y, Song L, et al. Clinical efficacy and safety of cox-maze IV procedure for atrial fibrillation in patients with aortic valve calcification. Frontiers in Cardiovascular Medicine. 2023;**10**:1092068

[25] Cheng YT, Huang YT, Tu HT, Chan YH, Chien-Chia WV, Hung KC, et al. Long-term outcomes of concomitant surgical ablation for atrial fibrillation. The Annals of Thoracic Surgery. 2023;**116**(2):297-305

[26] Kim HJ, Han KD, Kim WK, Cho YH, Lee SH, Je HG. Clinical benefits of concomitant surgical ablation for atrial

fibrillation in patients undergoing mitral valve surgery. Heart Rhythm. 2023;**20**(1):3-11

[27] Huffman MD, Malaisrie SC, Karmali KN. Concomitant Atrial Fibrillation Surgery for People Undergoing Cardiac Surgery. 2017;**2**(3):334-335

[28] Tjon Joek Tjien A, Akca F, Lam K, Olsthoorn J, Dekker L, Van Der Voort P, et al. Concomitant atrial fibrillation ablation in minimally invasive cardiac surgery. Annals of Cardiothoracic Surgery. 2024;**13**(1):91-98

[29] Bisleri G, Pandey AK, Verma S, Ali Hassan SM, Yanagawa B, Khandaker M, et al. Combined minimally invasive surgical and percutaneous catheter ablation of atrial fibrillation. Journal of the American College of Cardiology. 2023;**81**(6):606-619

[30] The SOLVD Investigators. Effect of enalapril on survival in patients with reduced left ventricular ejection fractions and congestive heart failure. New England Journal of Medicine. 1991;**325**(5):293-302

[31] Pedersen OD, Bagger H, Køber L, Torp-Pedersen C. Trandolapril reduces the incidence of atrial fibrillation after acute myocardial infarction in patients with left ventricular dysfunction. Circulation. 1999;**100**(4):376-380

[32] Cohn JN, Gianni T. A randomized trial of the angiotensin-receptor blocker valsartan in chronic heart failure. New England Journal of Medicine. 2001;**345**(23):1667-1675

[33] Young JB, Dunlap ME, Pfeffer MA, Probstfield JL, Cohen-Solal A, Dietz R, et al. Mortality and morbidity reduction with candesartan in patients with chronic heart failure and left ventricular systolic dysfunction: Results of the CHARM low-left ventricular ejection fraction trials. Circulation. 2004;**110**(17):2618-2626

[34] McMurray JJV, Packer M, Desai AS, Gong J, Lefkowitz MP, Rizkala AR, et al. Angiotensin–neprilysin inhibition versus enalapril in heart failure. The New England Journal of Medicine. 2014;**371**(11):993-1004

[35] Bakris GL, Agarwal R, Anker SD, Pitt B, Ruilope LM, Rossing P, et al. Effect of finerenone on chronic kidney disease outcomes in type 2 diabetes. The New England Journal of Medicine. 2020;**383**(23):2219-2229

[36] Filippatos G, Bakris GL, Pitt B, Agarwal R, Rossing P, Ruilope LM, et al. Finerenone reduces new-onset atrial fibrillation in patients with chronic kidney disease and type 2 diabetes. Journal of the American College of Cardiology. 2021;**78**(2):142-152

[37] Zannad F, McMurray JJV, Krum H, Van Veldhuisen DJ, Swedberg K, Shi H, et al. Eplerenone in patients with systolic heart failure and mild symptoms. The New England Journal of Medicine. 2011;**364**(1):11-21

[38] McMurray JJV, Solomon SD, Inzucchi SE, Køber L, Kosiborod MN, Martinez FA, et al. Dapagliflozin in patients with heart failure and reduced ejection fraction. The New England Journal of Medicine. 2019;**381**(21):1995-2008

[39] Anker SD, Butler J, Filippatos G, Ferreira JP, Bocchi E, Böhm M, et al. Empagliflozin in heart failure with a preserved ejection fraction. The New England Journal of Medicine. 2021;**385**(16):1451-1461

[40] Solomon SD, McMurray JJV, Claggett B, De Boer RA, DeMets D, Hernandez AF, et al. Dapagliflozin in

heart failure with mildly reduced or preserved ejection fraction. The New England Journal of Medicine. 2022;**387**(12):1089-1098

[41] Pandey AK, Okaj I, Kaur H, Belley-Cote EP, Wang J, Oraii A, et al. Sodium-glucose co-transporter inhibitors and atrial fibrillation: A systematic review and meta-analysis of randomized controlled trials. JAHA. 2021;**10**(17):e022222

[42] Kapelios CJ, Lund LH, Benson L, Dahlström U, Rosano GMC, Hauptman PJ, et al. Digoxin use in contemporary heart failure with reduced ejection fraction: An analysis from the Swedish Heart Failure Registry. European Heart Journal—Cardiovascular Pharmacotherapy. 2022;**8**(8):756-767

[43] Kotecha D, Bunting KV, Gill SK, Mehta S, Stanbury M, Jones JC, et al. Effect of digoxin vs bisoprolol for heart rate control in atrial fibrillation on patient-reported quality of life: The RATE-AF randomized clinical trial. Journal of the American Medical Association. 2020;**324**(24):2497

[44] Carlisle MA, Fudim M, DeVore AD, Piccini JP. Heart failure and atrial fibrillation, like fire and fury. JACC: Heart Failure. 2019;7(6):447-456

[45] Huizar JF, Ellenbogen KA, Tan AY, Kaszala K. Arrhythmia-induced cardiomyopathy. Journal of the American College of Cardiology. 2019;**73**(18):2328-2344

[46] Tolu-Akinnawo O, Ogwu OI, Akintunde A, Akata N, Okafor H. Tachycardia-induced cardiomyopathy in a young adult: The significance of early diagnosis and treatment. Cureus. 2023;**15**(2):e35531. Available from: https://www.cureus.com/articles/141501-tachycardia-induced-cardiomyopathy-in-a-young-adult-the-significance-of-early-diagnosis-and-treatment

[47] Kim DY, Kim SH, Ryu KH. Tachycardia induced cardiomyopathy. Korean Circulation Journal. 2019;**49**(9):808

[48] Giugliano RP, Ruff CT, Braunwald E, Murphy SA, Wiviott SD, Halperin JL, et al. Edoxaban versus warfarin in patients with atrial fibrillation. The New England Journal of Medicine. 2013;**369**(22):2093-2104

Chapter 8

# Standardizing Evidence-Based Care for Atrial Fibrillation Using Clinical Pathways – A Practical Approach

*Ashley Diaz, Daniel Bujnowski and Corey E. Tabit*

## Abstract

While atrial fibrillation remains the most common cardiac arrhythmia and cause of stroke, management of atrial fibrillation varies widely from institution to institution and from provider to provider despite the existence of widely-published, multi-society guidelines. Initial diagnostic workup, first-line anticoagulant choice, rate- vs. rhythm-control approaches, and timing of referral for ablation or left atrial appendage closure devices vary. Standardization of these and other care processes leads to more reproducible outcomes and overall improvement in patients' symptoms and quality of life. However, distilling this large volume of available evidence and guidelines into practical care algorithms which providers can use to guide care in the real world can be a daunting task. In this chapter, we will discuss the practical approach to building a clinical pathway for the management of atrial fibrillation in the Inpatient and Emergency Department settings including our approach to weighing available evidence, building provider consensus, designing and refining the pathway, initial pathway launch, sustaining the change, measuring success, and updating the pathway as new evidence emerges. This chapter will draw heavily from our 10 years of experience building clinical pathways at the University of Chicago with special focus on generalizable points that can be applied to readers' home institutions.

**Keywords:** clinical pathways, evidence-based medicine, external reporting, guidelines, process standardization

## 1. Introduction

With over 30 million people affected globally, Atrial Fibrillation (AF) is the most common cardiac arrhythmia and is associated with a higher risk of thrombosis, stroke, heart failure, cardiovascular death, and all-cause mortality [1–3]. AF prevalence increases with age and risk factors including male sex, smoking, diabetes, obesity, hypertension, and prior myocardial infarction, among others [4]. Its increasing prevalence in the United States and worldwide has led not only to an increase in disease-related hospital visits, but a greater cost burden on patients and hospital systems. Due to the prevalence of AF and its high cost, many health systems are developing clinical pathways to standardize the management of AF [5, 6]. In this chapter, we will discuss the history of clinical pathways, summarize available pathways for AF, and discuss our experience building clinical pathways for AF and other cardiovascular conditions at the University of Chicago with special focus on generalizable points that can be applied to readers' home institutions.

## 2. Origins of clinical pathways

### 2.1 Definition

Clinical pathways have been used since the 1980s to operationalize evidence-based guidelines and improve patient care. While authors have proposed slightly varying definitions, most authors agree that clinical pathways include a recommended care plan for a specific clinical problem with task-oriented objectives to reduce variation in care. The European Pathways Association defines clinical/care pathways as a complex intervention for the mutual decision making and organization of care processes for a well-defined group of patients during a well-defined period [7]. Adjoining their definition are five criteria which must be present to constitute their interpretation of a clinical pathway. These include a structured intervention, the implementation of current guidelines, the translation of the intervention into steps/goals for care, the use of a timeline or criteria to progress between the steps of care, and the end goal of standardizing some facet of patient care that is being examined. Other authors have further generalized this definition using less stringent parameters, such as Kinsman et al. who posit a clinical pathway to include the first criterion (a structured intervention) and any three of the remaining four criteria [8]. In brief, clinical pathways are timely guidelines employed by hospitals and patient care facilities aimed at standardizing processes with a goal of improving outcomes and efficiently allocating hospital resources.

### 2.2 Development and implementation

Various methods exist to create and implement clinical pathways into hospital systems, some of which have been reported in the literature. Wendel et al. explained in detail the successful development of a clinical pathway for treating COVID-19 during the recent pandemic throughout a large hospital system in Colorado [9]. The clinical pathway was disseminated through the hospital system through their electronic medical record (EMR) and thus was made rapidly available to healthcare providers. The newly created COVID-19 clinical pathway was used 21,099 times, with 81% of use taking place in the Emergency Department (ED). The pathway was easily found within the EMR under a clearly-marked "Pathways" tab, followed by selecting "COVID-19", which aided in user adoption. The pathway was also searchable within the EMR and the orders that it contained were easily selectable. Providers and nurses were notified of the new development of this clinical pathway via email, and any updates to the pathway were communicated to providers by listing the last date the pathway was updated.

Importantly, Wendel and colleagues leveraged their EMR to drive users to the pathway. In large hospital systems with many providers, effecting meaningful change to longstanding processes can be challenging. By leveraging the EMR and providing a clearly marked, easily identifiable, and simple location to find the pathway, the developers aided user adoption. Similarly, at the University of Chicago, all of our clinical pathways are located within a "Pathways" tab in our EMR which is then organized into sub-folders for Cardiovascular, Oncologic, Obstetric, Surgical, and other pathways. A simple and easily-intelligible organization system improves the user experience and aids in pathway adoption.

In one systematic review, 27 studies that showed positive outcomes from clinical pathways commonly reported implementation strategies such as "use of an implementation team, identification of evidence-practice gaps, audit and feedback, and education sessions" [10]. The implementation of the pathway is just as vital to its success as its development, and the quality of the clinical pathway is irrelevant if providers do not incorporate it in their daily practice. Within the literature, there is broad agreement that maximizing input from clinicians, patients, and managers is necessary to alleviate the inherent resistance a hospital system may experience toward rollout of a new care process in a clinical pathway [10].

#### *2.2.1 Hurdles to development*

The barriers to pathway development and implementation are many, and leaders must plan for these barriers well before launching a new pathway. Just a short list of internal and external barriers include financial costs to patients and hospitals, practice inertia of long engrained habits, inadequate staffing, difficulties with provider and patient adherence, and challenges in communicating and teaching new pathways to a healthcare team composed of different roles and individuals [11]. Jabbour et al. specifically examined roadblocks to development by interviewing healthcare team members in the ED and identified the greatest hurdles to implementing clinical pathways as problems with memory, attention, environmental context, behavior, and reinforcement [12]. Simon et al. cited problems with "clinician perceptions, potential benefits, anticipated barriers/challenges, potential facilitators, and necessary resources" as the greatest hurdles to implementing clinical pathways in community hospitals [13]. In our experience at the University of Chicago, we have found difficulty in implementing a new system when there are many stakeholders involved that might see financial benefit from certain aspects of the clinical pathway, such as increased traffic from the ED on consult services or increased follow up appointment requirements. Leaders would be well advised to identify all stakeholders in the clinical process contained in a proposed pathway and to include those stakeholders early in the planning process.

While clinical benefits from process standardization are well known, data on the financial aspects of clinical pathway implementation are less clear. Some authors have found significantly decreased costs for patients receiving care via a clinical pathway, citing reduced orders of diagnostic studies and reduced length of stay, which contribute to lower patient healthcare costs [14]. However, while any change to an established process can be challenging, there may be an explicit resistance to the implementation of clinical pathways from providers as they may fear the loss of autonomy when following a step-by-step method. Although this method may feel foreign to many physicians, displaying the evidence of its benefit to patients should be built into implementation strategies to reassure physicians and build support. Unsurprisingly, Kinsman et al. demonstrated an increase in provider usage of clinical pathways when providers were directly involved in the creation of the pathway [15]. As such, leaders should be mindful of the psychology of clinicians' approach to a new management strategy and plan accordingly during pathway rollout.

As clinical pathways typically differ operationally between institutions, the lack of interinstitutional uniformity makes it difficult to compare outcomes and effects on patient care. The inability to generalize all outcomes of certain clinical pathways due to institutional differences makes it difficult to know with certainty if implementing such a pathway will be successful. This, coupled with differences in geography, patient population, and socioeconomic backgrounds, makes it difficult to create operationalized multi-center clinical pathways and is the basis for the guidelines which we discuss later in this chapter.

### 2.3 Use in hospital systems

Hospital systems create clinical pathways to standardize care throughout an institution based on clinical practice guidelines and the local standard of care. Clinical pathways are typically institution-specific due to differences in patient populations, hospital resources, medication formularies, local standards, and core competences. Effective clinical pathways should be able to be utilized in 60–80% of applicable cases with the remainder of cases requiring a significant deviation due to each patient's individual medical situation [16]. Thus, the clinical pathways are a guide for the care of most patients with a particular medical condition but not a prescription for all patients. Clinical judgment and experience are most certainly still required to determine when the use of a pathway is appropriate for each patient and when deviation from the typical approach is reasonable and necessary.

While most patients will closely follow the algorithm of the clinical pathway, many will deviate from the pathway depending on the speed at which they meet the desired outcome. If the outcome of the clinical pathway is met faster than expected (positive variance), then patients will progress faster through the clinical pathway or their care will deviate from the standard algorithm. Inversely, if a patient develops a complication or takes longer to meet the expected outcome (negative variance), the plan of care must change accordingly from the standard clinical pathway. Analysis of these variations is essential to improving a clinical pathway and is typically measured with length of stay, complication rates, mortality rates, and cost analyses [17]. Analyzing the success of a clinical pathway in meeting such outcome measures allows for continued improvements to maximize the pathway's efficacy. It is necessary to analyze many different variables when examining the efficacy of a health system's clinical pathways. For example, a shorter length of hospital stay may not correlate with a more cost-effective hospital course if more expensive diagnostic methods or treatments were used. The entire treatment course (including inpatient, outpatient, home, and emergency care) must be examined to effectively analyze the effects of a clinical pathway on the patient and hospital system.

#### *2.3.1 Successes*

Clinical pathways have been shown to improve several metrics of care in medicine. Rotter et al. systematically reviewed 27 clinical trials which compared clinical pathways with typical interventions and found a reduction of in-hospital complications and improved documentation with the use of clinical pathways [10]. Numerous other publications report decreased lengths of hospital stay when clinical pathways are implemented in a healthcare institution [18]. Ban et al. reported decreased length of hospital stay and complication rates when using a clinical pathway for treatment of COPD exacerbations [19]. Other studies have also reported surgical-based clinical pathways to be more cost effective than typical treatments [20]. Our experience at the University of Chicago mirrors that of the published literature. We have seen substantial reductions in length of stay and costs for patients with AF, heart failure, myocardial infarction, pulmonary embolism, valvular heart disease, aortic aneurysm, and other cardiovascular conditions when our clinical pathways are used.

#### *2.3.2 Challenges*

While multiple studies have shown improvements in certain metrics with clinical pathways including decreased length of stay and lower in-hospital complications, the effects of clinical pathways on many outcomes are unclear. Rotter et al. found no difference between clinical pathways and typical interventions on readmission rates and mortality [10]. Another meta-analysis by Trimarchi et al. examined the effects of clinical pathways on quality of life [21]. While they found a reduced length of hospital stay in patients who were treated using clinical pathways, it did not correlate with any significant differences in quality of life and satisfaction. One possible explanation for these findings is that pathways governing inpatient care are unlikely to alter the care of patients at home or in the outpatient setting. Therefore, metrics such as hospital readmission or all-cause mortality may be difficult to affect with a disease-specific inpatient pathway.

Similarly, our experience at the University of Chicago mirrored these findings. Our clinical pathway for acute heart failure, while derived directly from the ACC/AHA guidelines did not reduce readmissions because the common causes for readmissions (medication and lifestyle non-adherence, progression of disease, other illnesses, substance abuse, etc.) occurred in the outpatient setting and therefore were not affected by the pathway [22, 23]. Similarly, while we found increased documentation of thromboembolic risk, increased use of appropriate anticoagulation, and improved heart rate and rhythm targets when providers used our AF pathway, we have not seen changes in outpatient metrics such as readmissions, medication compliance, or home heart rate control.

## 3. Atrial Fibrillation Better Care (ABC) and RACE pathways

### 3.1 Definition

The AF Better Care (ABC) and the Rate control, Anticoagulation, Cardioversion, Electrophysiology/antiarrhythmic medication (RACE) pathways are both published care algorithms for treatment of AF. The ABC pathway consists of three pillars, A for avoidance of stroke with anticoagulants, B for better symptom management, and C for cardiovascular and comorbidity risk management [24]. Use of all three pillars of the ABC pathway is associated with lower rates of all-cause mortality, thromboembolic events, acute coronary syndrome/percutaneous interventions, and advancement of heart failure [25]. Studies have found lower rates of complications as individuals adhere to more pillars of the ABC pathway. The RACE pathway closely follows the same pillars as the ABC pathway but is somewhat less studied in the literature; however, similar results would be expected based on their close similarities [26].

### 3.2 Adherence

Multiple clinical trials have compared adherence to the pillars of the ABC pathway with non-adherence in treating AF. Individuals who adhere to the tenants of the ABC pathway have significantly lower rates of all-cause mortality, thromboembolism, and major cardiovascular events [27, 28]. Adherence to increasing amounts of the three ABC pillars is also associated with lower rates of complications. Patel et al. analyzed a sample of 20,926 patients included in the ENGAGE AF-TIMI 48 trial and reported that 38% of patients were adherent to all three criteria of ABC [29]. Adherent individuals had significantly lower rates of stroke/systemic embolic events, major bleeding, major cardiac adverse events, CV hospitalization, CV death, and all-cause mortality [29].

### 3.3 Non-adherence

Most occurrences of non-adherence to the ABC and RACE pathways occur with the cardiovascular and comorbidity risk management pillar. In one clinical trial, 87% were adherent to the A pillar, 94% were adherent to B, and 47% to C [25]. In a 4013 patient prospective trial by Bucci et al., where 39% of participants were adherent to all three pillars of ABC, ABC non-adherent individuals tended to be older and had higher $CHA_2DS_2$-VASc scores [25].

Other studies have further examined non-adherence in patients with AF, specifically focusing on medication non-adherence. A large observational study consisting of over 12,000 patients reported that 6.3% of patients did not adhere to their medication regimens, meaning that they missed doses one or more times per week or were taking medications differently than prescribed ≥75% of the time. The study also found lower rates of adherence in racial and ethnic minorities, unmarried individuals, and having low health literacy among other socio-economic and demographic factors [30]. Conversely, patients with hypertension as well as those with an older age (65–84 years old) compared with those less than 65 years were less likely to be non-adherent to ABC [30].

### 3.4 Repercussions

Individuals who do not adhere to the principals of the ABC or RACE pathways are at a greater risk of major complications. AF is correlated with a three to fivefold increase in stroke risk after adjusting for other risk factors [31]. Furthermore, studies have reported a two to fivefold increased risk of systemic embolization, ischemic stroke, and TIA in patients with valvular AF compared with non-valvular AF (NVAF) [2, 32]. Valvular AF is often caused by mitral stenosis which is correlated with a 25% chance of mortality from systemic embolism [33]. AF can lead to stroke via thrombus formation through the stasis of blood due to uncoordinated myocyte activation, most commonly found in the left atrial appendage. Thrombus formation then can lead to embolism and consequently stroke. AF can also cause atrial remodeling, typically in the form of atrial hypertrophy which functions as a positive feedback loop and further increases the risk of future AF and thrombus formation [34]. We believe that adherence to the pillars of the ABC and RACE pathways is imperative and these pathways were considered heavily in the development of our own AF clinical pathway at the University of Chicago.

## 4. Standardized steps to build clinical pathways

### 4.1 Identifying scope and building multidisciplinary teams

A first step in creating a clinical pathway is to identify potential areas of improvement in the treatment, management, and overall workflow of a particular condition such as AF. Goals should be clearly demarcated and may include improving specific outcomes such as stroke reduction or readmissions, standardizing care such as documentation of risk scores, reducing variability of treatment such as guiding appropriate use of anticoagulants, or enhancing efficiency within the hospital system such as aiding providers in deciding between rate-control vs. rhythm-control strategies. We recommend ensuring that the chosen goals are consistent with established institutional goals and are reasonably feasible and sustainable with available resources. Close coordination with health system leadership is imperative to ensure that the chosen goals align with institutional priorities.

Once the goals have been outlined, areas of improvement can be workshopped. To do this, pathway creators must closely understand the mechanics of care processes in their current state. For example, if one goal is to increase the appropriate use of anticoagulation in patients with AF, pathway authors must understand which provider typically chooses the first-line anticoagulant (intern, resident, midlevel provider, attending physician, pharmacist, etc.) and which options are available at a particular institution. To improve usability, we recommend choosing targeted areas for improvement that are applicable to the majority of patients who present with the particular condition of interest, such as AF. Minimizing the need to deviate from the preset clinical pathway improves efficiency, timeliness of care received, and the delegation of hospital resources.

After identifying areas for improvement, we recommend assembling a multidisciplinary team of stakeholders who may be affected by the clinical pathway. Involve the individuals who directly carry out any of the planned changes in the clinical pathway, such as lab workers, patient transport, IT staff, physicians from multiple specialties, nurses, patients and their representatives, pharmacists, therapists, and procedural teams. Administrative staff can also be valuable contributors to the clinical pathway by supplying data collection, implementation support, and further monitoring. By involving everyone affected by the proposed clinical pathway, the multidisciplinary team can incorporate their diverse perspectives and, ultimately, foster a sense of inclusion that lessens resistance on different fronts. Excluding individuals affected by the new clinical pathway from the creation process breeds divisiveness, restricts valuable input, and decreases adherence to the pathway in the long term. This aspect of clinical pathway development and implementation is perhaps the most vital for lasting success and adherence and should not be overlooked. From our experience at the University of Chicago, we recommend including all stakeholders at an initial kick-off meeting, rather than adding stakeholders as the pathway development process progresses. Thus, stakeholders feel included in the process from the beginning rather than being surprised later that they were not approached beforehand.

### 4.2 Evidence review and mapping the care pathway

Once the stakeholders are engaged, a thorough review of current evidence-based guidelines, best practices, and relevant literature must be conducted. This step is crucial as it forms the foundation of the pathway by ensuring that it is based on current best practices. Critical appraisal, which involves evaluating the quality of evidence presented by using GRADE (Grading of Recommendations Assessment, Development and Evaluation) recommendations, is the first step in evidence review [35]. At the University of Chicago, we closely follow published multi-society guidelines in the development of our clinical pathways. For AF, we recommend close adherence to published guidelines from the American Heart Association, American College of Cardiology, Heart Rhythm Society, European Society of Cardiology, and others [36].

Once evidence has been properly assessed, step-by-step protocols can begin to take form at each stage of the management pathway. We recommend starting with broad themes and then filling in details in subsequent revisions. For example, a typical AF pathway would contain sections for initial stabilization, diagnostic testing, rate/rhythm control, anticoagulation management, screening for specific risk factors such as obstructive sleep apnea, discharge planning and post-acute care. In this stage, decision points where clinical judgment may influence the pathway should be identified and expanded upon to ensure flexibility while maintaining adherence to best practices.

### 4.3 Key performance indicators

At this stage, the logistics of implementing the proposed clinical pathway must be discussed and measurable outcomes that indicate the success of a pathway must be identified. Outcomes such as length of stay, complication rates, readmission rates, patient satisfaction, and adherence to protocols are all examples of possible measures. It is important to ensure that any chosen outcome metrics align with institutional priorities. We strongly advise discussing these metrics with institutional leadership early in the development process.

Moreover, important questions such as the expected volume of patients to be affected by a pathway and whether providers and facilities can reasonably perform the expected tasks in the new process are often-overlooked aspects to clinical pathway development. These types of logistics will need to be revisited throughout the entire pathway creation process; earlier consideration of these topics will save valuable time from meetings and revisions.

A successful clinical pathway will be evidence-based and incorporate updated guidelines. It will integrate the expert opinions of not only the institution's employees, but of those in other hospital systems [7]. Different expert perspectives on healthcare delivery will help root out institution-specific inefficiencies. Establishing key performance indicators to monitor pathway implementation and success will help institutional leaders judge the pathway's effectiveness over time.

### 4.4 Implementation strategy and evaluation

Timeline establishment and resource identification are essential pieces of implementation strategy. The importance of understanding available resources (and their limits) including personnel, funding, technology, and necessary infrastructure changes cannot be overstated. In addition, stakeholder recruitment and engagement as mentioned earlier continues to be essential during implementation of a clinical pathway. Clear and open communication channels are required to keep these vital stakeholders informed about the implementation plan, progress updates, and unforeseen challenges. This channel also allows for feedback solicitation, debate, and compromise, and improves buy-in and ownership from all involved parties. In addition, it is recommended to conduct an assessment of educational needs to determine training requirements of staff and provide training as needed in the forms of refresher courses, peer mentoring, and access to clinical pathway champions.

Next, working with IT staff to incorporate EMR integration (when available) makes the pathway more accessible by using alerts, reminders, or other forms of clinical decision support. Moreover, pilot testing of the pathway in select clinical areas or departments to identify workflow issues and gather frontline feedback is also recommended. Launching the pathway initially to a limited number of highly-engaged users allows leaders to respond to user feedback and provide useful updates before launching to an entire health system.

Setting and adhering to an official institution-wide launch date is a key aspect that should not be delayed. Although no clinical pathway will ever be perfect (especially at the time of initial launch), it is important to release the pathway at the pre-specified time, to take stock of what can be improved and workshopped for further iterations, and then release rapid updates when needed. By developing a comprehensive implementation strategy that addresses these elements, healthcare organizations can enhance the successful adoption and integration of clinical pathways into routine clinical practice. This approach not only improves consistency and quality of care but also supports the achievement of organizational goals related to patient outcomes and healthcare efficiency.

### 4.5 Monitoring/evaluating and updating clinical pathways

Defining key performance indicators as mentioned above aids in data collection and quality improvement. Soliciting feedback from stakeholders, including patients, is an essential part of the implementation strategy of a clinical pathway. This, along with a commitment from leadership to sustain necessary resources over time, is important to ensure survival of the clinical pathway. Sharing the success and lessons learned from each step across the organization is an adaptable part of the evaluation process not to be understated.

Updating clinical pathways involves the same series of steps discussed above such as identifying the scope of the intended improvement, building a multidisciplinary team, using evidence-based best practices and current literature to guide the change, identifying key performance indicators to measure success, solidifying an implementation strategy, effectively monitoring and evaluating the change, and documenting the finalized pathway. Frequent updates to existing pathways are necessary in order to incorporate new evidence, technologies, and guidelines, and to maintain pathway relevance. At the University of Chicago, we review and update all of our cardiovascular pathways every 6 months and will often release off-cycle updates if new evidence, guidelines, or technologies become available. As such, we intend for our clinical pathways to represent the current state-of-the-art in cardiovascular care, operationalized for our institution.

## 5. The atrial fibrillation clinical pathways at the University of Chicago

At our center, we have two complimentary AF clinical pathways in current use. The pathway used by the Emergency Department focuses on initial stabilization and triaging, while the pathway used by our Inpatient teams focuses on diagnostics and therapeutics specific to AF. Both were designed with input from members of the patient care team including cardiologists, primary care physicians, anesthesiologists, emergency medicine physicians, pharmacists, multidisciplinary nurses, social workers, physical therapists, IT staff, and hospital administrators. Including a variety of unique perspectives is essential to operationalize pathways to individual centers. While our methodology includes the same core tenants of the ABC and RACE pathways discussed above, it also addresses social and environmental risk factors, screening for obstructive sleep apnea, and several "cannot miss" items. We also include resources and pharmaceutical options to assist with smoking cessation which may help alleviate the increased risk of atrial fibrillation and thrombus formation seen in smokers [37].

### 5.1 The emergency department AF pathway

An example ED AF pathway is shown in **Figure 1**. This pathway is initiated when a patient enters our ED and their 12-lead EKG shows AF. Providers are immediately reminded to perform direct current cardioversion if the patient is hemodynamically

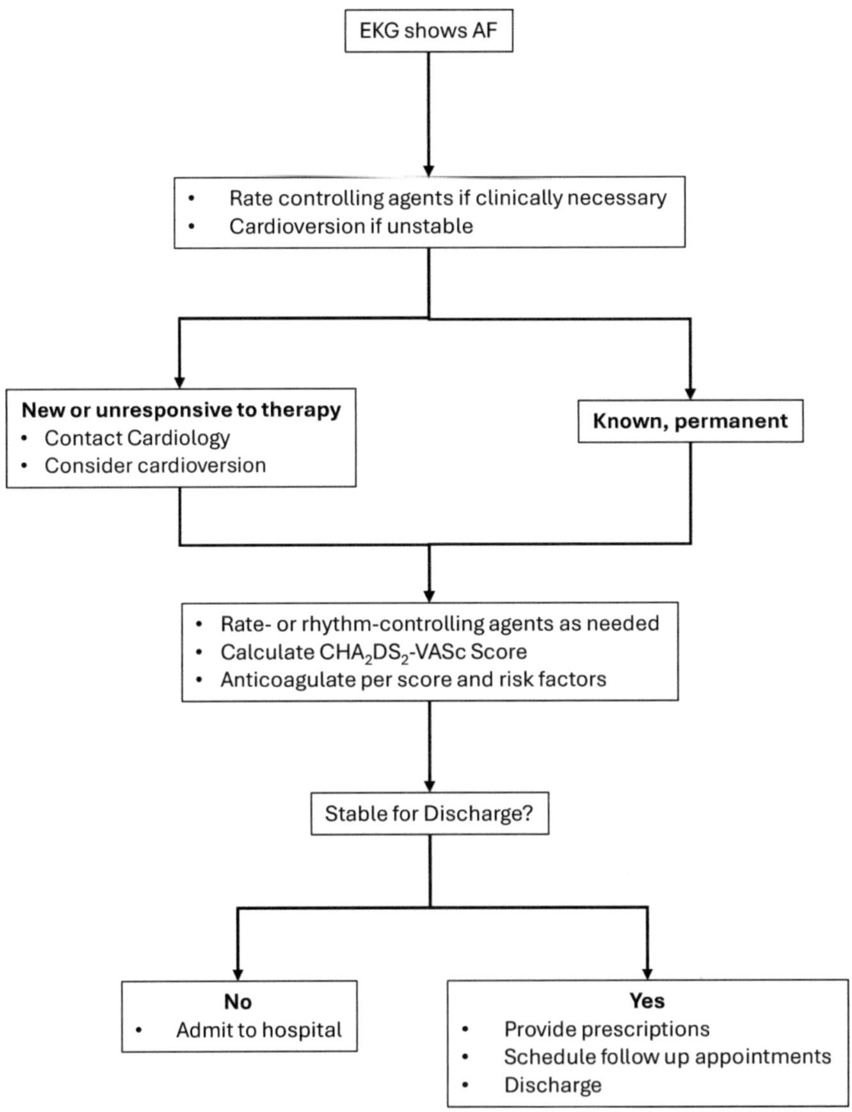


**Figure 1.**
*Emergency Department Atrial Fibrillation Pathway.*

unstable. Beta blockers, calcium channel blockers, and digitalis can be used for rate control and the providers are reminded to avoid the use of intravenous calcium channel blockers in patients with left ventricular systolic dysfunction as this can precipitate cardiogenic shock. Similarly, rapid administration of intravenous beta blockers can also precipitate shock. Our providers are warned of both of these items in the pathway and through frequent educational sessions.

For patients where AF is either newly diagnosed or unresponsive to initial therapies, our pathway recommends involvement of a cardiologist. At our center, we have a dedicated consult pager for this purpose in order to streamline communication between ED providers and the consulting cardiologists. The pathway outlines the process for obtaining one of these rapid consults in our center. It then lists criteria for direct current cardioversion (DCCV) in the ED including AF <48 hours, no history of mitral stenosis or prosthetic valves, and no history of stroke, TIA, or thromboembolism. If all criteria are met, DCCV is attempted in the ED and, if successful, the patient is typically discharged to follow up in the Cardiology clinic. For patients who do not meet criteria for DCCV in the ED, our pathway lists several options for rate control and initial anticoagulation based on the $CHA_2DS_2$-VASc score [36]. In our center, direct oral anticoagulants are used as first line therapy in the ED.

If the patient has been converted to sinus rhythm or has been adequately rate controlled, our ED AF pathway recommends discharge with close follow up in the Cardiology clinic. Providers are reminded to document the $CHA_2DS_2$-VASc score, prescribe anticoagulation, and ensure the patient is scheduled for a follow-up appointment before discharge from the ED. However, for patients who do not achieve adequate rate/rhythm-control in the ED, remain symptomatic from their AF, or who require hospitalization for another reason, our pathway recommends hospital admission and leads into our Inpatient AF Pathway discussed below.

### 5.2 The inpatient AF pathway

An example inpatient AF pathway is shown in **Figure 2**. Our inpatient AF clinical pathway begins with admission of the patient from the ED. It contains an admission order set which includes standard orders for telemetry monitoring, diet, and patient education. There is a separate option for entrance into the pathway for patients who are already admitted and are subsequently discovered to have AF, such as post-operative patients or those admitted for another reason. Upon pathway enrollment, we first perform diagnostic testing such as measuring serum thyrotropin and a digitalis assay (if the patient is taking digitalis), as well as various imaging procedures including echocardiography and chest radiography.

Next, the pathway advises the user to decide between a rate-control vs. rhythm-control strategy. Our pathway advises doing this within 12 hours of admission in order to facilitate timely cardioversion, when indicated, but this timeline may differ from institution to institution. To this end, we do advise stating clearly in the pathway when the provider should decide on a rate-control vs. rhythm-control approach as providers often delay this decision otherwise, in our experience. Our pathway then lists several options for rate controlling agents including beta blockers, calcium channel blockers, and digitalis, along with warnings to providers to avoid the use of intravenous calcium channel blockers in patients with left ventricular systolic dysfunction which can precipitate cardiogenic shock. We then list several options for cardioversion including electrical cardioversion and rhythm-controlling agents such

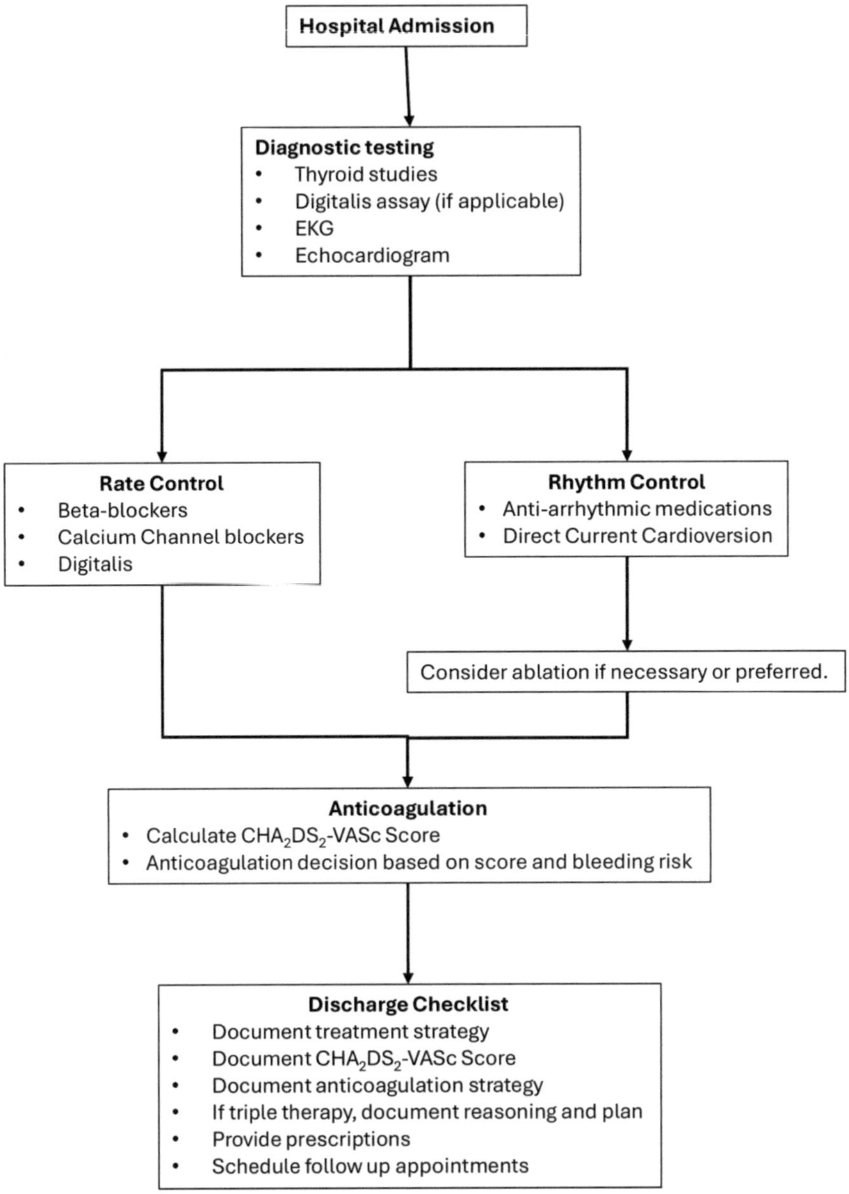


**Figure 2.**
*Inpatient Atrial Fibrillation Pathway.*

as amiodarone and others as well as imaging options for exclusion of atrial appendage thrombosis prior to cardioversion.

When a rhythm-control approach is preferred but unable to be achieved despite cardioversion and/or antiarrhythmic agents, our pathway recommends consultation with an electrophysiologist to consider catheter ablation. In general, this consultation is performed as an outpatient at our center if the patient is hemodynamically stable and is minimally symptomatic from the AF. However, for patients where more immediate rhythm-control is preferred (such as patients with low left ventricular ejection fractions, those with heart rates that are difficult to control, or those intolerant of rate-controlling or rhythm-controlling medications), ablation may be performed while the patient is admitted. Similarly, surgical MAZE procedure may be performed if the patient is undergoing cardiac surgery for another reason, such as significant valvular disease. Consideration of these therapies should always be individualized to each unique patient, placing emphasis on each patient's symptoms, goals, and life-expectancy. Such shared decision-making leads to patient-centered outcomes and minimization of unnecessary testing and procedures.

After the diagnostics and medical therapies above, our pathway moves to the differentiation of anticoagulants based on thromboembolic risk using the $CHA_2DS_2$-VASc score, after excluding rheumatic mitral stenosis or other severe valve disease as the cause of AF [38]. In patients with nonvalvular atrial fibrillation (NVAF) with a $CHA_2DS_2$-VASc score of 2 or higher, direct oral anticoagulants (DOAC) are the preferred method of anticoagulation at our center and our pathway lists several options which are approved for use in the United States and on formulary at our center. Available options of course will vary by locality. In some centers, warfarin may still be the most available option. In patients with $CHA_2DS_2$-VASc scores of 0 or 1, we recommend either no anticoagulation or aspirin depending on the patient's comorbidities, consistent with ACC/AHA guidelines [36]. For atrial fibrillation caused by mitral stenosis and other severe valvular diseases, termed valvular atrial fibrillation, warfarin is recommended as the standard of care.

Our pathway further provides guidance to providers to assess each patient's risk for bleeding before deciding on an anticoagulation strategy. If warfarin is used, measurement of the International Normalized Ratio (INR) within 1 week is recommended at our center but may vary with local standards. Typically, an INR goal of 2–3 is targeted in the absence of other factors that affect bleeding or thrombotic risk. For patients intolerant of anticoagulation, our pathway recommends evaluation for a left atrial appendage occlusion device which is typically done as an outpatient at our center but may vary based on local practice.

One important feature of our inpatient AF pathway is a Discharge Checklist, a list of items that must be completed by the provider before discharge. All of our cardiovascular pathways at the University of Chicago have this feature and items are customized to each disease. For AF, the provider must document the intended strategy of rate control or rhythm control and must similarly document the $CHA_2DS_2$-VASc score. Then, the provider must document the intended anticoagulation strategy (if any) and must document their reasoning when the prescribed anticoagulation strategy does not match the $CHA_2DS_2$-VASc score – for example, a patient with a $CHA_2DS_2$-VASc score of 5 where no anticoagulation is prescribed due to a recent history of life-threatening bleeding. In our center, we also include an item in the discharge checklist to ensure that all medications have been delivered to the patient by a clinical pharmacist and that all medication-related questions have been answered prior to discharge – this practice will vary in different localities. We specifically ask providers to justify instances where patients are discharged with "Triple Therapy" – aspirin, a P2Y12 inhibitor, and an anticoagulant – due to substantially elevated bleeding risk and limited additional clinical benefit [39].

Finally, at the time of discharge, our AF pathway includes a reminder to refer the patient for a sleep study if the patient has risk factors for obstructive sleep apnea. Patients are then scheduled for a follow up visit in the Cardiology clinic within 14 days and with their primary care provider within 30 days.

### 5.3 Sustaining the change

Soliciting feedback from all levels at our institution was an essential part of sustaining the change to pathway-directed AF care at the University of Chicago. Feedback mostly centered around the streamlined workflow and ensuring that all steps in the management of a patient with AF were included in the pathway. Many providers praised the pathway and felt it helped them remember when to perform critical tasks and how best to avoid pitfalls. This feedback was shared in presentations when describing the need and nuances of the clinical pathway to more providers throughout the hospital to encourage more adoption institution-wide.

## 6. Conclusion

Clinical pathways, although not novel and certainly not a perfect prescription for every single patient, complement clinical practice guidelines, disease-management programs, and clinical checklists or protocols. They operationalize clinical guidelines and current evidence for an individual center and help reduce variation in care. Frequent updates to incorporate new evidence and customization to meet specific institutional needs are critical to maintain pathway relevance. For local healthcare providers and policymakers, the decision to adopt clinical pathway strategies should also consider the anticipated costs and benefits of these interventions. It is important to recognize that developing and implementing clinical pathways requires significant resources. Ultimately, the potential cost savings achievable depend on the volume of cases addressed by the pathway. For patients with AF, we have had great success using clinical pathways at the University of Chicago. Our providers appreciate the clinical decision support, treatment options, critical warnings, and logistical help listed in our pathways. We hope this chapter serves as a guide for other healthcare leaders developing cardiovascular pathways at their own institutions.

## Acknowledgements

We would like to acknowledge the healthcare providers at the University of Chicago Medical Center for their support, feedback, and use of the clinical pathways discussed in this chapter. All authors have met the criteria for authorship on this chapter. There is no funding source to acknowledge.

## Conflict of interest

No conflicts of interest to disclose.

## Author details

Ashley Diaz[1], Daniel Bujnowski[1] and Corey E. Tabit[2*]

1 Duke University Hospital, Durham, NC, USA

2 University of Chicago Medicine, Chicago, IL, USA

*Address all correspondence to: ctabit@uchicagomedicine.org

## References

[1] Weng LC, Preis SR, Hulme OL, Larson MG, Choi SH, Wang B, et al. Genetic predisposition, clinical risk factor burden, and lifetime risk of atrial fibrillation. Circulation. 2018;**137**(10):1027-1038

[2] Wolf PA, Abbott RD, Kannel WB. Atrial fibrillation as an independent risk factor for stroke: The Framingham study. Stroke. 1991;**22**(8):983-988

[3] Fauchier L, Villejoubert O, Clementy N, Bernard A, Pierre B, Angoulvant D, et al. Causes of death and influencing factors in patients with atrial fibrillation. The American Journal of Medicine. 2016;**129**(12):1278-1287

[4] Amponsah MKD, Benjamin EJ, Magnani JW. Atrial fibrillation and Race – A contemporary review. Current Cardiovascular Risk Reports. 2013;**7**(5):336-345

[5] Kirchhof P. The future of atrial fibrillation management: Integrated care and stratified therapy. Lancet. 2017;**390**(10105):1873-1887

[6] Hindricks G, Potpara T, Dagres N, Arbelo E, Bax JJ, Blomström-Lundqvist C, et al. 2020 ESC guidelines for the diagnosis and management of atrial fibrillation developed in collaboration with the European Association for Cardio-Thoracic Surgery (EACTS): The task force for the diagnosis and management of atrial fibrillation of the European Society of Cardiology (ESC) developed with the special contribution of the European heart rhythm association (EHRA) of the ESC. European Heart Journal. 2021;**42**(5):373-498

[7] Latina R, Salomone K, D'Angelo D, Coclite D, Castellini G, Gianola S, et al. Towards a new system for the assessment of the quality in care pathways: An overview of systematic reviews. International Journal of Environmental Research and Public Health. 2020;**17**(22):8634

[8] Kinsman L, Rotter T, James E, Snow P, Willis J. What is a clinical pathway? Development of a definition to inform the debate. BMC Medicine. 2010;**8**:31

[9] Wendel SK, Bookman K, Holmes M, Wiler JL. Successful implementation of workflow-embedded clinical pathways during the COVID 19 pandemic. Quality Management in Healthcare. 2023;**32**(3):205

[10] Rotter T, Kinsman L, James E, Machotta A, Gothe H, Willis J, et al. Clinical pathways: Effects on professional practice, patient outcomes, length of stay and hospital costs. Cochrane Database of Systematic Reviews. 2010;**3**:CD006632

[11] Seckler E, Regauer V, Rotter T, Bauer P, Müller M. Barriers to and facilitators of the implementation of multi-disciplinary care pathways in primary care: A systematic review. BMC Family Practice. 2020;**21**:113

[12] Jabbour M, Newton AS, Johnson D, Curran JA. Defining barriers and enablers for clinical pathway implementation in complex clinical settings. Implementation Science. 2018;**13**(1):139

[13] Outram SM, Rooholamini SN, Desai M, Edwards Y, Ja C, Morton K, et al. Barriers and facilitators of high-efficiency clinical pathway implementation in community hospitals. Hospital Pediatrics. 2023;**13**(10):931-939

[14] Lanska DJ. The role of clinical pathways in reducing the economic burden of stroke. PharmacoEconomics. 1998;**14**(2):151-158

[15] Kinsman L, James E, Ham J. An interdisciplinary, evidence-based process of clinical pathway implementation increases pathway usage. Lippincott's Case Management. 2004;**9**(4):184-196

[16] Cheah J. Development and implementation of a clinical pathway programme in an acute care general hospital in Singapore. International Journal for Quality in Health Care. 2000;**12**(5):403-412

[17] Hipp R, Abel E, Weber RJ. A primer on clinical pathways. Hospital Pharmacy. 2016;**51**(5):416-421

[18] Hanna E, Schultz S, Doctor D, Vural E, Stern S, Suen J. Development and implementation of a clinical pathway for patients undergoing total laryngectomy: Impact on cost and quality of care. Archives of Otolaryngology – Head & Neck Surgery. 1999;**125**(11):1247-1251

[19] Ban A, Ismail A, Harun R, Abdul Rahman A, Sulung S, Syed MA. Impact of clinical pathway on clinical outcomes in the management of COPD exacerbation. BMC Pulmonary Medicine. 2012;**12**:27

[20] Pritts TA, Nussbaum MS, Flesch LV, Fegelman EJ, Parikh AA, Fischer JE. Implementation of a clinical pathway decreases length of stay and cost for bowel resection. Annals of Surgery. 1999;**230**(5):728-733

[21] Trimarchi L, Caruso R, Magon G, Odone A, Arrigoni C. Clinical pathways and patient-related outcomes in hospital-based settings: A systematic review and meta-analysis of randomized controlled trials. Acta Bio-Medica. 2021;**92**(1):e2021093

[22] Tabit CE, Coplan MJ, Spencer KT, Alcain CF, Spiegel T, Vohra AS, et al. Cardiology consultation in the emergency department reduces re-hospitalizations for low-socioeconomic patients with acute decompensated heart failure. The American Journal of Medicine. 2017;**130**(9):1112.e17-1112.e31

[23] Heidenreich PA, Bozkurt B, Aguilar D, Allen LA, Byun JJ, Colvin MM, et al. 2022 AHA/ACC/HFSA guideline for the Management of Heart Failure: A report of the American College of Cardiology/American Heart Association joint committee on clinical practice guidelines. Circulation. 2022;**145**(18):e895-e1032

[24] Proietti M, Romiti GF, Olshansky B, Lane DA, Lip GYH. Comprehensive management with the ABC (atrial fibrillation better care) pathway in clinically complex patients with atrial fibrillation: A *post hoc* ancillary analysis from the AFFIRM trial. Journal of the American Heart Association. 2020;**9**(10):e014932

[25] Bucci T, Proietti M, Shantsila A, Romiti GF, Teo WS, Park HW, et al. Integrated care for atrial fibrillation using the ABC pathway in the prospective APHRS-AF registry. JACC Asia. 2023;**3**(4):580-591

[26] Herzog E, Argulian E, Levy SB, Aziz EF. Pathway for the management of atrial fibrillation and atrial flutter. Critical Pathways in Cardiology. 2017;**16**(2):47-52

[27] Romiti GF, Proietti M, Bonini N, Ding WY, Boriani G, Huisman MV, et al. Adherence to the atrial fibrillation better care (ABC) pathway and the

risk of major outcomes in patients with atrial fibrillation: A *post-hoc* analysis from the prospective GLORIA-AF registry. eClinicalMedicine [Internet]. 2023;**55**:101757. Available from: https://www.thelancet.com/journals/eclinm/article/PIIS2589-5370(22)00486-2/fulltext [Accessed: June 15, 2024]

[28] Rivera-Caravaca JM, Roldán V, Martínez-Montesinos L, Vicente V, Lip GYH, Marín F. The atrial fibrillation better care (ABC) pathway and clinical outcomes in patients with atrial fibrillation: The prospective Murcia AF project phase II cohort. Journal of General Internal Medicine. 2023;**38**(2):315-323

[29] Patel SM, Palazzolo MG, Murphy SA, Antman EM, Braunwald E, Lanz HJ, et al. Evaluation of the atrial fibrillation better care pathway in the ENGAGE AF-TIMI 48 trial. Europace. 2022;**24**(11):1730-1738

[30] Reading SR, Black MH, Singer DE, Go AS, Fang MC, Udaltsova N, et al. Risk factors for medication non-adherence among atrial fibrillation patients. BMC Cardiovascular Disorders. 2019;**19**:38

[31] Kamel H, Okin PM, Elkind MSV, Iadecola C. Atrial fibrillation and mechanisms of stroke: Time for a new model. Stroke. 2016;**47**(3):895-900

[32] Benjamin EJ, Wolf PA, D'Agostino RB, Silbershatz H, Kannel WB, Levy D. Impact of atrial fibrillation on the risk of death: The Framingham heart study. Circulation. 1998;**98**(10):946-952

[33] Al Rawahi MN, Al-Maqbali JS, Al Noumani J, Al Alawi AM, Essebag V. Novel oral anticoagulants in patients with atrial fibrillation and moderate to severe mitral stenosis: A systematic review. Cureus. 2023;**15**(1):e33222

[34] De Jong AM, Maass AH, Oberdorf-Maass SU, Van Veldhuisen DJ, Van Gilst WH, Van Gelder IC. Mechanisms of atrial structural changes caused by stretch occurring before and during early atrial fibrillation. Cardiovascular Research. 2011;**89**(4):754-765

[35] What is GRADE? BMJ Best Practice [Internet]. Available from: https://bestpractice.bmj.com/info/toolkit/learn-ebm/what-is-grade/ [Accessed: June 28, 2024]

[36] Joglar JA, Chung MK, Armbruster AL, Benjamin EJ, Chyou JY, et al. 2023 ACC/AHA/ACCP/HRS guideline for the diagnosis and management of atrial fibrillation. Journal of the American College of Cardiology. 2024;**83**(1):109-279

[37] Arai H, Ueda S, Uchida K, Sakakibara F, Kinjo N, Nezu M, et al. Effect of current smoking on ischemic events in patients with atrial fibrillation taking vitamin K antagonist. International Journal of Cardiology Cardiovascular Risk and Prevention. 2022;**14**:200135

[38] Østergaard L, Olesen JB, Petersen JK, Nielsen LS, Kristensen SL, Schou M, et al. Arterial thromboembolism in patients with atrial fibrillation and CHA2DS2-VASc score 1: A nationwide study. Circulation. 2024;**149**(10):764-773

[39] Kumbhani DJ, Cannon CP, Beavers CJ, Bhatt DL, Cuker A, Gluckman TJ, et al. 2020 ACC expert consensus decision pathway for anticoagulant and antiplatelet therapy in patients with atrial fibrillation or venous thromboembolism undergoing percutaneous coronary intervention or with atherosclerotic cardiovascular disease. Journal of the American College of Cardiology. 2021;**77**(5):629-658

Chapter 9

# Anesthetic Considerations for Atrial Fibrillation Interventions: Surgical and Endovascular Approaches

*Larissa Kiwakyou, Anna Reichardt, Allen Ninh and Louise Sun*

## Abstract

Atrial fibrillation (AF) is the most common cardiac arrhythmia, impacting millions of people worldwide and leading to a significant increase in morbidity and mortality. In recent decades, there has been an exponential increase in both surgical and endovascular interventions to eliminate AF or reduce the risk of stroke through left atrial appendage occlusion. This chapter provides an overview of anesthetic considerations for atrial fibrillation interventions, intended for both anesthesiologists and the multidisciplinary teams involved in these procedures.

**Keywords:** atrial fibrillation, radiofrequency ablation, cryoablation, Cox-maze, pulmonary vein isolation, left atrial appendage occlusion, anesthesia

## 1. Introduction

### 1.1 Pathophysiology and classification of atrial fibrillation

Atrial fibrillation (AF) is the most common arrhythmia worldwide, affecting approximately 50 million people globally. It is associated with a 1.5- to 2-fold higher risk of death, a 2.4-fold higher risk of stroke, as well as cognitive impairment, myocardial infarction, heart failure, chronic kidney disease, and increased health care utilization costs [1]. The incidence of AF increases with age, affecting approximately one in four individuals over age 40 and one in three over age 55, and its prevalence continues to increase worldwide [1–3].

Atrial fibrillation (AF) occurs when atrial electrical impulses no longer originate from the sinoatrial note but instead arise from ectopic foci, most commonly the pulmonary veins, creating reentrant circuits with chaotic, uncoordinated atrial contraction and leading to atrial remodeling [1]. Structural remodeling in the form of atrial dilation and fibrosis promotes persistent arrhythmias, as an enlarged atrium increases the physical area that can sustain abnormal circuits and myocyte fibrosis alters electrical conduction patterns. Electrical remodeling in the form of shortened atrial refractory periods further reinforces the arrhythmia [4].

Atrial fibrillation has been categorized by duration into paroxysmal, persistent, long-standing persistent, and permanent AF. Paroxysmal AF is a continuous episode lasting between 30 seconds and 7 days, while persistent AF is an episode between 7 days and 12 months in duration. Long-standing persistent AF is an episode lasting longer than 12 months where rhythm control continues to be pursued by the patient and clinician. If a decision is made to no longer pursue rhythm control, it is termed permanent AF [4].

Atrial fibrillation has also historically been categorized as valvular or non-valvular based on the presence or absence of mitral stenosis, however such terminology is now considered obsolete [1]. Post-operative atrial fibrillation is another common distinction, referring to new-onset atrial fibrillation following surgery, with cardiac surgery being the most common [5].

Recently, the 2023 ACC/AHA/ACCP/HRS Guideline for the Diagnosis and Management of Atrial Fibrillation proposed a new classification system using stages that recognize AF as a progressive continuum of disease (**Table 1**). The purpose of this new system is to promote greater focus on prevention, risk factor modification, screening and therapy.

## 1.2 Management strategies

In AF, both rate- and rhythm-control strategies can be effective; the choice to pursue one or the other should be made using shared decision-making process that considers the patient's specific comorbidities and preferences. Rate control is typically achieved through pharmacologic therapy using beta blockers, nondihydropyridine calcium channel blockers, or digoxin. However, in cases refractory to medication,

| **Duration-based classification** [4] | |
|---|---|
| Paroxysmal | Continuous AF lasting 30 seconds to 7 days |
| Persistent | Continuous AF lasting >7 days to <12 months |
| Long-standing persistent | Continuous AF lasting >12 months in which rhythm control is being pursued |
| Permanent | AF in which no further attempts at rhythm control are being pursued |
| **Stage-based classification (2023 guidelines)** [1] | |
| Stage 1: At risk for AF | Presence of modifiable and non-modifiable risk factors associated with AF (e.g. obesity, HTN, OSA) |
| Stage 2: Pre-AF | Presence of structural or electrical findings that further predispose to AF (e.g. atrial enlargement, frequent atrial ectopy) |
| Stage 3: AF | Four substages described:<br>• Paroxysmal AF (3A): Intermittent, terminates <7 days after onset<br>• Persistent AF (3B): Continuous AF >7 days requiring intervention<br>• Long-standing persistent AF (3C): Continuous AF >1 year<br>• Successful AF ablation (3D): freedom from AF after ablation |
| Stage 4: Permanent AF | AF in which no further attempts at rhythm control are being pursued |

**Table 1.**
*Atrial fibrillation classifications. AF, atrial fibrillation; HTN, hypertension; OSA, obstructive sleep apnea.*

atrioventricular (AV) nodal ablation may be pursued where complete heart block is intentionally created, and a permanent pacemaker is then used to control the ventricular rate [1].

Restoration of sinus rhythm may be more beneficial than rate control in patients with reduced left ventricular function. Additionally, patients with structural heart disease such as mitral stenosis and hypertrophic cardiomyopathy may unable to tolerate the loss of sinus rhythm [6]. Antiarrhythmic drugs (AADs) commonly used to achieve sinus rhythm include Class III antiarrhythmics (amiodarone, sotalol, dofetilide, and ibutilide) and Class I antiarrhythmics (flecainide and propafenone). Patients requiring acute rhythm control may undergo electrical or chemical cardioversion; in those with hemodynamically unstable AF, synchronized direct current cardioversion (DCCV) is recommended as the most rapid and effective treatment [1].

In patients with refractory AF or those unable to tolerate medical management, cardiac ablation procedures to achieve complete electrical isolation of the pulmonary veins can be performed to restore sinus rhythm [1, 7]. In recent decades, both surgical and percutaneous catheter ablation procedures have become well-established, evidence-based treatment options for the termination of AF and prevention of recurrence; in select patients, ablation may even be pursued as a first-line approach to rhythm control [8]. Cardiac ablation for AF management is a multidisciplinary effort requiring collaboration between electrophysiologists, cardiac surgeons, and anesthesiologists. Thus, an understanding of both key procedural and anesthetic considerations is needed to ensure procedure success and optimal patient outcomes.

## 2. Preoperative evaluation for patients undergoing atrial fibrillation procedures

Those undergoing AF ablation may range from young, otherwise healthy patients with paroxysmal AF to older patients with multiple comorbidities, or those with congenital heart disease and complex prior surgical repairs. Patients undergoing left atrial appendage occlusion (LAAO) device placement are often those at high risk for bleeding due to frailty and frequent falls, prior major bleeds, or coagulation disorders [9]. A comprehensive preoperative assessment should be performed on all patients presenting for atrial fibrillation procedures, including a detailed medical history assessing for neurologic, cardiovascular, pulmonary and other comorbidities, functional status, medications such as antiarrhythmics and anticoagulants, and a history of prior surgeries and anesthetics.

Atrial fibrillation (AF) is associated with several conditions relevant to the anesthetic plan and periprocedural safety. These conditions include hypertension, diabetes mellitus, smoking, physical inactivity, obesity, alcohol use and obstructive sleep apnea (OSA), and need to be evaluated preoperatively [4]. Valvular heart diseases that often predispose patients to AF also have structural and hemodynamic consequences that require tailored anesthetic regimens to maintain cardiac output, rhythm, and end organ perfusion. The preoperative evaluation should therefore include a thorough assessment for cardiac conditions such as mitral stenosis. Cardiac workup may include arrythmia event monitors, transthoracic echocardiography (TTE), cardiac magnetic resonance imaging, or cardiac catheterization. Additional testing should be directed by the history and physical examination.

As atrial thrombus is a contraindication to AF ablation or LAAO device placement, patients who are at risk for this require imaging to exclude the presence of thrombus.

Appropriate imaging modalities include transesophageal echocardiography (TEE), cardiac computed tomography (CT), or intraprocedural intracardiac echocardiography (ICE). Current guidelines for patients undergoing AF ablation note that such imaging may be used within 48 hours prior to the procedure to rule out atrial thrombus and is reasonable for patients with risk factors for stroke or increased risk of thrombus who have not been therapeutically anticoagulated for 3 weeks or longer [4].

If TEE is planned for the procedure, the patient should also be evaluated for any history of dysphagia, esophageal strictures, or surgeries on the upper gastrointestinal tract as these may impact the ability to safely perform TEE or necessitate the use of a smaller probe. Studies such as esophagogastroduodenoscopy should be reviewed if available; patients with a concerning history may require evaluation by a gastroenterologist for preoperative planning.

The patient's prior surgical history should be reviewed. For procedures involving transseptal puncture, such as catheter ablation and LAAO device placement, history of any prior interventions on the interatrial septum such as atrial septal defect repair should be elicited. It is also important to determine whether the patient has had prior sternotomy, as this can increase the risk of complications should reentry into the chest be necessary.

All pertinent studies should be reviewed, including electrocardiogram (ECG), echocardiogram evaluating for valvular lesions and ventricular function. Relevant labs include coagulation studies such as PTT and INR, electrolytes, markers of renal function, and baseline hemoglobin and hematocrit. Due to the risk of complications requiring blood transfusions, patients should have an active type and screen with cross-matched blood available. Female patients of childbearing age should have a pregnancy test prior to the procedure. This is particularly important for catheter ablation and LAAO device placement due to the risk of radiation exposure during the procedure.

As patients are often on systemic anticoagulation to reduce the risk of thromboembolism, medication history should include the type of anticoagulation, timing of the last dose taken, and any missed or held doses. Patients may also be on antiarrhythmics; as there are currently no established recommendations on management of AADs during ablation procedures, these may be continued or held perioperatively per the discretion of the electrophysiology and interventional cardiology teams [4]. Medication history should also include assessment for use of sodium-glucose cotransporter-2 (SGLT2) inhibitors and glucagon-like peptide-1 (GLP-1) receptor agonists. SGLT2 inhibitors are now often prescribed as part of goal-directed medical therapy for heart failure or treatment of DM, and GLP-1 receptor agonists for those with DM or obesity. As all of these conditions are also associated with AF, the anesthesiologist caring for this patient population can expect to encounter these medications with increasing frequency. Given their relative novelty, guidelines as to their optimal management are still being developed, but they have implications for anesthetic management including concerns for euglycemic ketoacidosis with SGLT2 inhibitors and delayed gastric emptying with GLP-1 receptor agonists.

## 3. Anesthesia considerations in the electrophysiology laboratory

Catheter ablation and LAAO procedures are frequently performed in locations remote from the operating room. Special considerations must be taken when providing anesthesia in the electrophysiology (EP) and cardiac catheterization laboratories, including physical distance from operating rooms and surgical support, limited access to the patient during procedures, radiation exposure, and variable levels of staff familiarity with patients under general anesthesia (GA) [10]. Due to the risk of complications requiring surgical intervention, which may include cardiopulmonary bypass in extreme cases, these procedures should be performed at hospitals with appropriate surgical, perfusionist, and critical care support [4].

The arrangement of anesthesia equipment in the EP labs may be different from what anesthesiology providers are accustomed to, as the intraoperative use of fluoroscopy equipment and procedural display screens may result in the anesthesia machine, medication cart and other equipment being positioned away from the patient. This may require extensions on IV fluid lines, an extended ventilator circuit, and careful monitoring to ensure there is enough slack to avoid inadvertent disconnections. Importantly, the configuration of the EP lab may limit access to the patient's airway, so planning for appropriate airway management equipment is critical.

As fluoroscopy is often used during these procedures, all members of the team must be aware of the risk of radiation exposure and take appropriate protective measures. There is a paucity of literature on radiation exposure to anesthesiologists during EP or structural heart procedures, however studies examining radiation exposure to anesthesiologists in the neurointerventional suite and interventional echocardiographers during transcatheter edge-to-edge mitral valve repair and LAAO device placement suggest that providers who operate at the head of the table may be exposed to radiation doses exceeding that of the interventionists [11, 12].

Risks of radiation exposure include malignancies, radiation-induced cataracts, and reproductive issues. Recommended protection includes lead aprons and gowns, lead thyroid shields, radiation-proof glasses, and dosimeters to monitor cumulative radiation exposure. Lead shields can provide an additional layer of protection, and providers should attempt to maintain distance from the C-arm as the intensity of radiation decreases by the square of the distance from the source. If close proximity to the patient is required, such as during urgent airway management, the anesthesia provider should request that fluoroscopy be briefly halted.

## 4. Catheter ablation for atrial fibrillation

### 4.1 Background

Catheter ablation is recommended for improving AF symptoms and reducing recurrence in patients with symptomatic paroxysmal or persistent AF who have failed conventional medical management. Catheter ablation a Class IA indication for rhythm control in patients with symptomatic AF who have been unable to tolerate or unsuccessful with AADs, and in select patients with symptomatic paroxysmal AF, catheter ablation is also a Class I indication as first-line therapy [1].

The goal of AF ablation is to electrically isolate the pulmonary veins from the remainder of the left atrium. Mapping is used to construct an accurate model of the patient's left atrium to allow accurate navigation of the catheters within the chamber; this is typically performed using a multielectrode mapping catheter which constructs a three-dimensional shell of the left atrium via electroanatomical mapping systems [4]. Once the chamber has been mapped, an ablation catheter is used to create a thermal injury leading to cell death, fibrosis, and electrical isolation. Ablation is performed using either a radiofrequency current to heat and denature cellular proteins or cryogenic energy to freeze the tissue. A third modality, pulsed field ablation, is an emerging non-thermal technique that is still under investigation but shows promising efficacy and safety profiles [4].

Radiofrequency ablation (RFA) is the original technique used in catheter ablation, in which the pulmonary vein ostia is circumscribed one point at a time using radiofrequency current applied from the open tip of the ablation catheter [13]. The tip of the catheter is irrigated with saline to cool the tissue interface and allow higher application of energy; this may result in patients receive more than a liter of intravascular fluid from irrigation alone [10]. RFA is a complex technique as the catheter tip must be manipulated around the circumference of each pulmonary vein ostium. In contrast, cryoablation uses a balloon-tipped catheter which is inserted into the pulmonary vein and filled with liquid nitrogen to cool the tissue, creating a circumferential lesion from a single catheter position. The FIRE and ICE randomized trial in 2016 showed non-inferiority of cryoablation compared to RFA in both efficacy and safety, and both methods are currently in use [13].

### 4.2 Preoperative anticoagulation and antiarrhythmic drug management

Studies on the vitamin K agonist (VKA) warfarin and direct acting oral anticoagulants (DOACs) have shown that uninterrupted oral anticoagulation during catheter ablation reduces the risk of thromboembolic events without significantly increasing the risk of major bleeding, and current guidelines support uninterrupted anticoagulation for patients on these agents. A minimally interrupted DOAC anticoagulation strategy, in which a single dose is skipped the day of the procedure, may be reasonable however evidence for this approach is less robust [4].

Management of antiarrhythmic drugs (AADs) is less well-defined due to a lack of definitive evidence on periprocedural continuation of AADs [4]. The patient will be instructed to hold or continue any AADs at the discretion of the electrophysiologist.

### 4.3 Choice of anesthetic technique

Sedation and anesthesia techniques for AF ablation procedures range from proceduralist-supervised conscious sedation to GA with endotracheal intubation. The choice of technique is influenced by patient comorbidities, patient and proceduralist preferences, and institutional practices. In patients undergoing RFA, studies have noted a measurable increase in catheter stability and a lower incidence of pulmonary vein (PV) reconnection when the ablation is performed under GA compared to conscious sedation [14, 15]. In a study comparing GA to sedation by an anesthesia provider for RFA procedure, ablation time was 5 minutes shorter under GA compared to sedation, although there was a higher cost and longer duration of time under anesthesia in the GA group [16].

Factors to consider when choosing an anesthetic approach include anticipated procedure duration, patient cooperation and ability to remain motionless for prolonged periods of time, risk for airway obstruction and respiratory depression, and type of ablation energy being employed. As AF ablation procedures may last for several hours and success is dependent on catheter stability, a patient who is unable to comfortably lie still or who coughs frequently may be more appropriate for GA from a procedural perspective. From a patient safety perspective, those with increased risk for respiratory depression (such as patients with OSA or unfavorable airways) or who cannot safely tolerate periods of hypoventilation (such as those with right ventricular dysfunction or pulmonary hypertension), GA with controlled ventilation may be the safest choice. The type of ablation energy is also an important factor, as RFA can be more painful than cryoablation and may require a deeper plane of anesthesia [17]. Of note, studies showing similar long-term outcomes between conscious sedation and GA have been in patients undergoing cryoablation [18].

### 4.4 Intraoperative management and considerations

Upon arrival to the room, the patient will often be requested to initially sit upright on the table so that the patches and electrodes required for mapping and ablation can be applied by the EP laboratory staff. In addition to the standard anesthetic monitors for oxygenation, ventilation, circulation and temperature, a specialized esophageal temperature probe or cooling device may be employed to reduce the risk of esophageal injury in RFA procedures. A depth of anesthesia monitor with processed EEG should be considered in cases where GA is administered, particularly where a total intravenous anesthetic technique (TIVA) is employed.

Invasive blood pressure monitoring with an arterial line should be considered in patients who need close hemodynamic monitoring, such as those with reduced cardiac function, stenotic valvular lesions, or poor tolerance of rapid ventricular response, and for those requiring frequent lab draws or arterial blood gasses. As left atrial access for the ablation requires the proceduralist to perform a transseptal puncture, close hemodynamic monitoring with an arterial line is also beneficial in the event of complications such as pericardial effusion and tamponade.

The transseptal puncture for left atrial access is commonly performed under echocardiographic visualization; if ICE is not used during the procedure, a TEE may need to be placed to provide guidance during the procedure.

Large-bore peripheral IV access (two peripheral IVs of size 18 g or larger) is usually sufficient for AF ablation procedures. Central venous catheterization is generally not required unless indicated for patient comorbidities, as emergent central access for fluid and medication administration can be achieved using the venous sheaths that are routinely placed during the procedure.

After placement of appropriate monitors, GA can be induced with a short-acting opioid such as fentanyl, a sedative-hypnotic such as propofol, and a depolarizing muscle relaxant. Unlike ablation procedures for sympathetically mediated arrhythmias like ventricular tachycardia, where GA can interfere with arrhythmia induction during the mapping process, patients undergoing AF ablation can be placed under GA immediately since the ablation is based on the anatomic location of the pulmonary veins.

Endotracheal intubation is generally used. In select cases, a laryngeal mask airway may also be used, although this is less common as minimizing movement from respiratory variation is better accomplished with controlled rather than spontaneous ventilation modes. Various ventilatory modes have been employed to reduce respiratory variation and improve catheter stability, including high-frequency low-tidal volume ventilation, high-frequency jet ventilation (HFJV), and periods of apnea. Jet ventilation should be used with caution in patients with pulmonary hypertension and those at risk for right-ventricular dysfunction and/or pneumothorax [19, 20].

General anesthesia can be maintained with volatile agents, IV anesthetics, or a combination of both. If HFJV is used, a TIVA is appropriate as volatile agents cannot be reliably used to maintain anesthesia. The anesthetic plan should incorporate prophylaxis for postoperative nausea and vomiting, for patient comfort as well as minimizing the risk of groin hematoma in the postoperative period.

For procedures performed under sedation, various regimens can be employed including a propofol or dexmedetomidine infusion and small boluses of fentanyl and/or midazolam. Care must be taken to ensure patient comfort while avoiding respiratory depression. The provider must be prepared to convert to general anesthesia at any point during the procedure should the need arise, such as inability to achieve adequate depth of sedation without respiratory depression, frequent patient coughing, or procedural complications requiring surgical intervention.

The choice of vasoactive agents depends primarily on patient comorbidities. Both phenylephrine and norepinephrine are commonly used vasopressors for ablation procedures. In select patients with severe pulmonary hypertension, vasopressin may be appropriate. Patients may also receive cardioactive agents from the procedural team for arrhythmia induction and to evaluate efficacy of the ablation. Isoproterenol is a beta-1 agonist used to increase intrinsic pacemaker activity and evaluate pulmonary vein connections; this may be infused at a rate of up to 30 mcg/min and can cause systemic hypotension requiring vasopressor support. Patients who are awake may also experience flushing, nausea, dizziness, headache, sweating, tremors, and blurred vision. Adenosine is an atrioventricular nodal blocking agent used to unmask arrhythmias; it can cause a transient sinus pause lasting several seconds. As it also acts on bronchial smooth muscle, there have been reports of it triggering bronchospasm particularly in patients with a history of reactive airway disease [21]. Anesthesia providers should be aware of when these agents are administered and prepared to support patient hemodynamics.

Heparin is administered prior to the transseptal puncture to reduce the risk of thromboembolic events, and is titrated to achieve an activated clotting time (ACT) of >300 until all catheters have been removed from the left side of the heart.

At the end of the procedure, protamine may be administered slowly to minimize the risk of protamine reaction, which may range from moderate hypotension due to histamine release to anaphylaxis. Alternatively, the proceduralist may opt to wait until the ACT decreases to <200–250 s, at which point the sheaths can be removed without reversal of the heparin [4]. Smooth emergence from anesthesia is important to reduce the risk of developing a hematoma at the groin access sites.

Volume management during AF ablation is crucial, particularly in patients with heart failure. In addition to fluids administered by the anesthesia provider, patients often receive multiple liters of fluid from continuous irrigation of RFA catheters. It is therefore important to monitor total fluid intake and diurese if an excessive amount of fluid has been administered. For this reason, foley catheter placement should be considered for cases that are anticipated to be prolonged.

### 4.5 Postoperative considerations

Patients may be recovered from anesthesia in the EP laboratory, a post-anesthesia care unit (PACU), or the intensive care unit. A period of bed rest must be observed after sheath removal; this often is for four or more hours, although efforts are being made to safely reduce the duration of bed rest to facilitate same-day discharge. While patients have typically been admitted for one or more nights to monitor for complications, this is associated with increased health care costs and resource utilization, and efforts are being made to develop and implement same-day discharge protocols [4].

Pain management strategies during recovery include local anesthetic infiltration at the sites of vascular access with supplemental IV and enteral analgesics such as acetaminophen and opioids. While patients may experience some discomfort at the access sites or in the back after remaining supine for a prolonged period of time, severe groin or back pain should alert providers to the possibility of a retroperitoneal hematoma or other vascular injury and should be promptly evaluated.

Postoperatively, it is recommended that patients remain on anticoagulation for at least 2 months regardless of their baseline risk of thromboembolism due to left atrium stunning, endothelial stunning, and an inflammatory state that can occur after ablation. Those at low risk for stroke may be eligible to discontinue anticoagulation after 2 months, however evidence to guide anticoagulation management outside this period is lacking [4]. Patients are often prescribed a short-term course of proton pump inhibitors to reduce the risk of esophageal injury, as gastroesophageal reflux is thought to contribute to atrio-esophageal fistula formation [4].

### 4.6 Procedure complications

Knowledge of potential complications in the intraoperative and immediate postoperative period will enable rapid diagnosis and management. Overall rates of complications from AF catheter ablation range from 2.5 to 8%, with vascular access injury such as groin hematoma and retroperitoneal bleeds being most common. Of note, female patients suffer higher rates of complications. The most common life-threatening complication is cardiac tamponade, which occurs in 0.4–1.3% of cases, some requiring emergent surgical intervention [4]. Other major complications include thromboembolism, air embolism, and phrenic nerve palsy.

Any episode of unexplained acute intraoperative hypotension should alert to the possibility of tamponade or hemorrhage and prompt the use of echocardiography to look for pericardial fluid and fluoroscopy to assess for decreased excursion of the cardiac silhouette (both seen in tamponade). In addition, angiography should be performed to rule out vascular extravasation while supporting the patient's hemodynamics with vasoactive medications and volume expansion [4, 22]. Treatment of cardiac tamponade typically involves emergent pericardiocentesis and reversal of heparinization with protamine, although protamine administration needs to be balanced with the risk of clotting the pericardial catheter [4]. If the bleeding is unable to be controlled, emergent surgical intervention needs to be performed.

Complications that typically present with a greater time delay (on the order of weeks) include esophageal injury, and pulmonary vein stenosis, although delayed cardiac tamponade has also been observed. Delayed thromboembolic events may be seen, as patients remain at elevated risk for the first 2 weeks after ablation [4].

Atrioesophageal fistula (AEF) is life-threatening and requires immediate intervention. In a worldwide survey on AEF after AF ablation, the most common presenting symptoms were fever, chest pain, odynophagia, and neurologic events [23]. Treatment involves urgent surgical or endoscopic treatment, as mortality ranges from 83 to 100% without surgical repair [4].

## 5. Percutaneous left atrial appendage occlusion

### 5.1 Background

For patients with atrial fibrillation, stroke due to thrombus formation within the left atrial appendage (LAA) remains a significant source of morbidity and mortality. Anticoagulation is a mainstay for stroke prevention, however, patients with a prohibitively high bleeding risk or contraindication to anticoagulation may benefit from closure of the LAA. Percutaneous LAAO involves accessing the left atrium via the venous system through a transseptal puncture and deployment of the occlusion device within the left atrium under ultrasound guidance.

Current LAAO devices in use in the United States are the Watchman (Boston Scientific), the Amplatzer Cardiac Plug (ACP) and Amulet (St. Jude Medical) and the LARIAT (SentreHEART, Inc.). The Watchman, ACP, and Amulet are endocardial self-expanding nitinol devices with hooks to anchor them within the LAA; the Watchman is shaped as a basket with a membrane-covered base facing outwards toward the left atrium while the ACP and Amulet consist of a cylinder that sits within the body of the LAA and a broader disk to occlude the appendage orifice. The LARIAT is an epicardial device that requires both epicardial and endocardial access for placement, as the suture wire used to externally close the LAA is guided into position by an endocardial balloon and epicardial guide wire [9].

### 5.2 Choice of anesthetic technique

Left atrial appendage occlusion (LAAO) devices require ultrasound guidance for positioning within the LAA and confirmation of complete appendage occlusion. These procedures are typically performed under GA with TEE guidance, although a 2021 study comparing GA with conscious sedation in Amplatzer Amulet placement showed that this procedure could be safely performed under conscious sedation with TEE [24]. Endocardial LAAO with guidance from ICE instead of TEE is an area of active exploration, especially as 3D ICE becomes available. While TEE currently remains the imaging modality of choice, anesthesia providers can expect to see an increasing number of these cases performed with ICE in the coming years which may lead to a shift away from GA toward monitored anesthesia care or conscious sedation [25].

Additional considerations in selecting the anesthetic technique are similar to that for catheter ablation procedures, including the need for immobility during critical portions of the procedure (such as the transseptal puncture), avoidance of respiratory depression and airway obstruction, and the patient's ability to tolerate lying flat for a prolonged period of time. Patient comorbidities should be carefully taken into consideration and the anesthetic plan tailored accordingly to optimize both procedural success and patient safety.

### 5.3 Anesthetic management and considerations

In addition to standard anesthetic monitors, invasive arterial blood pressure monitoring should be considered due to the possibility of arrhythmias and hemodynamic instability in the event of complications such as pericardial effusion or vascular injury. If ICE is not being used, TEE guidance is required to evaluate the LAA and guide the transseptal puncture and device deployment. Vascular access should include one to two large bore peripheral IVs; central venous access is generally not required as long as there is adequate peripheral access for resuscitation in the event of tamponade or hemorrhage. Cross-matched blood products should be available in the event of emergency.

Maintenance of general anesthesia can be performed with a volatile, intravenous, or combined anesthetic technique. The airway is typically secured with an endotracheal tube to facilitate the use of TEE throughout the case. Heparin is administered after the transseptal puncture to reduce the risk of intraoperative thrombus and embolic stroke. The heparin may be reversed with protamine at the conclusion of the procedure, or the ACT may be allowed to normalize without reversal.

### 5.4 Postoperative considerations

In most cases, patients are extubated at the end of the procedure. Early postoperative neurologic assessment is routinely performed. For postoperative pain management, local anesthetic may be administered at the vascular access sites by the interventionalist, and standard enteral and parenteral analgesics can be administered as needed. Patients can be recovered in a post-anesthesia care unit, during which they must observe several hours of bedrest to reduce the risk of groin hematoma. As with catheter ablation procedures, they are typically monitored overnight for development of pericardial effusion and other complications. Patients who have undergone LARIAT placement may have a pigtail catheter left in the pericardial space which can be removed the following day [26].

As patients remain at risk for thrombus formation until the device has undergone complete endothelialization, postoperative antithrombotic therapy is recommended with interval evaluation by TEE to assess for device stability and any residual flow in the LAA. For the Watchman device, warfarin and aspirin are administered for at least 45 days; if the interval TEE shows no thrombus or significant leak, patients may then be transitioned to dual anti-platelet therapy for 6 months and then to aspirin alone thereafter [9, 26].

Despite the belief that postoperative antithrombotic therapy was not required for the LARIAT when the extracardiac device was first introduced, anticoagulation is now recommended for the first few months due to risk of thrombus formation at the suture site or partial re-opening of the appendage [9, 26].

### 5.5 Procedure complications

Complications of endovascular LAAO device placement include pericardial effusion, vascular injury and major bleeding, air embolism, stroke, and device embolization. For the LARIAT procedure, additional risks associated with the combined endovascular and epicardial technique include perforation of the right ventricle or LAA, epicardial vessel injury, and postoperative pericarditis or Dressler syndrome [26].

## 6. Surgical and hybrid ablation for atrial fibrillation

### 6.1 Background

Epicardial surgical ablation for AF can be performed as a stand-alone procedure or concurrently with other cardiac surgery. The strongest recommendations for surgical ablation currently exist for patients undergoing cardiac surgery for other indications: per the 2023 ACC/AHA/ACCP/HRS Guideline for the Diagnosis and Management of Atrial Fibrillation, concomitant surgical ablation is a Class IIa recommendation in patients with AF undergoing cardiac surgery [1]. The 2024 EHRA/HRS/APHRS/LAHRS Expert Consensus Statement on Catheter and Surgical Ablation of Atrial Fibrillation provides further granularity, recommending concomitant surgical ablation for all patients with paroxysmal or persistent AF undergoing surgery with an open left atrium and in patients undergoing surgery with a closed left atrium if they have been unsuccessful with or intolerant of AAD therapy [4]. Several studies have shown the efficacy and safety of concomitant AF ablation and LAA exclusion or excision during cardiac surgical procedures, and concomitant AF surgery is associated with improved long-term survival as well as a decreased risk of stroke [4, 27, 28]. The STS 2023 guidelines recommend surgical ablation for AF during non-emergent first-time mitral valve surgery as a class IA recommendation and during non-mitral surgeries as a class IB recommendation. Additionally, the 2023 guidelines give Class IA recommendation to exclude the LAA during all non-emergent first-time cardiac surgeries in those with AF [27].

Stand-alone surgical ablation can be considered in patients with symptomatic persistent AF who have either had prior unsuccessful catheter ablation or who are unable to achieve control with AAD therapy and prefer a surgical approach; there is currently limited evidence for those with paroxysmal AF [4]. The 2023 ACC/AHA/ACCP/HRS Guidelines provide a Class IIb recommendation for hybrid surgical ablation in patients with refractory, symptomatic persistent AF, noting increased freedom from atrial arrhythmias at 12 months. However, this must be weighed against the risk of major procedural complications including stroke, bleeding, and pericardial effusion [1].

Surgical ablation typically involves isolation of the pulmonary veins and the posterior left atrial well; additional lesion sets may be performed in both the left and right atria with the most complete approach being the Cox maze procedure. First developed in 1987 by Dr. James Cox, the operation has evolved through several iterations to the Cox maze IV procedure, which replaces earlier cut-and-sew techniques with RFA and cryoablation and can be performed either via sternotomy or right mini thoracotomy. While the Cox maze IV is highly effective, it requires bilateral atriotomies and therefore must be done on cardiopulmonary bypass with placement of an aortic cross-clamp and cardioplegic arrest [29].

In the early 2000s, thoracoscopic maze procedures were developed as a minimally invasive surgical solution for atrial fibrillation [30]. Video-assisted thoracoscopy (VATS) is used to enter the pericardium from the pleural space and isolate the pulmonary veins under direct visualization with RFA, followed by ligation of the left atrial appendage [31]. To minimize re-entrant circuits, additional epicardial ablation lines are performed to approximate the ablation lines of the Cox-Maze IV procedure; a variety of lesions sets are possible [32].

Hybrid ablation is a newer approach which combines both epicardial and endocardial ablation techniques and is performed in concert with cardiac surgeons and interventional electrophysiologists. The surgical and percutaneous catheter ablations may be performed as a single-stage approach in which both are performed during the same procedure, sequentially with the epicardial surgical ablation performed first followed by the endocardial portion during the same hospital admission, or as a two-stage approach with the endocardial ablation performed 2–4 months after the epicardial ablation [33].

The epicardial portion of the hybrid ablation can be performed either thoracoscopically or through a subxiphoid incision [4]. Initial thoracoscopic approaches used bilateral VATS, however a unilateral approach via left thoracoscopic access has been associated with a shorter hospital length of stay and no significant difference in freedom from AF at 1 year when compared to the bilateral approach [34]. In what is termed the hybrid convergent procedure, a subxiphoid incision is made to allow catheter access to the posterior LA wall [4].

The endocardial phase is performed using techniques described in earlier sections of this chapter and involves an assessment of the epicardial lesion integrity, ablation of any remaining gaps, and placement of additional lines in the right atrium [35].

For patients with AF undergoing cardiac surgery for other indications, the optimal lesion set to target for ablation will depend on whether the surgery requires a left atriotomy. For patients undergoing open LA procedures, the biatrial Cox-Maze IV procedure is preferred, while PVI and lesions targeting isolation of the posterior wall should be performed in those who would not otherwise have a left atriotomy [28].

### 6.2 Preoperative assessment

In addition to the preoperative considerations for patients with AF discussed earlier in this chapter, there are additional factors to evaluate when preparing patients for thoracoscopic approaches. Due to the use of lung isolation, it is necessary to assess for the presence of lung disease or severe heart disease that could preclude tolerance of one-lung ventilation. This includes evaluating for a history of smoking, restrictive or obstructive lung disease, and prior lung surgeries including resection. Pulmonary function tests including spirometry and a 6-mintue walk test may be obtained to further assess pulmonary function. Attention should be given to the airway exam and any chest imaging, including chest radiographs or CT scans, to guide choice of technique for lung isolation.

### 6.3 Choice of anesthetic technique

General anesthesia is required for patients undergoing surgical AF ablation, whether performed as a stand-alone procedure or concomitant to other cardiac surgery. Anesthetic induction agents are determined by patient characteristics and comorbidities as well as the anesthesia provider's preference. For maintenance of anesthesia, both volatile and intravenous anesthetics can be used. For stand-alone ablation procedures, anesthetic management should prioritize the use of shorter-acting agents to facilitate rapid emergence and extubation in the operating. When the ablation is performed concomitant to other cardiac surgery, the patient's primary cardiac pathology should be considered when formulating the anesthetic plan.

Lung isolation is required during thoracoscopic approaches to allow access to the pericardium. This can be achieved with either a double-lumen endotracheal tube (DLT) or a bronchial blocker placed through a single lumen endotracheal tube, depending on provider preference and patient factors such as airway anatomy. Fiberoptic bronchoscopy should be used to confirm appropriate tube or blocker positioning both on initial airway placement and after final patient positioning [36]. DLTs are still considered the gold standard for lung isolation as they provide excellent lung isolation in addition to access to the non-ventilated lung for bronchoscopy, suction, and application of continuous positive airway pressure when needed. However, they can be difficult to position in patients with unfavorable airway anatomy, may cause airway trauma due to their larger external diameter and are not suitable for prolonged use in the intensive care unit should the patient need to remain intubated postoperatively [37]. If a DLT is used, intravenous dexamethasone may be prophylactically administered during the anesthetic to reduce the incidence of sore throat and hoarseness postoperatively [38].

## 6.4 Intraoperative management and considerations

During the surgery, the patient will often be in supine position with arms tucked in, allowing for rapid conversion to sternotomy in case of emergency. Attention should be given to positioning to avoid brachial plexus stretch injuries, as the arms may be tucked more posteriorly to the patient's sides to allow for thoracoscopic port placement while in the supine position. External defibrillation pads should be placed on the patient prior to surgery both in case of hemodynamically significant cardiac arrhythmias and for planned external electrical cardioversion after the procedure is completed. These procedures are typically performed with cardiopulmonary bypass (CPB) standby, and a fully primed CPB machine and perfusionist should be immediately available in the event of complications requiring CPB such as cardiac or vascular perforation.

Due to rapid hemodynamic changes during surgical manipulation of the heart and pulmonary vein clamping, an arterial line is recommended for continuous blood pressure monitoring; this additionally allows for monitoring arterial blood gasses during one-lung ventilation. Large bore peripheral IV access is required for resuscitation should significant bleeding occur. Central access may be obtained at the discretion of the anesthesiologist for vasoactive medication administration and in the event of emergent CPB initiation. Crossmatched blood should be readily available.

Intraoperative TEE is utilized to rule out presence of intracardiac thrombus prior to LAA ligation and electrical cardioversion. As the left circumflex (LCx) coronary artery courses immediately inferior to the LAA, it is at risk for injury during LAA ligation; it is important to monitor the left ventricle for new anterolateral and inferolateral wall motion abnormalities during this period. TEE is also used to ensure the adequacy of the LAA ligation, as leaving a residual stump can result in future thromboembolic events [4]. To minimize the risk for esophageal injury and subsequent AEF formation, the TEE probe should be withdrawn from the left atrium during radiofrequency ablation [39].

Should hypoxia be encountered during one-lung ventilation, several maneuvers may be attempted. The patient should be placed on 100% inspired oxygen while confirming the position of the endotracheal tube and rapidly assessing for any ventilator or circuit issues. Should hypoxia persist, the surgeon should be informed and the nonventilated lung should be re-expanded. This may be achieved with intermittent two-lung ventilation or application of CPAP to the nonventilated lung at a pressure 5–10 cm $H_2O$ after initial reinflation [40]. However, even partial re-expansion of the lung with CPAP may interfere with surgical visualization during thoracoscopy. In extreme cases, the procedure may need to be aborted or performed via an alternative approach.

Transient hypoxia, reduced end-tidal $CO_2$ on capnography, and hypotension may also be encountered when pulmonary vein isolation is performed using a RF bipolar clamp device, as clamping the pulmonary veins temporarily reduces venous return to the left atrium from that lung. This is most evident if performed on pulmonary veins draining a ventilated lung. While the abrupt change in oxygenation and hemodynamics can be alarming to those unfamiliar with this procedure, it usually resolves promptly after the clamp is released and can be temporized with 100% inspired oxygen and judicious vasoactive support to avoid rebound hypertension after clamp release.

### 6.5 Postoperative considerations

Patients undergoing an uncomplicated stand-alone VATS PVI can often be extubated at the end of the case and recovered in the postoperative anesthesia care unit. However, these surgeries should only be performed at institutions with critical care capabilities as patients may require ICU admission in the event of conversion to sternotomy with cardiopulmonary bypass or other intraoperative complications. If postoperative ventilation is needed in a patient with a DLT, exchange to a single-lumen tube should be performed when safe to do so.

Despite the smaller incisions associated with thoracoscopic surgery, patients can still experience significant postoperative pain. As inadequate analgesia can increase the risk of postoperative pulmonary complications and negatively impact patient satisfaction, the anesthesiologist plays an important role in perioperative pain management. Multimodal analgesia options include acetaminophen, dexamethasone, non-steroidal anti-inflammatory drugs (if not contraindicated), and regional anesthesia techniques including paravertebral, erector spinae fascial plane, and serratus anterior fascial plane blocks. If a regional local anesthetic is not used, systemic lidocaine may be considered. Gabapentinoids can be continued in patients who have been on them preoperatively, and ketamine may be used in select patients [41].

### 6.6 Procedure complications

Significant bleeding due to injury to the pulmonary veins or other cardiovascular structures may require conversion to thoracotomy, initiation of CPB, and even sternotomy. Additional complications associated with surgical ablation include the recurrence of atrial fibrillation and atrial tachycardias, the need for permanent pacemaker placement, stroke, phrenic nerve palsy, AEF, pericardial effusion and hemothorax [4]. As the LAA is typically ligated during these procedures, LCx coronary artery injury is possible, and the team should be vigilant for ST-segment changes on the ECG and new wall motion abnormalities in the LCx territory on intraoperative TEE.

## 7. Conclusion

The management of AF has evolved significantly over the years, with both catheter and surgical ablation techniques playing a pivotal role in achieving rhythm control, preventing AF recurrence, and improving patient quality of life. Percutaneous options for closure of the LAA additionally offers freedom from long-term anticoagulation and reduced risk of embolic stroke in those unable to tolerate or take systemic anticoagulation. Advances in energy delivery, such as the use of non-thermal energy in pulsed field ablation, continue to be pursued to improve safety and efficacy of these procedures. While this chapter primarily focuses on the management of patients presenting for procedures targeted at rhythm control, the new classification of AF as a disease continuum highlights the importance of patient management at all stages of this disease. As anesthesiologists are intimately involved in patients' perioperative care, recognition and optimization of AF risk factors is important not only for patients undergoing ablation procedures but all those presenting for anesthetic care.

## Conflict of interest

The authors declare no conflict of interest.

## Author details

Larissa Kiwakyou, Anna Reichardt, Allen Ninh and Louise Sun*
Division of Cardiothoracic Anesthesiology, Department of Anesthesiology
Perioperative and Pain Medicine, Stanford University, Palo Alto, California, USA

*Address all correspondence to: sunl@stanford.edu

## References

[1] Joglar JA et al. 2023 ACC/AHA/ACCP/HRS guideline for the diagnosis and management of atrial fibrillation: A report of the American College of Cardiology/American Heart Association joint committee on clinical practice guidelines (in eng). Circulation. 2024;**149**(1):e1-e156. DOI: 10.1161/CIR.0000000000001193

[2] Boriani G, Vitolo M, Lane DA, Potpara TS, Lip GY. Beyond the 2020 guidelines on atrial fibrillation of the European Society of Cardiolog (in eng). European Journal of Internal Medicine. 2021;**86**:1-11. DOI: 10.1016/j.ejim.2021.01.006

[3] Lloyd-Jones DM et al. Lifetime risk for development of atrial fibrillation: The Framingham heart study (in eng). Circulation. 2004;**110**(9):1042-1046. DOI: 10.1161/01.CIR.0000140263.20897.42

[4] Tzeis S, Gerstenfeld EP, Kalman J, Saad EB, Sepehri Shamloo A, Andrade JG, et al. 2024 European Heart Rhythm Association/Heart Rhythm Society/Asia Pacific Heart Rhythm Society/Latin American Heart Rhythm Society expert consensus statement on catheter and surgical ablation of atrial fibrillation. Europace. 30 Mar 2024;**26**(4):euae043. DOI: 10.1093/europace/euae043. PMID: 38587017; PMCID: PMC11000153

[5] Lopes LA, Agrawal DK. Post-operative atrial fibrillation: Current treatments and etiologies for a persistent surgical complication (in eng). Journal of Surgery and Research. 2022;**5**(1):159-172. DOI: 10.26502/jsr.10020209

[6] Darby AE, Dimarco JP. Management of atrial fibrillation in patients with structural heart disease (in eng). Circulation. 2012;**125**(7):945-957. DOI: 10.1161/CIRCULATIONAHA.111.019935

[7] Hindricks G et al. 2020 ESC guidelines for the diagnosis and management of atrial fibrillation developed in collaboration with the European Association for Cardio-Thoracic Surgery (EACTS): The task force for the diagnosis and management of atrial fibrillation of the European Society of Cardiology (ESC) developed with the special contribution of the European Heart Rhythm Association (EHRA) of the ESC (in eng). European Heart Journal. 2021;**42**(5):373-498. DOI: 10.1093/eurheartj/ehaa612

[8] Parameswaran R, Al-Kaisey AM, Kalman JM. Catheter ablation for atrial fibrillation: Current indications and evolving technologies (in eng). Nature Reviews Cardiology. 2021;**18**(3):210-225. DOI: 10.1038/s41569-020-00451-x

[9] Casu G et al. ANMCO/AIAC/SICI-GISE/SIC/SICCH consensus document: Percutaneous occlusion of the left atrial appendage in non-valvular atrial fibrillation patients: Indications, patient selection, staff skills, organisation, and training (in eng). European Heart Journal Supplements: Journal of the European Society of Cardiology. 2017;**19**(Suppl. D):D333-D353. DOI: 10.1093/eurheartj/sux008

[10] Dooley N, Lowe M, Ashley EMC. Advances in management of electrophysiology and atrial fibrillation in the cardiac catheter laboratory: Implications for anaesthesia (in eng). BJA Education. 2018;**18**(11):349-356. DOI: 10.1016/j.bjae.2018.08.001

[11] McNamara DA et al. Comparison of radiation exposure among interventional

echocardiographers, interventional cardiologists, and sonographers during percutaneous structural heart interventions (in eng). JAMA Network Open. 2022;**5**(7):e2220597. DOI: 10.1001/jamanetworkopen.2022.20597

[12] Anastasian ZH, Strozyk D, Meyers PM, Wang S, Berman MF. Radiation exposure of the anesthesiologist in the neurointerventional suite (in eng). Anesthesiology. 2011;**114**(3):512-520. DOI: 10.1097/ALN.0b013e31820c2b81

[13] Kuck K, Brugada J, Albenque J. Cryoballoon or radiofrequency ablation for atrial fibrillation (in eng). The New England Journal of Medicine. 2016;**375**(11):1100-1101. DOI: 10.1056/NEJMc1609160

[14] Kuno S et al. Impact of general anesthesia on ablation catheter stability during pulmonary vein isolation based on a novel measurement approach (in eng). Scientific Reports. 2023;**13**(1):17204. DOI: 10.1038/s41598-023-44450-7

[15] Di Biase L et al. General anesthesia reduces the prevalence of pulmonary vein reconnection during repeat ablation when compared with conscious sedation: Results from a randomized study (in eng). Heart Rhythm. 2011;**8**(3):368-372. DOI: 10.1016/j.hrthm.2010.10.043

[16] Yokokawa M et al. A comparison of clinical outcomes and cost of radiofrequency catheter ablation for atrial fibrillation with monitored anesthesia care versus general anesthesia (in eng). Journal of Cardiovascular Electrophysiology. 2022;**33**(8):1714-1722. DOI: 10.1111/jce.15582

[17] Attanasio P et al. Pain reactions during pulmonary vein isolation under deep sedation: Cryothermal versus radiofrequency ablation (in eng). Pacing and Clinical Electrophysiology. 2016;**39**(5):452-457. DOI: 10.1111/pace.12840

[18] Wasserlauf J et al. Moderate sedation reduces lab time compared to general anesthesia during cryoballoon ablation for AF without compromising safety or long-term efficacy (in eng). Pacing and Clinical Electrophysiology. 2016;**39**(12):1359-1365. DOI: 10.1111/pace.12961

[19] Babapoor-Farrokhran S, Alzubi J, Port Z, Khraisha O, Mainigi SK. Utility of high-frequency jet ventilation in atrial fibrillation ablation (in eng). Innovations in Cardiac Rhythm Management. 2021;**12**(7):4590-4593. DOI: 10.19102/icrm.2021.120708

[20] Osorio J et al. High-frequency low-tidal volume ventilation improves long-term outcomes in AF ablation: A multicenter prospective study (in eng). JACC: Clinical Electrophysiology. 2023;**9**(8 Pt 2):1543-1554. DOI: 10.1016/j.jacep.2023.05.015

[21] Salter B, O'Donnell T, Weiner M, Fischer G. Adenosine and bronchospasm: Vigilance in the electrophysiology suite (in eng). Journal of Cardiothoracic and Vascular Anesthesia. 2015;**29**(2):410-411. DOI: 10.1053/j.jvca.2013.09.002

[22] Malladi V, Naeini PS, Razavi M, Collard CD, Anton JM, Tolpin DA. Endovascular ablation of atrial fibrillation (in eng). Anesthesiology. 2014;**120**(6):1513-1519. DOI: 10.1097/ALN.0000000000000261

[23] Tilz RR et al. A worldwide survey on incidence, management, and prognosis of oesophageal fistula formation following atrial fibrillation catheter ablation: The POTTER-AF study (in eng). European Heart Journal.

2023;**44**(27):2458-2469. DOI: 10.1093/eurheartj/ehad250

[24] Piayda K et al. Clinical outcomes of patients undergoing percutaneous left atrial appendage occlusion in general anaesthesia or conscious sedation: Data from the prospective global Amplatzer Amulet occluder observational study (in eng). BMJ Open. 2021;**11**(3):e040455. DOI: 10.1136/bmjopen-2020-040455

[25] Diaz JC et al. Intracardiac echocardiography-guided left atrial appendage occlusion (in eng). Arrhythmia & Electrophysiology Review. 2024;**13**:e03. DOI: 10.15420/aer.2023.29

[26] Husain Z et al. Anesthetic management of patients undergoing percutaneous endocardial and epicardial left atrial appendage occlusion (in eng). Seminars in Cardiothoracic and Vascular Anesthesia. 2017;**21**(4):291-301. DOI: 10.1177/1089253217714581

[27] Wyler von Ballmoos MC, Hui DS, Mehaffey JH, Malaisrie SC, Vardas PN, Gillinov AM, et al. The Society of Thoracic Surgeons 2023 clinical practice guidelines for the surgical treatment of atrial fibrillation. The Annals of Thoracic Surgery. Aug 2024;**118**(2):291-310. DOI: 10.1016/j.athoracsur.2024.01.007. Epub 2024 Jan 27. PMID: 38286206

[28] Badhwar V et al. The Society of Thoracic Surgeons 2017 clinical practice guidelines for the surgical treatment of atrial fibrillation (in eng). The Annals of Thoracic Surgery. 2017;**103**(1):329-341. DOI: 10.1016/j.athoracsur.2016.10.076

[29] Ruaengsri C, Schill MR, Khiabani AJ, Schuessler RB, Melby SJ, Damiano RJ. The Cox-maze IV procedure in its second decade: Still the gold standard? (in eng). European Journal of Cardio-Thoracic Surgery. 2018;**53**(Suppl. 1):i19-i25. DOI: 10.1093/ejcts/ezx326

[30] Geuzebroek GS, Bentala M, Molhoek SG, Kelder JC, Schaap J, Van Putte BP. Totally thoracoscopic left atrial maze: Standardized, effective and safe (in eng). Interactive Cardiovascular and Thoracic Surgery. 2016;**22**(3):259-264. DOI: 10.1093/icvts/ivv358

[31] Wolf RK et al. Video-assisted bilateral pulmonary vein isolation and left atrial appendage exclusion for atrial fibrillation (in eng). The Journal of Thoracic and Cardiovascular Surgery. 2005;**130**(3):797-802. DOI: 10.1016/j.jtcvs.2005.03.041

[32] Abo-Salem E et al. Surgical treatment of atrial fibrillation (in eng). Journal of Cardiovascular Electrophysiology. 2015;**26**(9):1027-1037. DOI: 10.1111/jce.12731

[33] Vroomen M, Pison L. Hybrid ablation for atrial fibrillation: A systematic review (in eng). Journal of Interventional Cardiac Electrophysiology. 2016;**47**(3):265-274. DOI: 10.1007/s10840-016-0183-9

[34] Pong T et al. Hybrid ablation for atrial fibrillation: Safety & efficacy of unilateral epicardial access (in eng). Seminars in Thoracic and Cardiovascular Surgery. 2023;**35**(2):277-286. DOI: 10.1053/j.semtcvs.2022.03.003

[35] Cox JL et al. A hybrid maze procedure for long-standing persistent atrial fibrillation (in eng). The Annals of Thoracic Surgery. 2019;**107**(2):610-618. DOI: 10.1016/j.athoracsur.2018.06.064

[36] Elsayed HH, Moharram AA. Tailored anaesthesia for thoracoscopic surgery promoting enhanced recovery: The state of the art (in eng). Anaesthesia Critical Care & Pain Medicine. 2021;**40**(2):100846. DOI: 10.1016/j.accpm.2021.100846

[37] Patel M, Wilson A, Ong C. Double-lumen tubes and bronchial blockers (in eng). BJA Education. 2023;**23**(11):416-424. DOI: 10.1016/j.bjae.2023.07.001

[38] Park SH, Han SH, Do SH, Kim JW, Rhee KY, Kim JH. Prophylactic dexamethasone decreases the incidence of sore throat and hoarseness after tracheal extubation with a double-lumen endobronchial tube (in eng). Anesthesia and Analgesia. 2008;**107**(6):1814-1818. DOI: 10.1213/ane.0b013e318185d093

[39] Sun Z, Fu P, Odo N, Patel V, Sharma G, Agarwal S. Anesthetic management of total thoracoscopic left atrial maze procedure for chronic atrial fibrillation-A single-institution experience (in eng). Journal of Cardiothoracic and Vascular Anesthesia. 2019;**33**(7):1801-1808. DOI: 10.1053/j.jvca.2019.02.034

[40] Karzai W, Schwarzkopf K. Hypoxemia during one-lung ventilation: Prediction, prevention, and treatment (in eng). Anesthesiology. 2009;**110**(6):1402-1411. DOI: 10.1097/ALN.0b013e31819fb15d

[41] Hamilton C, Alfille P, Mountjoy J, Bao X. Regional anesthesia and acute perioperative pain management in thoracic surgery: A narrative review (in eng). Journal of Thoracic Disease. 2022;**14**(6):2276-2296. DOI: 10.21037/jtd-21-1740

Chapter 10

# Different Type of Ablation Procedures for Atrial Fibrillation

*Mehmet Ozgeyik, Ozge Turgay Yildirim and Mehmet Hakan Uzun*

## Abstract

Atrial fibrillation (AF) is a prevalent cardiac arrhythmia associated with significant health risks and costs. Catheter ablation has proven effective for managing AF, offering superior outcomes compared to anti-arrhythmic drugs, particularly for maintaining sinus rhythm and reversing arrhythmia-induced cardiomyopathy. AF's pathophysiology involves disorganized atrial electrical activity, often initiated by ectopic beats from the pulmonary veins and sustained by atrial substrate remodeling. Ablation targets these ectopic foci and substrates with various techniques such as radiofrequency, cryoablation, laser balloon ablation, high-intensity focused ultrasound, electroporation, and hybrid ablation. Each technique has unique mechanisms, procedures, and efficacy profiles. Comparative studies, like the FIRE and ICE trial, demonstrate comparable efficacy between radiofrequency and cryoablation, while emerging methods like electroporation show promise. Continuous advancements in ablation technology aim to improve safety and long-term outcomes for AF patients.

**Keywords:** atrial fibrillation, catheter ablation, cryoablation, electroporation ablation, hybrid ablation, pulmonary vein isolation, radiofrequency ablation

## 1. Introduction

Atrial fibrillation (AF) is the most common sustained cardiac arrhythmia encountered in clinical practice, affecting millions of individuals worldwide. It is associated with significant morbidity, mortality, and healthcare costs. Ablation procedures have emerged as a cornerstone in the management of AF, offering the potential for symptom relief and rhythm control in patients who do not respond adequately to pharmacological therapy. In recent years, results from studies on long-term follow-up of catheter ablation have shown that catheter ablation is a safe and superior alternative to anti-arrhythmic drugs (AADs) in maintaining sinus rhythm [1]. In addition, a new clinical entity named "arrhythmia-induced cardiomyopathy" has been described in numerous studies, showing that AF may cause and/or worsen cardiomyopathy and reduce ventricular functions, and this functional deterioration may be reversed by catheter ablation [2–4]. In light of these findings, current guidelines have been updated with recommendations for AF catheter ablation in various clinical contexts.

## 2. Overview of atrial fibrillation

### 2.1 Epidemiology

Atrial fibrillation (AF) affects approximately 1–2% of the general population, with prevalence increasing with age. It is estimated that the lifetime risk of developing AF is 1 in 4 for individuals over 40 years of age. Well-known risk factors of AF development are advanced age, increased body mass index, genetic predisposition, history of smoking, hypertension, diabetes mellitus, obstructive sleep apnea, heart failure, and myocardial infarction [5]. The prevalence of AF in patients with Asian and African-American ancestry is found to be lower than in patients with European ancestry in the United States [6]. Even though the situation has been attributed to worse access to healthcare services and consequent under-detection of AF in these populations, recent studies have shown that patients with European ancestry have increased single-nucleotide polymorphism, which increases predisposition to AF, compared to patients with African-American ancestry [7, 8]. In another recent study, more than 100 genetic foci have been identified, which are associated with an increased risk of AF development [9]. Further studies are needed to expand our understanding of genetic factors to identify patients at risk of developing AF.

### 2.2 Pathophysiology

Atrial fibrillation (AF) is characterized by disorganized atrial electrical activity and ineffective atrial contraction. The pathogenesis involves complex interactions between triggers, such as ectopic beats from the pulmonary veins, and a vulnerable atrial substrate, which are often related to structural remodeling and fibrosis. The importance of ectopic beats in initiating AF arising from myocardial cells protruding toward pulmonary venous endothelium, called myocyte sleeves, has first been identified by Haissaguerre et al. [10]. Due to electrical properties and complex extracellular architecture in myocyte sleeves, these ectopic beats may trigger micro reentry and initiate AF [11]. In sustaining AF, substrates in atrial tissues play an important part. Risk factors, such as hypertension and genetic disposition, facilitate the development of substrates by causing remodeling in local cellular and extracellular architecture, impairing normal anisotropic conduction, shortening the refractory period, and increasing conduction time in the atria. This results in increased susceptibility to conduct ectopic beats and creates a reentry circuit within these substrates [12]. Electroanatomic isolation of pulmonary veins and atrial substrates has shown to be an effective treatment method in managing paroxysmal AF and has significantly increased success rates of rhythm control therapies [13]. Further research into technical aspects of electroanatomic mapping and durable lesion delivery in AF ablation has shown promising results, with novel technical methods obtaining U.S. food and drug administration (FDA) approval in the use of catheter ablation procedures.

### 2.3 Clinical presentation and diagnosis

Patients with AF may present with palpitations, dyspnea, fatigue, or may be asymptomatic. Diagnosis is confirmed through electrocardiography (ECG), showing an irregularly irregular rhythm with the absence of distinct P waves. Establishing clinical diagnosis requires at least 30 seconds of AF or the presence of AF during the entire 12-lead ECG strip [14–16]. After establishing diagnosis, initial assessment requires obtaining a detailed medical history and performing a targeted physical examination. Basic laboratory tests and transthoracic echocardiography should be performed in accordance with current guidelines to detect concomitant predisposing modifiable and non-modifiable risk factors [14–16]. An individualized strategy for thromboembolic risk management and rhythm and/or rate management is required to improve quality of life (QoL) and reduce complications related to AF [14–16].

## 3. Indications for ablation in AF

Ablation is indicated in patients with symptomatic paroxysmal or persistent AF who are refractory to or intolerant of anti-arrhythmic drugs. It is also considered in select patients with heart failure, where rhythm control is deemed beneficial. In addition, there are two important guidelines for indication of AF ablation (**Tables 1** and **2**).

### 3.1 Patient selection criteria

- Symptomatic AF despite anti-arrhythmic therapy.
- Patient preference for a non-pharmacological approach.
- Left atrial anatomy suitable for ablation.
- Absence of contraindications such as uncontrolled infection or thrombus.

### 3.2 Benefits and risks

- Benefits include symptom relief, potential reduction in AF burden, and improvement in quality of life.
- Risks involve procedural complications such as cardiac tamponade, stroke, and pulmonary vein stenosis.

## 4. Types of ablation procedures

### 4.1 Radiofrequency ablation (RFA)

- *Mechanism*: Utilizes high-frequency electrical energy to create thermal lesions, disrupting arrhythmogenic foci.
- *Procedure*: Performed via catheterization, with electrodes delivering radiofrequency energy to targeted areas within the atria.
- *Efficacy*: Success rates range from 60 to 80% for paroxysmal AF, with higher recurrence rates in persistent AF.

Radiofrequency (RF) electrical current is frequently used for ablation procedures. Catheter-tip irrigation can cool the catheter tip and surrounding tissues, concentrating

| Recommendations | Class[a] | Level[b] |
|---|---|---|
| Rhythm control therapy is recommended for symptom and QoL improvement in symptomatic patients with AF. | I | A |
| For the decision on AF catheter ablation, it is recommended to take into consideration the procedural risks and the major risk factors for AF recurrence following the procedure and discuss them with the patient. | I | B |
| Repeated PVI procedures should be considered in patients with AF recurrence provided the patient's symptoms were improved after the initial PVI. | IIa | B |
| AF catheter ablation for PVI is recommended for rhythm control after one failed or intolerant class I or III AAD, to improve symptoms of AF recurrences in patients with: | I | |
| • Paroxysmal AF | | A |
| • Persistent AF without major risk factors for recurrence | | A |
| • Persistent AF with major risk factors for recurrence | | B |
| AF catheter ablation for PVI should be considered for rhythm control after one failed or intolerant to beta-blocker treatment to improve symptoms of AF recurrences in patients with paroxysmal and persistent AF. | IIa | B |
| AF catheter ablation for PVI should/may be considered as first-line rhythm control therapy to improve symptoms in selected patients with symptomatic patients, as an alternative to AAD class I or III, considering patient choice, benefit and risk. | | |
| • Paroxysmal AF episodes | IIa | B |
| • Persistent AF without major risk factors for AF recurrence | IIb | C |
| AF catheter ablation: | | |
| • Is recommended to reverse LV dysfunction in AF patients when tachycardia-induced cardiomyopathy is highly probable, independent of their symptom status. | I | B |
| • Should be considered in selected AF patients with HF with reduced LVEF to improve survival and reduce HF hospitalization. | IIa | B |
| Complete electrical isolation of the pulmonary veins is recommended during all AF catheter-ablation procedures. | I | A |
| If the patient has a history of CTI-dependent AFL or if typical AFL is induced at the time of AF ablation, delivery of a CTI lesion may be considered. | IIb | B |
| Use of additional ablation lesions beyond PVI (low voltage areas, lines, fragmented activity, ectopic foci, rotors, and others) may be considered but is not well established. | IIb | B |
| Weight loss is recommended in obese patients with AF, particularly those who are being evaluated to undergo AF ablation. | I | B |
| Strict control of risk factors and avoidance of triggers are recommended as part of a rhythm control strategy. | I | B |

*AAD = anti-arrhythmic drug, AF = atrial fibrillation, AFL = atrial flutter, CTI = cavotricuspid isthmus, HF = heart failure, LV = left ventricular, LVEF = left ventricular ejection fraction, PVI = pulmonary vein isolation.*
*a: Class of recommendation.b: Level of evidence. (Definition for the significance of color entries can be found in 2020 ESC guideline).*

**Table 1.**
*Recommendations in 2020 ESC guidelines for atrial fibrillation catheter ablation.*

temperature increases deeper in the tissue (**Figure 1**). This reduces the risk of char or coagulum formation compared to non-irrigated catheters [17]. In the past, ablation was performed using an open irrigation catheter in power-controlled mode, and 25–30 Watt were used around the pulmonary veins (PVs) and posterior left atrium, and

| Recommendations | Class[a] | Level[b] |
|---|---|---|
| In a patient with symptomatic AF in whom antiarrhythmic drugs have been ineffective, contra-indicated, not tolerated or not preferred, and continued rhythm control is desired, catheter ablation is useful to improve symptoms. | 1 | A |
| In selected patients (generally younger with few comorbidities) with symptomatic paroxysmal AF in whom rhythm control is desired, catheter ablation is useful as first-line therapy to improve symptoms and to reduce progression to persistent AF. | 1 | A |
| In patients with symptomatic or clinically significant AFL, catheter ablation is useful for improving symptoms. | 1 | A |
| In patients who are undergoing ablation for AF, ablation of additional clinically significant supraventricular arrhythmias can be useful to reduce the likelihood of future arrhythmia. | 2a | B-NR |
| In patients (other than younger with few comorbidities) with symptomatic paroxysmal or persistent AF who are being managed with a rhythm-control strategy, catheter ablation as first line therapy can be useful to improve symptoms. | 2a | B-NR |
| Catheter ablation for symptomatic AF provides intermediate economic value compared with antiarrhythmic drug therapy. | Cost value statement: Intermediate | B-R |
| In selected* patients with asymptomatic or minimally symptomatic AF, catheter ablation may be useful for reducing progression of AF and its associated complications. | 2b | B-NR |

**Younger patients with few comorbidities and a moderate to high burden of AF or persistent AF and AFL.AAD = anti-arrhythmic drug, AF = atrial fibrillation, AFL = atrial flutter a: Class of recommendation.b: Level of evidence, NR: non-randomized, R: randomized. (Definition for the significance of color entries can be found in 2023 ACC/AHA/ACCP/HRS guidelines).*

**Table 2.**
*2023 ACC/AHA/ACCP/HRS guidelines for atrial fibrillation catheter ablation.*

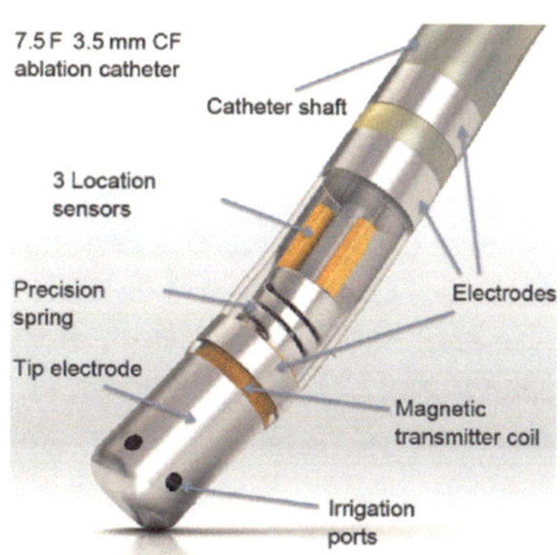


**Figure 1.**
*Schematic view of the contact force RF catheter.*

up to 30–35 Watt on the septum and anterior atrium. The irrigation flow is manually adjusted (10–60 mL/minute) to maintain temperatures below 45°C during RF application. RF energy is applied for 30–60 seconds initially or 60–120 seconds at sites showing significant effects, such as changes in PV activation pattern or isolation. While most centers prefer irrigated-tip catheters, 8-mm solid-tip catheters can also be used for atrial fibrillation (AF) ablation. Energy levels up to 50–70 W are applied with target temperatures of 50–55°C. Power is reduced on the posterior atrial wall when using non-irrigated catheters. However, in recent years, "High Power Short Duration (HPSD)" technique has been used in most of the centers. In this technique, an irrigated-tip catheter is used with 50 W and 30 mL/min flow. Ablation points were performed at the posterior wall and anterior wall for 10–12 and 15–20 seconds, respectively. HPSD technique allows physicians to avoid extracardiac organ damage [18–21]. Microbubbles detected on intracardiac echocardiography signals with non-irrigated catheters indicate excessive tissue heating and guide energy delivery titration. Before ablation, the position of the esophagus is determined using contrast swallow, intracardiac echocardiography (ICE), CT, MR, or a radiopaque nasogastric tube. Esophageal temperature monitoring is used but does not fully prevent esophageal injury due to its mobility during the procedure. Chest pain serves as a nonspecific marker for esophageal heating. Specialized RF ablation catheters allowing single-shot circumferential PV ablation have been developed. For example, the high-density mesh ablator (HDMA; Bard Electrophysiology, Lowell, MA) features 36 bipoles for high-density mapping and ablation. It achieves isolation in 88% of PVs in clinical trials [22–24]. Another example is the pulmonary vein ablation catheter (PVAC; Ablation Frontiers, Medtronic, Minneapolis, MN), which is a non-irrigated decapolar circular mapping and ablation catheter delivering bipolar and unipolar RF energy circumferentially or segmentally. Clinical studies report acute PV electrical isolation rates of 88–100%, with the absence of arrhythmia relapse in 83% of patients at 6 months [25–27].

### 4.2 Cryoablation

- *Mechanism*: Uses extreme cold to create tissue necrosis, similar to RFA but with different biophysical properties.

- *Procedure*: Typically involves the use of a balloon catheter to achieve pulmonary vein isolation (PVI).

- *Efficacy*: Comparable to RFA, with a potentially lower risk of pulmonary vein stenosis.

Pulmonary vein (PV) isolation using cryoablation became practical due to balloon catheters (Arctic Front, Medtronic, CryoCath and PolarX, Boston Scientific, St. Paul, MN, USA) designed for single-shot ostial PV ablation, emphasizing crucial tissue contact for complete isolation (**Figure 2**). Confirmation of PV occlusion by the balloon is ensured before ablation using PV angiography distal to the balloon or color Doppler with intracardiac echocardiography (**Figure 3**) [28]. Verification of PV electrical isolation necessitates a circular mapping catheter due to the balloon's lack of mapping capability. Typically, one to three 4-minute cryoablation applications are applied per vein. During cryoballoon ablation of right-sided veins, transient phrenic nerve palsy affects approximately 7% of patients. Continuous phrenic nerve pacing during cryoablation is recommended for prompt freezing cessation upon phrenic capture loss. Clinical studies report acute PV isolation rates of 93% (84–98%) and atrial fibrillation (AF) freedom in 71% (42–86%) of patients at 3–33 months [29–32]. The incidence of PV stenosis and esophageal fistula is minimal, though esophageal inflammation can occur. Focal cryoablation with a 6- or 8-mm catheter is used for PV connections not addressed by the balloon and for ablation near the esophagus on the

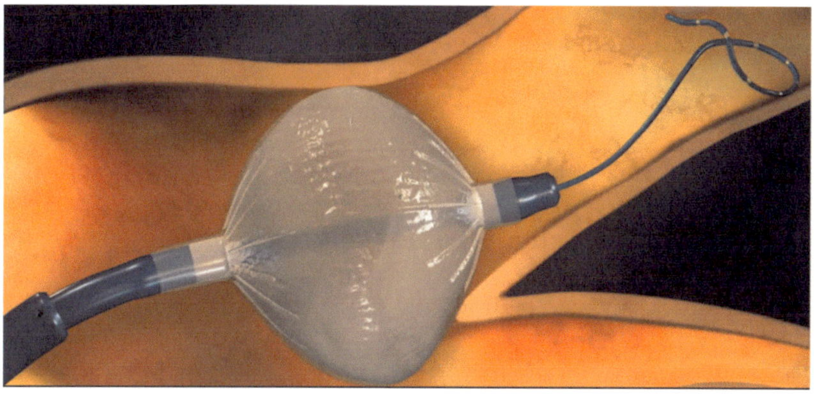

**Figure 2.**
*Schematic view of the cryoballoon ablation catheter.*

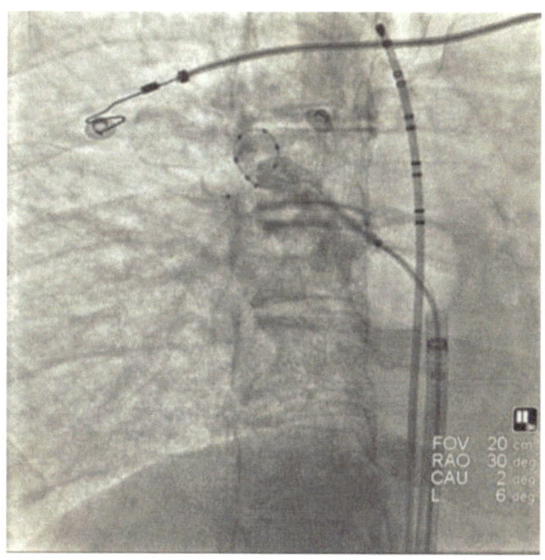


**Figure 3.**
*Fluoro image of the cryoballoon ablation catheter.*

posterior wall, as well as for more distal PV ablation when proximal isolation with radiofrequency ablation is unfeasible.

### 4.3 Laser balloon ablation

- *Mechanism*: Employs laser energy delivered through a balloon catheter to achieve precise lesions.
- *Procedure*: The balloon is inflated in the pulmonary vein ostium, and laser energy is applied circumferentially.
- *Efficacy*: Demonstrates good outcomes in achieving PVI, with an evolving role in clinical practice.

Light amplification by stimulated emission of radiation (laser) is being investigated as an alternative to RF energy for PV isolation using balloon catheters. Experimental evidence has shown that laser energy produces transmural coagulation necrosis [33–35]. In a recent clinical trial, a balloon catheter delivering laser energy through an optical fiber allowed direct endoscopic visualization of the treated area and achieved a reported success rate of 91% in acute PV isolation. After 1 year, 60% of patients remained free from arrhythmia following a single procedure [36]. It was noted that the ablation plane with all balloon catheters was more distal than initially anticipated, starting from the PV ostia and leaving the antral region without ablation [37].

### 4.4 High-intensity focused ultrasound (HIFU)

- *Mechanism*: Utilizes focused ultrasound waves to create deep, precise thermal lesions.
- *Procedure*: Performed endocardially or epicardially, though its use is less common due to technological challenges.
- *Efficacy*: Promising, but limited by current device limitations and procedural complexity.

High-intensity focused ultrasound (HIFU) energy uses ultrasound to create thermal injury delivered by a balloon-type catheter. The mechanism by which the lesion is created is a combination of coagulation necrosis and acoustic cavitation, where vibration, hyperthermia, and pressure changes lead to cellular death. Initial experience with HIFU revealed challenges, including the need for multiple applications to achieve pulmonary vein (PV) isolation, resulting in lengthy procedures. Concerns also arose regarding collateral structure damage, raising safety issues [38]. Recently, results from a clinical trial using a third generation of HIFU balloons have been published. This latest catheter version defocuses ultrasound to broaden the energy zone closer to the balloon-tissue interface, with lower energy density. It features a central lumen, allowing the insertion of a hexapolar spiral mapping catheter to monitor PV potentials and confirm isolation during ablation. In this trial involving 22 patients, acute PV isolation was achieved in 81% of PVs, and this increased to 90% with the use of a steerable sheath. Following one procedure, 71% of patients remained free from arrhythmia. Despite observing elevated esophageal temperatures in 25% of HIFU applications, no esophageal injury was reported. Further studies are needed to evaluate the safety and effectiveness of this HIFU modality in AF ablation.

### 4.5 Electroporation ablation (PFA)

- *Mechanism*: Involves the application of pulsed electrical fields to induce cell membrane permeability and cell death.
- *Procedure*: Emerging technology with ongoing research to refine safety and efficacy.
- *Efficacy*: Early studies suggest a potential for effective ablation with minimal collateral damage.

Pulsed-field ablation (PFA) represents a novel approach to treating AF by utilizing high-energy electrical pulses to induce irreversible electroporation of cardiac tissue. Unlike radiofrequency ablation, which relies on heat to create lesions, PFA works through the creation of nanopores in cell membranes, disrupting cellular integrity and leading to programmed cell death (apoptosis). This mechanism aims to create durable lesions that interrupt the abnormal electrical pathways responsible for AF maintenance.

The procedure for PFA involves the insertion of specialized catheters into the heart's atria under fluoroscopic or 3D mapping system guidance (**Figure 4**). Once positioned, the catheters deliver precisely controlled sequences of high-voltage electrical pulses. These pulses are designed to create targeted lesions in the myocardial tissue, particularly around the pulmonary veins and other critical areas involved in AF initiation and perpetuation. Real-time monitoring and mapping techniques help ensure accurate lesion formation and procedural safety.

Clinical studies investigating PFA have demonstrated promising outcomes. High rates of pulmonary vein isolation, a crucial target in AF ablation, have been reported with PFA, often achieved in a shorter procedural time than traditional methods. The ability of PFA to consistently create effective lesions may contribute to improved long-term success rates in maintaining sinus rhythm for patients with AF. In a study, 607 patients were compared with PFA and RF ablation. PFA was non-inferior to RF ablation with respect to documented atrial tachycardia in 1 year after 3-month blanking period [39].

One of the significant advantages of PFA is its potential to reduce collateral damage to adjacent structures, such as the esophagus and phrenic nerve, which can be at risk during thermal-based ablation techniques. By minimizing unintended tissue injury, PFA may enhance the safety profile of AF ablation procedures. Additionally, the non-thermal nature of PFA could mitigate the risk of thromboembolic events associated with heat-based ablation methods.

Despite its promise, PFA is not without challenges. Further research is needed to establish its long-term safety profile and efficacy compared to conventional ablation methods. Concerns include potential complications such as thromboembolic events and phrenic nerve injury, which require careful monitoring and refinement of procedural techniques. In the PULSED AF Pivotal Trial, PFA was shown to be effective at 1 year in 66.2% for paroxysmal AF and 55.1% for persistent AF. Only one patient had a primary safety endpoint (0.7%). This shows us that PFA seems safe and durable [40]. Furthermore, the combined 1-year results of the IMPULSE, PEFCAT, and PEFCAT-II studies showed that the 1-year freedom from any atrial arrhythmia was $78.5 \pm 3.8$ [41].

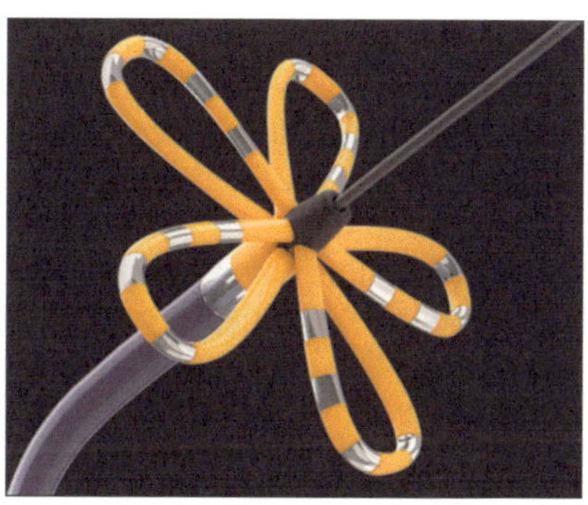

**Figure 4.**
*An example of electroporation ablation catheter.*

Ongoing research and clinical experience will be crucial in defining the role of PFA within the treatment algorithm for AF. Continued innovation in catheter design, energy delivery optimization, and patient selection criteria will likely further enhance the efficacy and safety of PFA. Ultimately, PFA holds the potential to improve outcomes and quality of life for patients with AF, offering a promising alternative to traditional ablation methods.

### 4.6 Epicardial left atrial appandage ligation (LARIAT) system

- *Mechanism:* The LARIAT system is designed to treat atrial fibrillation by closing off the left atrial appendage (LAA)

- *Procedure:* The procedure using the LARIAT system is minimally invasive and typically performed in a catheterization lab or an operating room. It involves the following steps:

    - A catheter is guided to the heart through a vein in the patient's leg or neck.

    - A small looped suture device (LARIAT snare) is then advanced through the catheter and positioned around the base of the LAA.

    - The looped suture is tightened to ligate (tie off) the LAA from the rest of the atrium, closing it off.

    - Over time, the LAA tissue that is cut off from blood flow may eventually shrink and seal off completely.

- *Efficacy:*

    - Stroke prevention

    - Minimally invasive

    - Preserves atrial function

    - Electrical isolation of LAA

Atrial fibrillation (AF) significantly increases the risk of stroke and other thromboembolic events due to the formation of blood clots in the left atrial appendage (LAA). The LARIAT system, a novel device, has emerged as a promising solution for LAA closure, particularly in patients undergoing atrial fibrillation ablation. The LAA is prone to clot formation, which can dislodge and cause stroke. The LAA is the predominant source of thromboemboli in AF patients, contributing to over 90% of left atrial thrombi in non-valvular AF. In addition, some patients have non-pulmonary vein foci that contribute to AF, such as the LAA. In the LARIAT procedure, the LAA is electrically isolated from the left atrium, helping the physician to keep the patient in sinus rhythm.

The LARIAT (SentreHEART, Inc.) system is a percutaneous, non-implant device designed to occlude the LAA by delivering a pre-tied suture loop around its base,

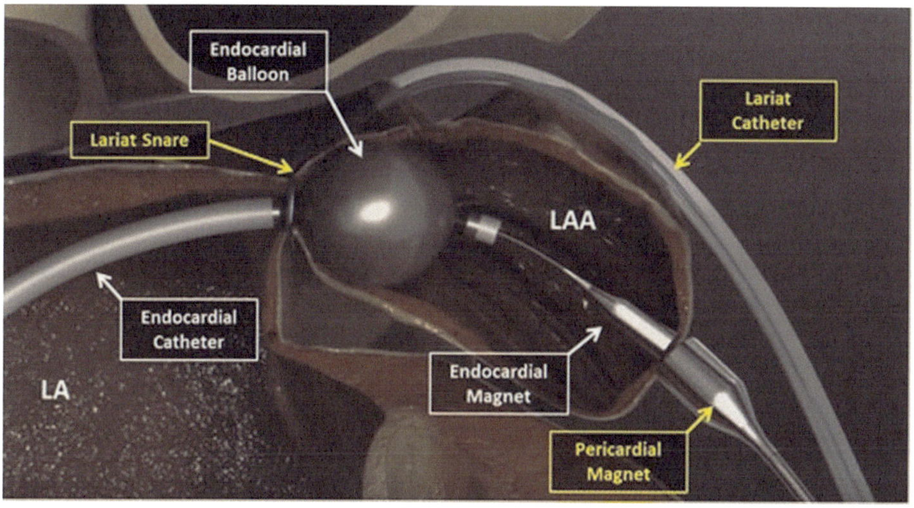


**Figure 5.**
*Schematic view of the LARIAT system.*

effectively isolating it from the left atrium (**Figure 5**). The procedure involves two main components:

1. *Transseptal puncture*: A catheter is advanced through the interatrial septum to gain access to the left atrium.

2. *Epicardial access*: A second catheter is introduced, a subxiphoid, to access the pericardial space, providing an epicardial approach to the LAA.

These two catheters are then used to guide the LARIAT suture delivery device to the base of the LAA. The suture is deployed, tightened, and secured, resulting in the complete exclusion of the LAA from systemic circulation.

Studies have demonstrated the efficacy and safety of the LARIAT system in reducing stroke risk in AF patients. Key benefits include:

- *Non-permanent*: Unlike other LAA occlusion devices (e.g., Watchman), the LARIAT does not leave a permanent implant, reducing the risk of device-related complications.

- *Stroke reduction*: Effective isolation of the LAA significantly reduces the risk of thromboembolic events.

- *Anticoagulation free*: Patients can often discontinue anticoagulation therapy, reducing bleeding risk.

In addition to stroke reduction, in the EXCLUDE LAA study, electrical LAA isolation was compared with RF and the LARIAT system. The persistence of electrical isolation after LARIAT was higher than RF isolation [42]. In the LAALA-AF registry, the primary outcome of freedom from AF at 1 year was higher in the LARIAT+RF group than only the RF group ($p = 0.002$). In addition, more patients in the RF group underwent repeat ablation because of AF recurrence [43].

The LARIAT system is indicated for patients with non-valvular atrial fibrillation who are at high risk for stroke and have contraindications to long-term anticoagulation therapy. It is contraindicated in patients with pericarditis, extensive pericardial adhesions, or anatomical variations that preclude safe access to the LAA.

While the LARIAT system offers numerous benefits, potential complications include:

- *Pericardial effusion*: Accumulation of fluid in the pericardial space.
- *Cardiac tamponade*: Severe compression of the heart due to pericardial effusion.
- *Access site complications*: Issues related to vascular access, including hematoma and infection.

The LARIAT system represents a significant advancement in the management of atrial fibrillation, providing a viable option for LAA closure in patients unsuitable for long-term anticoagulation. Its non-implant nature and effective stroke risk reduction make it a valuable tool in the electrophysiologist's arsenal. In addition, electrical isolation of LAA offers a more persistent sinus rhythm if LAA is responsible for AF recurrence.

### 4.7 Hybrid ablation

- *Mechanism*: Combines surgical and catheter-based techniques to enhance lesion formation and efficacy.
- *Procedure*: Often involves thoracoscopic surgery followed by catheter ablation, particularly in persistent AF.
- *Efficacy*: Shows promise in achieving durable rhythm control, especially in challenging cases.

Hybrid ablation combines the expertise of both cardiac surgeons and electrophysiologists to target AF from multiple angles. Unlike conventional catheter ablation performed solely by electrophysiologists, hybrid ablation involves a coordinated effort between a cardiac surgeon and an electrophysiologist working together in a hybrid operating room. This collaboration allows for a more comprehensive treatment approach, addressing the arrhythmia from inside and outside the heart simultaneously.

The procedure typically begins with the surgical component, where the cardiac surgeon accesses the heart through a small incision in the chest. This allows them to directly address certain aspects of the arrhythmia, such as removing the left atrial appendage (a common site of blood clot formation in AF patients) and creating lesions on the outside of the heart.

Following the surgical phase, the patient undergoes catheter ablation, where an electrophysiologist uses specialized catheters to navigate through blood vessels to the heart. This phase involves mapping the heart's electrical activity and delivering targeted energy to destroy or isolate the abnormal electrical pathways responsible for AF.

### 4.8 Advantages of hybrid ablation

1. *Enhanced success rates:* By combining surgical and catheter-based approaches, hybrid ablation aims to improve the likelihood of restoring normal heart rhythm compared to standalone procedures.

2. *Comprehensive treatment:* It allows for a more thorough treatment of AF by addressing both endocardial (inside the heart) and epicardial (outside the heart) aspects, potentially reducing the risk of recurrence.

3. *Patient selection:* Hybrid ablation is often considered for patients with persistent or longstanding persistent AF who have not responded well to medications or traditional catheter ablation alone.

While hybrid ablation offers promising outcomes, it is essential to note that, like any medical procedure, it carries risks such as infection, bleeding, or damage to surrounding structures. Patient selection and a thorough assessment of individual factors are crucial in determining candidacy for this approach.

Studies evaluating hybrid ablation have shown encouraging results in terms of improving quality of life, reducing AF burden, and decreasing the need for long-term medications. However, long-term data on efficacy and safety are still evolving as researchers continue to refine techniques and patient selection criteria.

Hybrid ablation represents a significant advancement in the treatment of atrial fibrillation, offering a tailored approach that combines the strengths of surgical and catheter-based interventions. As technology and techniques evolve, hybrid ablation holds promise for improving outcomes and quality of life for patients with persistent forms of AF. However, close collaboration between cardiac surgeons and electrophysiologists, along with careful patient selection and ongoing research, will continue to shape its role in managing this challenging condition. In a single center 10-year outcome study, non-paroxysmal AF patients went hybrid AF ablation, and survival from AF recurrence was 47.5% at 5 years follow-up. Complications occurred in %12.5 of patients [44]. In a meta-analysis, hybrid ablation offers good results for persistent AF patients, and 69% of patients were free from atrial arrhythmias [45].

## 5. Comparative efficacy and safety of ablation techniques

Success and complication rates vary among the different ablation techniques. Generally, RFA and cryoablation are the most commonly performed and well-studied, with established safety profiles and efficacy. Emerging techniques like electroporation and laser ablation offer potential advantages but require further validation.

The first multi-center and randomized study to compare efficacy and safety of RF and cryoballoon ablations is the FIRE AND ICE trial [46]. In this trial, a total of 762 patients were enrolled. Three hundred seventy-eight patients were assigned to cryoballoon ablation, and 384 were assigned to RF ablation. The mean length of follow-up was 1.5 years, and the main measure of effectiveness was defined as clinical failure (recurrence of atrial fibrillation, the occurrence of atrial flutter or tachycardia, use of anti-arrhythmic drugs, or repeat ablation), and was observed in 138 patients in the cryoballoon group and 143 patients in the radiofrequency group (with 1-year Kaplan-Meier event rate estimates of 34.6% and 35.9%, respectively; hazard ratio, 0.96; 95% confidence interval [CI], 0.76–1.22; $P < 0.001$ for non-inferiority). The primary safety measure was observed in 40 patients in the cryoballoon group and 51 patients in the radiofrequency group (with 1-year Kaplan-Meier event rate estimates of 10.2 and 12.8%, respectively; hazard ratio, 0.78; 95% CI, 0.52 to 1.18; $P = 0.24$) [46]. These results showed that cryoballoon ablation was non-inferior to RF ablation in terms of efficacy of treatment, with no statistically significant difference in safety between the two groups.

In another non-inferiority study, freedom from AF recurrence, safety endpoints and procedural times were compared between Cryoballoon and RF AF ablation [47]. Comparing Cryoballoon and RF ablations, the results indicated similar freedom from atrial fibrillation recurrence, with no statistically significant difference in safety between the groups. One-year freedom from atrial tachyarrhythmia, as defined by continuous rhythm monitoring, was 53.9, 52.2, and 51.7% for CF-RF, Cryo-4, and Cryo-2, respectively (P = 0.87). Additionally, 1-year freedom from symptomatic atrial tachyarrhythmia defined by continuous rhythm monitoring was 79.1, 78.2, and 73.3% for CF-RF, Cryo-4, and Cryo-2, respectively (P = 0.26). The reduction in atrial fibrillation burden varied slightly: 99.3% with CF-RF, 99.9% with Cryo-4, and 98.4% with Cryo-2 (P = 0.36). The occurrence of serious adverse events was 2.6% in the CF-RF group, 5.3% in the Cryo-4 group, and 6.0% in the Cryo-2 group, with no significant difference between the groups (P = 0.24). Furthermore, the RF ablation group had a significantly longer procedural duration but significantly shorter fluoroscopy exposure than the cryoballoon groups [47].

In a study comparing hybrid versus RF ablation in persistent AF, freedom from atrial tachyarrhythmias or anti-arrhythmic drug use was higher in the RF ablation group compared with the hybrid ablation group (89 vs. 41%, P = 0.002) (48). In safety terms, one patient required pericardiocentesis due to pericarditis, and one femoral arteriovenous fistula occurred in the hybrid ablation group (48). There were no deaths, strokes, need for pacemaker implantation, or conversions to sternotomy, and the number of (serious) adverse events was comparable between groups (21 vs. 14%, P = 0.685) [48].

A meta-analysis by Eranki et al. on four randomized trials compared freedom from AF durations. In these trials, 233 patients underwent hybrid ablation, and 189 underwent catheter ablation. Significantly more patients in the hybrid ablation group experienced major postoperative complications, with an odds ratio of 5.14 (95% CI 1.70–15.54, P < 0.01). A single death was reported in the hybrid ablation cohorts, while there were no deaths in the catheter ablation cohort [49].

In recent years, the number of studies comparing efficacy and safety of PFA with RF ablation has continually increased. A study conducted by Reddy VY et al. enrolled 607 patients and randomized 305 patients into the PFA group and 302 patients into the RF ablation group. At the 1-year mark, the primary efficacy endpoint, where no events occurred, was achieved in 204 patients (estimated probability, 73.3%) who underwent PFA and 194 patients (estimated probability, 71.3%) who underwent RF ablation. The difference between the two groups was 2.0 percentage points, with a 95% Bayesian credible interval of −5.2 to 9.2 and a posterior probability of non-inferiority greater than 0.999 (50). Regarding the primary safety endpoint, events occurred in six patients (estimated incidence, 2.1%) treated with PFA and four patients (estimated incidence, 1.5%) treated with RF ablation. The between-group difference was 0.6 percentage points, with a 95% Bayesian credible interval of −1.5–2.8 and a posterior probability of non-inferiority greater than 0.999 [50].

A literature review and indirect treatment comparison by Maccioni et al. reviewed three PFA studies enrolling 497 patients and six cryoballoon ablation studies enrolling 1113 patients and found that PFA was associated with significantly lower major adverse event risk ([95% confidence interval (CI) −5.8, −2.8]; risk ratio 0.16 [95% CI 0.07, 0.45]) (51). Meta-analyzes confirmed these findings, with major adverse events for PFA [0.4% (95% CI 0.0, 1.3)] vs. CBA [5.6% (95% CI 2.6, 8.6)] [51].

## 6. Conclusion

Ablation procedures have revolutionized the management of atrial fibrillation, offering significant benefits to selected patients. Continuous advancements in technology and technique hold promise for further improving outcomes and expanding the role of ablation in AF management. Although there are various AF ablation methods suitable for use in clinical practice, each method has its own advantages and disadvantages. In light of this, it should not be forgotten that procedural risks can be minimized by individualizing ablation strategy according to anatomical variations and the type of the planned procedure.

## Author details

Mehmet Ozgeyik[1*], Ozge Turgay Yildirim[1] and Mehmet Hakan Uzun[2]

1 Eskisehir City Hospital, Health Sciences University, Eskisehir, Turkey

2 Kutahya City Hospital, Kutahya Health Sciences University, Kutahya, Turkey

*Address all correspondence to: mehmetozgeyik@hotmail.com

## References

[1] Arbelo E, Brugada J, Blomstrom-Lundqvist C, Laroche C, Kautzner J, Pokushalov E, et al. On the behalf of the ESC EHRA Atrial Fibrillation Ablation Long-term Registry Investigators. Contemporary management of patients undergoing atrial fibrillation ablation: In-hospital and 1-year follow-up findings from the ESC-EHRA atrial fibrillation ablation long-term registry. European Heart Journal. 2017;**38**:1303–1316

[2] Qin D, Mansour MC, Ruskin JN, Heist EK. Atrial fibrillation-mediated cardiomyopathy. Circulation: Arrhythmia and Electrophysiology. 2019;**12**(12):e007809. DOI: 10.1161/CIRCEP.119.007809. Epub 2019 December 12

[3] Di Biase L, Mohanty P, Mohanty S, Santangeli P, Trivedi C, Lakkireddy D, et al. Ablation versus amiodarone for treatment of persistent atrial fibrillation in patients with congestive heart failure and an implanted device: Results from the AATAC multicenter randomized trial. Circulation. 2016;**133**:1637-1644

[4] Marrouche NF, Brachmann J, Andresen D, Siebels J, Boersma L, Jordaens L, et al. CASTLE-AF Investigators. Catheter ablation for atrial fibrillation with heart failure. The New England Journal of Medicine. 2018;**378**:417–427

[5] Kornej J, Börschel CS, Benjamin EJ, Schnabel RB. Epidemiology of atrial fibrillation in the 21st century: Novel methods and new insights. Circulation Research. 2020;**127**(1):4-20. DOI: 10.1161/CIRCRESAHA.120.316340. Epub 2020 June 18

[6] Borzecki AM, Bridgers DK, Liebschutz JM, Kader B, Kazis LE, Berlowitz DR. Racial differences in the prevalence of atrial fibrillation among males. Journal of the National Medical Association. 2008;**100**:237-245

[7] Soliman EZ, Alonso A, Goff DC Jr. Atrial fibrillation and ethnicity: The known, the unknown and the paradox. Future Cardiology. 2009;**5**:547-556

[8] Roberts JD, Hu D, Heckbert SR, Alonso A, Dewland TA, Vittinghoff E, et al. Genetic investigation into the differential risk of atrial fibrillation among black and white individuals. JAMA Cardiology. 2016;**1**:442-450

[9] Zhang J, Johnsen SP, Guo Y, Lip GYH. Epidemiology of atrial fibrillation: Geographic/ecological risk factors, age, sex, genetics. Cardiac Electrophysiology Clinics. 2021;**13**(1):1-23. DOI: 10.1016/j.ccep.2020.10.010. Epub 2021 January 8

[10] Haissaguerre M, Jais P, Shah DC, Takahashi A, Hocini M, Quiniou G, et al. Spontaneous initiation of atrial fibrillation by ectopic beats originating in the pulmonary veins. The New England Journal of Medicine. 1998;**339**:659-666

[11] Hocini M, Ho SY, Kawara T, Linnenbank AC, Potse M, Shah D, et al. Electrical conduction in canine pulmonary veins: Electrophysiological and anatomic correlation. Circulation. 2002;**105**:2442-2448

[12] Staerk L, Sherer JA, Ko D, Benjamin EJ, Helm RH. Atrial fibrillation: Epidemiology, pathophysiology, and clinical outcomes. Circulation Research. 2017;**120**(9):1501-1517. DOI: 10.1161/CIRCRESAHA.117.309732

[13] Loring Z et al. Procedural patterns and safety of atrial fibrillation ablation: Findings from get with the guidelines-atrial fibrillation. Circulation: Arrhythmia and Electrophysiology. 2020;**13**(9):e007944

[14] Hindricks G, Potpara T, Dagres N, Arbelo E, Bax JJ, Blomström-Lundqvist C, et al. ESC Scientific Document Group. 2020 ESC guidelines for the diagnosis and management of atrial fibrillation developed in collaboration with the European Association for Cardio-Thoracic Surgery (EACTS): The task force for the diagnosis and management of atrial fibrillation of the European Society of Cardiology (ESC) developed with the special contribution of the European Heart Rhythm Association (EHRA) of the ESC. European Heart Journal. 2021;**42**(5): 373-498. DOI: 10.1093/eurheartj/ehaa612. Erratum in: Eur Heart J. 2021 Feb 1;42(5):507. doi: 10.1093/eurheartj/ehaa798. Erratum in: Eur Heart J. 2021 Feb 1;42(5):546-547. doi: 10.1093/eurheartj/ehaa945. Erratum in: Eur Heart J. 2021 Oct 21;42(40):4194. doi: 10.1093/eurheartj/ehab648

[15] Joglar JA, Chung MK, Armbruster AL, Benjamin EJ, Chyou JY, Cronin EM, et al. Peer Review Committee Members. 2023 ACC/AHA/ACCP/HRS guideline for the diagnosis and management of atrial fibrillation: A report of the American College of Cardiology/American Heart Association Joint Committee on clinical practice guidelines. Circulation. 2024;**149**(1):e1-e156. DOI: 10.1161/CIR.0000000000001193. Epub 2023 November 30. Erratum in: Circulation. 2024 Jan 2;149(1):e167. doi: 10.1161/CIR.0000000000001207. Erratum in: Circulation. 2024 Feb 27;149(9):e936. doi: 10.1161/CIR.0000000000001218. Erratum in: Circulation. 2024 Jun 11;149(24):e1413. doi: 10.1161/CIR.0000000000001263

[16] Andrade JG, Aguilar M, Atzema C, Bell A, Cairns JA, Cheung CC, et al. Members of the Secondary Panel. The 2020 Canadian Cardiovascular Society/Canadian Heart Rhythm Society comprehensive guidelines for the management of atrial fibrillation. The Canadian Journal of Cardiology. 2020; **36**(12):1847-1948. DOI: 10.1016/j.cjca.2020.09.001. Epub 2020 October 22

[17] Macle L, Jais P, Weerasooriya R, et al. Irrigated-tip catheter ablation of pulmonary veins for treatment of atrial fibrillation. Journal of Cardiovascular Electrophysiology. 2002;**13**:1067-1073

[18] Knotts RJ, Barbhaiya CR. High-power, short-duration ablation for atrial fibrillation: Pros and cons. Progress in Cardiovascular Diseases. 2021;**66**:86-91. DOI: 10.1016/j.pcad.2021.06.005

[19] Naniwadekar A, Dukkipati SR. High-power short-duration ablation of atrial fibrillation: A contemporary review. Pacing and Clinical Electrophysiology. 2021;**44**(3):528-540. DOI: 10.1111/pace.14167. Epub 2021 January 31

[20] Junarta J, Rodriguez S, Ullah W, Siddiqui MU, Riley JM, Patel A, et al. Comparison of very high-power short-duration, high-power short-duration, and low-power long-duration radiofrequency ablation for atrial fibrillation: A systematic review and network meta-analysis. Pacing and Clinical Electrophysiology. 2023;**46**(12): 1609-1634. DOI: 10.1111/pace.14879. Epub 2023 November 16

[21] Xu M, Yang Y, Zhang D, Jiang W. Meta-analysis of high power short duration in atrial fibrillation ablation - A superior efficient ablation strategy. Acta Cardiologica. 2022;**77**(1):14-32. DOI: 10.1080/00015385.2021.1939512. Epub 2021 July 5

[22] Meissner A, Plehn G, Van Bracht M, et al. First experiences for pulmonary vein isolation with the high-density mesh ablator (HDMA): A novel mesh electrode catheter for both mapping and radiofrequency delivery in a single unit. Journal of Cardiovascular Electrophysiology. 2009;**20**:359-366

[23] Pratola C, Notarstefano P, Artale P, et al. Radiofrequency ablation of paroxysmal atrial fibrillation by mesh catheter. Journal of Interventional Cardiac Electrophysiology. 2009;**25**: 135-140

[24] Arruda MS, He DS, Friedman P, et al. A novel mesh electrode catheter for mapping and radiofrequency delivery at the left atrium-pulmonary vein junction: A single-catheter approach to pulmonary vein antrum isolation. Journal of Cardiovascular Electrophysiology. 2007; **18**:206-211

[25] Fredersdorf S, Weber S, Jilek C, et al. Safe and rapid isolation of pulmonary veins using a novel circular ablation catheter and duty-cycled RF generator. Journal of Cardiovascular Electrophysiology. 2009;**20**:1097-1101

[26] Wijffels MC, Van Oosternhout M, Boersma LV, et al. Characterization of in vitro and in vivo lesions made by a novel multichannel ablation generator and a circumlinear decapolar ablation catheter. Journal of Cardiovascular Electrophysiology. 2009;**20**:1142-1148

[27] Boersma LV, Wijffels MC, Oral H, et al. Pulmonary vein isolation by duty cycled bipolar and unipolar radiofrequency energy with a multielectrode ablation catheter. Heart Rhythm. 2008;**5**:1635-1642

[28] Siklody CH, Minners J, Allgeier M, et al. Cryoballoon pulmonary vein isolation guided by transesophageal echocardiography: Novel aspects on an emerging ablation technique. Journal of Cardiovascular Electrophysiology. 2009; **20**:1197-1202

[29] Chun KR, Schmidt B, Metzner A, et al. The 'single big cryoballoon' technique for acute pulmonary vein isolation in patients with paroxysmal atrial fibrillation: A prospective observational single centre study. European Heart Journal. 2009;**30**: 699-709

[30] Malmborg H, Lonnerholm S, Blomstrom-Lundqvist C. Acute and clinical effects of cryoballoon pulmonary vein isolation in patients with symptomatic paroxysmal and persistent atrial fibrillation. Europace. 2008;**10**: 1277-1280

[31] Van Belle Y, Janse P, Rivero-Ayerza MJ, et al. Pulmonary vein isolation using an occluding cryoballoon for circumferential ablation: Feasibility, complications, and short-term outcome. European Heart Journal. 2007;**28**: 2231-2237

[32] Neumann T, Vogt J, Schumacher B, et al. Circumferential pulmonary vein isolation with the cryoballoon technique results from a prospective 3-center study. Journal of the American College of Cardiology. 2008;**52**:273-278

[33] Fried NM, Tsitlik A, Rent KC, et al. Laser ablation of the pulmonary veins by using a fiberoptic balloon catheter: Implications for treatment of paroxysmal atrial fibrillation. Lasers in Surgery and Medicine. 2001;**28**:197-203

[34] Lemery R, Veinot JP, Tang AS, et al. Fiberoptic balloon catheter ablation of pulmonary vein ostia in pigs using photonic energy delivery with diode laser. Pacing and Clinical Electrophysiology. 2002;**25**:32-36

[35] Reddy VY, Houghtaling C, Fallon J, et al. Use of a diode laser balloon ablation catheter to generate circumferential pulmonary venous lesions in an open thoracotomy caprine model. Pacing and Clinical Electrophysiology. 2004;**27**: 52-57

[36] Reddy VY, Neuzil P, Themistoclakis S, et al. Visually-guided balloon catheter ablation of atrial fibrillation: Experimental feasibility and first-in-human multicenter clinical outcome. Circulation. 2009;**120**:12-20

[37] Phillips KP, Schweikert RA, Saliba WI, et al. Anatomic location of pulmonary vein electrical disconnection with balloon-based catheter ablation. Journal of Cardiovascular Electrophysiology. 2008;**19**:14-18

[38] Schmidt B, Antz M, Ernst S, et al. Pulmonary vein isolation by high-intensity focused ultrasound: First-in-man study with a steerable balloon catheter. Heart Rhythm. 2007;**4**:575-584

[39] Reddy VY, Gerstenfeld EP, Natale A, Whang W, Cuoco FA., Patel C, et al. ADVENT Investigators. Pulsed field or conventional thermal ablation for paroxysmal atrial fibrillation. The New England Journal of Medicine. 2023; **389**(18):1660–1671

[40] Verma A, Haines DE, Boersma LV, Sood N, Natale A, Marchlinski FE, et al. PULSED AF Investigators. Pulsed field ablation for the treatment of atrial fibrillation: PULSED AF pivotal trial. Circulation. 2023;**147**(19):1422–1432

[41] Reddy VY, Dukkipati SR, Neuzil P, Anic A, Petru J, Funasako M, et al. Pulsed field ablation of paroxysmal atrial fibrillation: 1-year outcomes of IMPULSE, PEFCAT, and PEFCAT II. JACC: Clinical Electrophysiology. 2021; 7(5):614-627

[42] Parikh V, Rasekh A, Mohanty S, Yarlagadda B, Atkins D, Bommana S, et al. Exclusion of electrical and mechanical function of the left atrial appendage in patients with persistent atrial fibrillation: Differences in efficacy and safety between endocardial ablation vs epicardial LARIAT ligation (the EXCLUDE LAA study). Journal of Interventional Cardiac Electrophysiology: An International Journal of Arrhythmias and Pacing. 2020;**57**(3):409-416

[43] Lakkireddy D, Sridhar Mahankali A, Kanmanthareddy A, Lee R, Badhwar N, Bartus K, et al. Left atrial appendage ligation and ablation for persistent atrial fibrillation: The LAALA-AF registry. JACC: Clinical Electrophysiology. 2015; **1**(3):153-160. DOI: 10.1016/j.jacep.2015.04.006

[44] Pannone L, Mouram S, Della Rocca DG, Sorgente A, Monaco C, Del Monte A, et al. Hybrid atrial fibrillation ablation: Long-term outcomes from a single-centre 10-year experience. Europace: European Pacing, Arrhythmias, and Cardiac Electrophysiology: Journal of the Working Groups on Cardiac Pacing, Arrhythmias, and Cardiac Cellular Electrophysiology of the European Society of Cardiology. 2023;**25**(5): euad114. DOI: 10.1093/europace/euad114

[45] Shrestha S, Plasseraud KM, Makati K, Sood N, Killu AM, Contractor T, et al. Hybrid convergent ablation for atrial fibrillation: A systematic review and meta-analysis. Heart Rhythm O2. 2022;**3**(4):396-404. DOI: 10.1016/j.hroo.2022.05.006

[46] Kuck KH, Brugada J, Fürnkranz A, Metzner A, Ouyang F, Chun KR, et al.; FIRE and ICE Investigators. Cryoballoon or radiofrequency ablation for

paroxysmal atrial fibrillation. The New England Journal of Medicine. 2016; **374**(23):2235-2245. DOI: 10.1056/NEJMoa1602014. Epub 2016 April 4

[47] Andrade JG, Champagne J, Dubuc M, Deyell MW, Verma A, Macle L, et al. CIRCA-DOSE Study Investigators. Cryoballoon or radiofrequency ablation for atrial fibrillation assessed by continuous monitoring: A randomized clinical trial. Circulation. 2019;**140**(22):1779-1788. DOI: 10.1161/CIRCULATIONAHA.119.042622. Epub 2019 October 21

[48] van der Heijden CAJ, Weberndörfer V, Vroomen M, Luermans JG, Chaldoupi SM, Bidar E, et al. Hybrid ablation versus repeated catheter ablation in persistent atrial fibrillation: A randomized controlled trial. JACC: Clinical Electrophysiology. 2023;**9**(7 Pt 2):1013-1023. DOI: 10.1016/j.jacep.2022.12.011. Epub 2023 January 18

[49] Eranki A, Wilson-Smith AR, Williams ML, Flynn CD, Manganas C. Hybrid convergent ablation versus endocardial catheter ablation for atrial fibrillation: A systematic review and meta-analysis of randomised control trials and propensity matched studies. Journal of Cardiothoracic Surgery. 2022; **17**(1):181. DOI: 10.1186/s13019-022-01930-7

[50] Reddy VY, Gerstenfeld EP, Natale A, Whang W, Cuoco FA, Patel C, et al. ADVENT Investigators. Pulsed field or conventional thermal ablation for paroxysmal atrial fibrillation. The New England Journal of Medicine. 2023; **389**(18):1660-1671. DOI: 10.1056/NEJMoa2307291. Epub 2023 August 27

[51] Maccioni S, Sharma R, Lee DD, Haltner A, Khanna R, Vijgen J. Comparative safety of pulsed field ablation and cryoballoon ablation technologies for pulmonary vein isolation in patients with paroxysmal atrial fibrillation: A critical literature review and indirect treatment comparison. Advances in Therapy. 2024;**41**(3): 932-944. DOI: 10.1007/s12325-023-02765-x. Epub 2024 January 8

Chapter 11

# New Insights into Cardiac Ablation

*Shriya Sharma, Rohan M. Goswami, Juan Leoni and Jose Ruiz*

## Abstract

Catheter ablation has emerged as a significant treatment approach to treat symptoms and regulate heart rate or rhythm. This review highlights the evolution of catheter ablation, focusing on its applications in atrial fibrillation (AF). Radiofrequency (RF) catheter ablation has become a primary treatment option due to its high success rate and minimal adverse effects. Using three-dimensional (3D) reconstruction and mapping systems enhances precision in targeting arrhythmogenic substrates.

**Keywords:** catheter ablation, arrhythmia, mapping, radiofrequency, pulmonary vein, PFA

## 1. Introduction

Catheter ablation involves using an electrode catheter to eliminate specific small areas of heart tissue or the conduction system, which are crucial in causing or perpetuating cardiac arrhythmias. In addition to antiarrhythmic medications, catheter ablation provides an effective and potentially curative treatment for patients with complex congenital heart disease, focusing on the source of underlying arrhythmias. The use of 3D reconstruction from MRI or computed tomography is beneficial for understanding heart anatomy, pinpointing the target chamber, and assisting in access planning [1].

Due to its high success rate and minimal adverse effects, radiofrequency (RF) catheter ablation has emerged as a primary treatment option for numerous arrhythmias. In this procedure, one or more electrode catheters are introduced percutaneously through the vasculature to contact cardiac tissues. A diagnostic study is conducted to understand the mechanism of the arrhythmia, and then an ablation catheter is positioned adjacent to the arrhythmogenic substrate. Radiofrequency energy, reaching up to 50 W, is delivered in the form of a continuous, unmodulated sinusoidal waveform, typically for 60 seconds. The application of energy is well tolerated by a mildly sedated patient and results in the creation of a small, well-defined lesion (5 mm). This process involves the destruction of tissue critical for arrhythmogenesis, such as an accessory pathway, and its subsequent replacement with scar tissue, effectively eliminating the arrhythmia [2].

RF catheter ablation has become a primary treatment choice for various arrhythmias due to its high success rate and minimal adverse effects. Electrode catheters are inserted percutaneously through blood vessels to reach the heart tissues. A diagnostic study is performed to understand the arrhythmia mechanism, followed by positioning an ablation catheter near the area causing the arrhythmia. Radiofrequency energy,


IntechOpen

typically delivered at up to 50 W in a continuous, unmodulated sinusoidal waveform for around 60 seconds, is used. This energy application is well tolerated by patients under mild sedation and leads to the creation of a small, well-defined lesion (5 mm). This process involves the destruction of tissue responsible for causing arrhythmias, such as an accessory pathway, and its replacement with scar tissue, effectively eliminating arrhythmia [2].

## 2. AF ablation

The development of AF from sporadic and brief occurrences to more sustained forms is a typical progression seen in many affected individuals. However, the specific patterns of this progression can vary significantly among individuals.

While some patients may experience a rapid progression, others may have rare and brief episodes for an extended period. Nevertheless, there is a general trend toward AF progression in all patients. It remains unclear whether AF itself contributes to this progression, prompting the question of whether early AF ablation could be a viable strategy to slow down or halt AF progression [3].

Catheter ablation has become an essential strategy for controlling the rhythm in AF and is the most performed cardiac ablation procedure globally. According to current guidelines, this procedure is recommended for symptomatic patients with paroxysmal or persistent AF who do not respond well to or cannot tolerate antiarrhythmic medications. In some cases, it may also be considered as an initial treatment for asymptomatic patients. Although data from large studies suggest that AF ablation may reduce mortality, heart failure, and stroke risk, evidence from randomized controlled trials is not conclusive. Pulmonary vein isolation, achieved through either point-by-point radiofrequency or cryoballoon techniques, remains primary method in AF ablation. The primary objectives in managing patients with AF include symptom improvement, heart rate or rhythm control, and reducing the risk of stroke [4].

Achieving electrical isolation through circumferential ablation of the pulmonary veins constitutes a fundamental aspect in most AF ablation procedures. This method entails creating a series of radiofrequency lesions, implemented point by point, encircling the two left and two right PVs. This can be achieved either through a singular circumferential lesion surrounding each set of PVs or by incorporating lesions between ipsilateral PVs, resulting in a figure-eight lesion set. The confirmation of PV isolation is commonly conducted using a circular multipolar electrode catheter. The primary tools used for this procedure are irrigated radiofrequency ablation catheters, often used with an electroanatomic mapping system [5].

### 2.1 The SARA trial

Although several studies have demonstrated superiority of catheter ablation over anti-arrhythmic drugs (AAD) in patients with paroxysmal AF, the Study of Ablation Versus Antiarrhythmic Drugs in Persistent Atrial Fibrillation (SARA) study is the first multicenter, randomized controlled trial conceived to specifically evaluate patients with persistent AF. In this study, catheter ablation was demonstrated to be superior to rhythm control at mid-term follow-up, with a significant QoL improvement. Of note, the ablation approach was PV isolation-only in most cases, with a very low proportion of additional substrate modification. This adds evidence to the hypothesis that limited ablation may be effective in a well-selected population with persistent AF.

This study included 146 patients with persistent drug-refractory AF. The primary endpoint, sustained episodes of AF (>24 hours) after a three-month blanking period, showed that the catheter ablation group had a significantly higher proportion of patients free of sustained AF episodes at 12 months compared to the AAD group (70.4 vs. 43.7%). Additionally, the catheter ablation group demonstrated a higher probability of remaining free of any AF recurrence (>30 seconds) and a lower need for electrical cardioversion. Patients with early recurrences were at a higher risk of reaching the primary endpoint. Quality of life scores did not significantly differ between groups. Complication rates were low in both the catheter ablation group (6.1%) and the AAD group (4.7%). The SARA study concludes that catheter ablation is superior to AAD for rhythm control in patients with persistent AF [6].

## 3. Mapping

Cardiac mapping involves the precise maneuvering of a mapping or ablation catheter within the targeted region, searching for the site where radiofrequency or cryothermal ablation can effectively treat the arrhythmia.

Techniques for mapping, such as ultra-high-density mapping, isochronal late activation mapping, and ripple mapping, have improved the identification of arrhythmogenic substrates. These advancements not only offer the potential for procedural success but also contribute to minimizing the duration of ablation procedures and reducing the risk of hemodynamic compromise. Sophisticated mapping and ablation techniques, such as epicardial and intramyocardial approaches, enable operators to accurately pinpoint arrhythmogenic substrates [7].

The utilization of a 3D electroanatomic mapping system helps to achieve multiple objectives in catheter ablation procedures. Firstly, it facilitates the localization of catheters without the need for radiographs. Secondly, it calculates and displays 3D representations of electrical activation sequences (activation maps) and local voltage distributions (voltage maps). Thirdly, it visually presents the anatomy of a heart chamber in three dimensions through sequential catheter localization [8].

The superimposition of 3D electroanatomic maps onto the reconstructed surfaces of every cardiac structure enhances the visualization and understanding of the procedure. This operates on a point-by-point basis, requiring a stable arrhythmia and thorough exploration of all relevant sites to generate a comprehensive 3D reconstruction of the activation sequence associated with any arrhythmia. Incomplete mapping may lead to inconclusive maps and unsuccessful ablation attempts [8].

The mapping system consists of an acquisition module linked to a computer capable of concurrently analyzing diverse signals: 32 bipolar electrograms from the basket catheter, 16 bipolar/unipolar electrogram signals, a 12-lead ECG, and a pressure signal. It generates real-time color-coded activation maps, with the electrograms and activation maps presented on a computer monitor. The recorded signals are storable for later offline analysis. Activation marks are automatically generated using algorithms based on peak or slope and manual editing of activation times is performed, as necessary (**Figure 1**) [9].

Challenges may arise in cases involving a chronically volume-overloaded or scarred myocardium, potentially hindering successful catheter ablation even with precise 3D mapping. The implementation of irrigated tip catheter with increased lesion depth has positively impacted the capacity to produce transmural lesions, addressing certain limitations. However, issues persist in scenarios with restricted

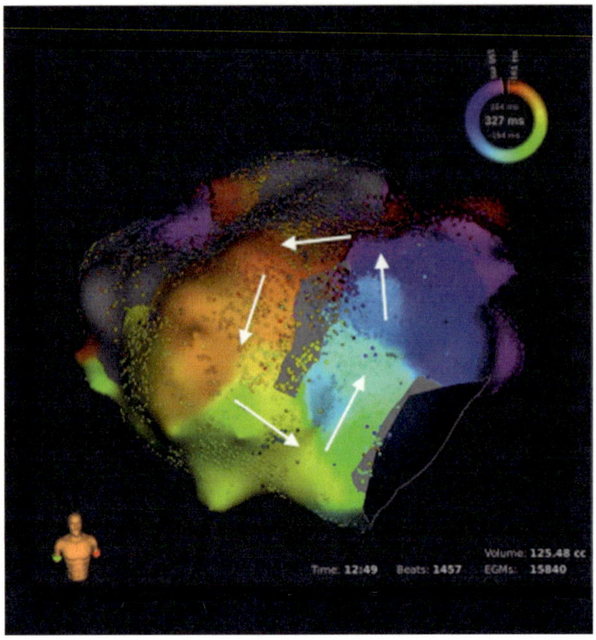


**Figure 1.**
*Example of three-dimensional maps acquired using the RHYTHMIA™ system. Left atrial re-entry on the anterior and septal aspect of the mitral annulus; arrows display the direction of rotation around a small area of scar (grey) [1].*

catheter-tissue contact, such as in extensively dilated atrial chambers, or when variations in blood flow impact lesion formation [8].

## 4. Mapping systems

Achieving seamless, transmural lesions in a beating heart is challenging and demands reliable 3D navigation to mitigate potential complications such as pulmonary vein stenosis, perforation, or nerve injuries. Electroanatomical-mapping systems (EAMs) have been devised to aid catheter ablation procedures with reduced radiation exposure compared to fluoroscopy. These systems track intracardiac electrodes in 3D maps, enhancing navigation during ablation. However, conventional mapping systems struggle to detect localized AF drivers due to their sequential spatiotemporal characteristics, intermittent firing, and spatial variability. Consequently, advanced mapping tools have been developed to visualize and comprehend AF-maintaining drivers more effectively [10].

The widely utilized 3D mapping systems include CARTO by Biosense Webster and EnSite Precision by Abbott. Boston Scientific's Rhythmia system, recently introduced, has significantly contributed to the advancement of high-density mapping for complex arrhythmias [11].

### 4.1 The CARTO system

The CARTO system, initially introduced in 1996, employs magnetic fields for electroanatomical navigation and geometry reconstruction. This system utilizes ultralow magnetic fields ranging from 0.05 to 0.2 gauss ($5 \times 10^{-5}$ to $5 \times 10^{-6}$ Tesla) for triangulation. Three magnetic generators placed beneath the operating table allow continuous measurement of the catheter's distance, facilitating precise localization of its tip in space.

Recent advancements in the CARTO system include the capability to visualize non-dedicated catheters (non-magnetic) through impedance-based navigation, utilizing six skin patches like the NavX system. However, these non-dedicated catheters cannot be utilized for geometry construction or local information tagging on maps. Additionally, the CARTO system offers intracardiac echocardiography-based 3D reconstruction and integration of rotational angiography or fluoroscopy views.

The developments in the CARTO system involve automated annotation of radiofrequency application locations with adequate contact force and the integration of fluoroscopic views/movies [10].

### 4.2 The EnSite NavX system

The EnSite system comprises three pairs of skin patches along with a system reference patch, utilizing impedance-based localization and tracking methods. These patches, when placed on the patient's skin, establish electrical fields along three perpendicular axes. By emitting low-power currents of 350 mA at 8 kHz frequency through the three pairs of patches, a 3D electrical field centered around the heart is formed.

For anatomical reference, the EnSite system employs either the system reference patch on the patient's body or an intracardiac electrode, enhancing compensation for cardiac and respiratory motion artifacts. The latest version, the EnSite Precision cardiac mapping system, combines the benefits of hybrid impedance and magnetic field technologies, offering significantly improved precision and accuracy compared to earlier versions.

The Precision system necessitates an additional magnetic field source, termed the EnSite Precision field frame, and two extra sensors on the patient. This frame, affixed beneath the patient's table, generates a weak magnetic field like the CARTO system's location pad [11].

### 4.3 The RHYTHMIA system

The RHYTHMIA system introduces cutting-edge 3D mapping technology characterized by exceptionally high resolution, employing both magnetic and impedance-based localization methods. It utilizes a unique multipolar basket-like catheter equipped with small non-circular electrodes to optimize the recording of electrocardiograms and anatomical reconstruction.

This specialized catheter design enhances the system's capability to reject "far-field" signals and capture "near-field" local potentials, even at minimal amplitudes. Consequently, mapping is expedited, definitions are precise, and the signal-to-noise ratio is notably high, resulting in fewer artifacts. Additionally, the system incorporates an intelligent algorithm that analyzes wave propagation, automatically identifying areas of blockage with remarkable reliability [10].

## 5. Advantages of RFA

The advantages of using radiofrequency lesions in the treatment of certain arrhythmias stem from the small size of these lesions. This approach has proven phenomenally successful in addressing arrhythmias with a focal origin or those dependent on a narrow isthmus for maintenance. The effectiveness of ablation is particularly in cases where arrhythmias have anatomically based or directed substrates, such as accessory pathways and atrioventricular nodal re-entry tachycardia (AVNRT).

Accessory pathways, anomalous connections between the atria and ventricles, are commonly found along the mitral or tricuspid valve annulus. The key to successful ablation in such cases lies in precise lesion placement. Fluoroscopically guided by an electrode catheter in the coronary sinus, the ablation catheter's position is directed along the mitral annulus. The bipolar electrogram, specifically the relative amplitude of atrial and ventricular components, recorded by the ablation catheter, aids in positioning relative to the annulus. Identifying the earliest atrial or ventricular activation during pathway conduction assists in locating the pathway along the annulus. In cases of AVNRT, where the target for catheter ablation is in the posteroseptum, the procedure becomes more predictable. Ablation can be guided solely by anatomical landmarks relative to His bundle and coronary sinus catheter positions using fluoroscopy. Alternatively, an approach involving both anatomic and electrogram considerations may be employed. This combination enhances the precision and effectiveness of the ablation procedure in treating specific arrhythmias [11, 12].

## 6. Contraindications

- Unstable angina
- Bloodstream infection
- Acute worsening of congestive heart failure not due to the arrhythmia
- Significant tendency for excessive bleeding
- Acute blood clot in the veins of the lower extremities if femoral vein cannulation is desired
- Presence of a mass or blood clot within the heart

## 7. Timeline of innovations in treating cardiac rhythm disorders

The evolution of strategies for managing heart rhythm disorders has seen significant advancements over time. From surgical antiarrhythmic techniques to the introduction of implantable cardioverter-defibrillators, the landscape of treatment options has expanded. Direct current catheter ablation emerged as a milestone, offering a minimally invasive approach to correct arrhythmias. RFA further revolutionized the field, providing precise and effective treatment with improved outcomes. More recently, pulsed-field ablation has emerged as a promising innovation, offering a non-thermal alternative with potential advantages in safety and efficacy. These progressive developments highlight the ongoing efforts to refine and enhance the management of heart rhythm disorders (**Figure 2**).

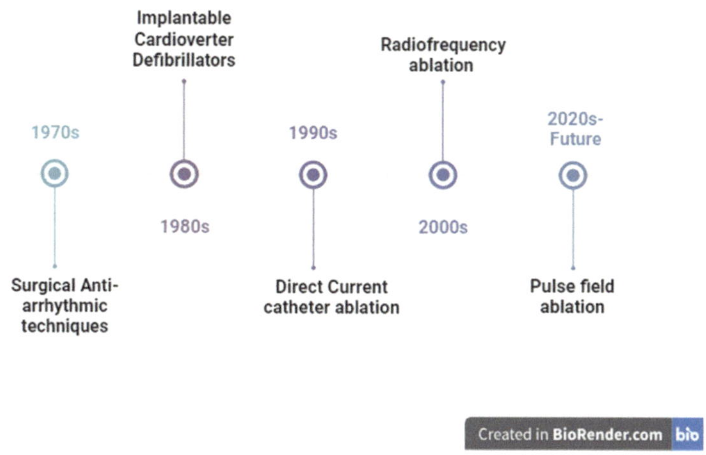


**Figure 2.**
*Evolution of strategies for managing heart rhythm disorders.*

## 8. Special populations

Patient populations at the highest risk but greatest benefit from ablative therapies are those with advanced heart failure. In the setting of patients with progressive cardiac dysfunction from ischemic, non-ischemic, valvular, or inherited disorders, the burden of arrhythmias and the detrimental effect on myocyte performance can be profound. Our center has developed a model to identify high-risk patients in a multi-disciplinary fashion through a combination of specialties: transplant cardiology, cardiothoracic anesthesia, cardiac surgery, and electrophysiology. The utility of each of these providers is to identify high-risk patients, provide high-quality care in the operative theater, and consider the use of left ventricular assist devices for the maintenance of hemodynamic stability. We have previously published this using extracorporeal membrane oxygenation and percutaneous axillary mechanical circulatory support in high-risk ventricular tachycardia ablations [13]. Furthermore, the role of a multi-disciplinary approach in high-risk patients has been further advanced due to recent data from large trials such as CASTLE-HTx demonstrating increased freedom from transplant, durable ventricular assist device, or death in this population [14]. Based on center and surgical comfort, application of early ECMO, percutaneous support, or a combination may allow for appropriate anesthetic dose, stimulation attempts, and longer duration of ablation to achieve a more sustained outcome – without sacrificing cerebral and end-organ perfusion.

## 9. Advancements in technology

### 9.1 High-power, short-duration (HPSD) ablation

HPSD ablation is becoming a new option for treating AF instead of using traditional settings with lower power and longer duration. There is concern about the safety of using higher power RF energy, especially on the posterior wall of the heart. Recent animal studies suggest that using 50 watts of energy for 5 seconds works better than lower power, longer duration ablations and has fewer complications.In a small study with humans using contact force-sensing catheters, using 50 watts of energy for about 11 seconds at each spot led to great results without any issues.

The very high-power short-duration (vHPSD) mode uses 90 watts for up to 4 seconds and automatically adjusts the power if it gets too hot. On the other hand, the conventional power temperature-controlled mode uses less than 50 watts and adjusts the water flow and power based on temperature feedback to keep it at the right temperature. To monitor the temperature in real-time, there are six sensors in the catheter's tip that measure the temperature where it touches the tissue, and three microelectrodes provide detailed electrical signals to map the endocardial surface better and find any conduction gaps. The 3D electroanatomical mapping system helps with this and can reduce the need for using fluoroscopy during the procedure [15].

According to the Multicenter Q-FFICIENCY Trial, temperature-controlled paroxysmal AF ablation using the innovative QDM catheter in very high-power short-duration (vHPSD) mode (90 W, ≤4 seconds), either alone or in combination with conventional power temperature-controlled mode (25–50 W), has proven to be highly efficient and effective in treating atrial fibrillation (AF). This approach maintains safety standards without compromising on efficacy (**Figure 3**) [17].

## 9.2 Pulsed field ablation (PFA)

Pulsed field ablation (PFA) stands as a nonthermal innovative technology for treating cardiac arrhythmias, particularly AF. Instead, it employs high-amplitude pulsed electrical fields to induce tissue ablation via irreversible electroporation, a process that boosts cell membrane permeability, ultimately leading to cell death. Unlike conventional thermal ablation methods, PFA achieves tissue ablation through

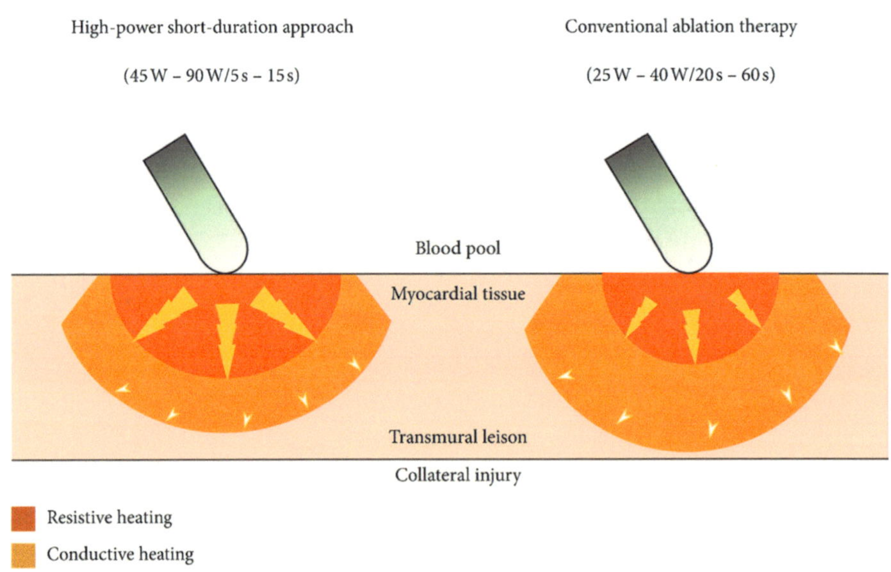


**Figure 3.**
*Comparison between HPSD approach and conventional ablation therapy. Lesion dimensions of radiofrequency ablation and heating distribution in myocardial tissue are demonstrated. HPSD approach and conventional ablation therapy could create comparable lesion size. HPSD approach results in an ablation lesion that is heated directly from the catheter during the resistive phase (red part), while, in conventional ablation therapy, myocardial tissue is largely heated because of conductive heating (golden yellow part) [16].*

microsecond-duration high-amplitude electrical pulses, targeting the myocardium by electroporating the sarcolemmal membrane.

A lesion is typically created with 3–4 PFA deliveries, each completed within one heartbeat. The high-voltage electric fields generate irreversible electroporation without significant heating, which allows the produced heat to dissipate through conduction and convection, making it a nonthermal ablation method. This mechanism targets cell membranes while sparing the extracellular matrix. Success with PFA depends on electrode proximity to the target tissue rather than physical contact. Different regions within the heart have varying sensitivities to electroporation, with the ventricular endocardium being more susceptible than the epicardium. PFA is tissue specific – the myocardium is highly vulnerable to injury, surrounding structures such as the esophagus, phrenic nerves, pulmonary veins, and coronary arteries which are relatively resistant. This specificity broadens its therapeutic potential and could improve safety during AF ablation procedures. The rapid vein isolation achievable in seconds suggests that PFA could significantly shorten procedure durations to less than an hour, marking a notable advancement in AF ablation techniques (**Figure 4**) [19].

In large animal studies, biphasic PFA multipolar endocardial catheters were found to safely create lasting linear and circular atrial ablations. Reddy et al. conducted three multicenter PFA studies (IMPULSE, PEFCAT, and PEFCAT II) focusing on patients with paroxysmal atrial fibrillation undergoing pulmonary vein isolation. Among 121 patients, PFA alone achieved acute pulmonary vein isolation in all cases. Follow-up remapping after approximately three months showed durable pulmonary vein isolation in most patients, particularly when using the optimized biphasic energy PFA waveform. Pulmonary vein remapping, performed in 110 patients at 93.0 ± 30.1 days, demonstrated durable PVI in 84.8% of pulmonary veins (64.5% of patients) and 96.0% of pulmonary veins (84.1% of patients) treated with the optimized biphasic energy PFA waveform. Furthermore, the one-year estimates for freedom from any atrial arrhythmia were promising, with the entire study population showing a rate of 78.5±3.8% and the optimized biphasic energy energy waveform cohort showing a slightly higher rate of 84.5±5.4% [20].

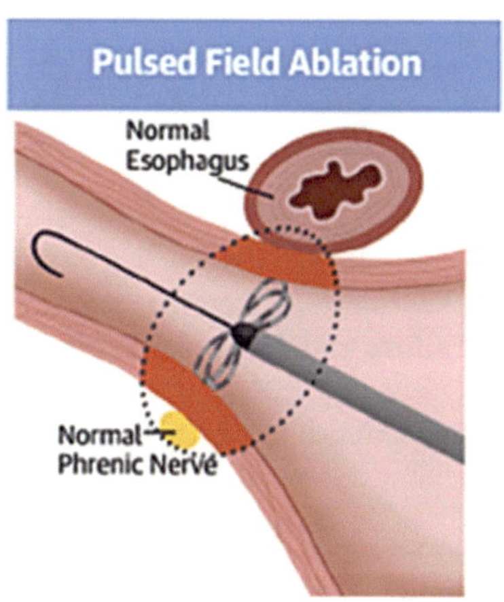


**Figure 4.**
*Pulsed field ablation for pulmonary vein isolation in atrial fibrillation [18].*

## 10. Conclusion

Radiofrequency catheter ablation techniques have dramatically impacted the treatment of cardiac arrhythmias. Initially, surgical approaches were employed, but more recently, catheter ablation has emerged as a crucial and increasingly prominent method for managing these conditions. In the case of most supraventricular arrhythmias, the efficacy of medical treatment with antiarrhythmic drugs is often poor. Moreover, these drugs are associated with issues such as poor or irregular effectiveness, bothersome and occasionally severe side effects, the potential for proarrhythmia, excessive costs, and inconvenience. Advancements in catheter ablation technology, including HPSD ablation and PFA, have significantly influenced the management of cardiac arrhythmias, particularly AF. These innovative techniques offer promising alternatives to traditional approaches, providing more effective and safer options for patients. Future goals for optimizing patient outcomes are utilizing innovative methods and technology to provide ablative options to a larger group of patients.

## Highlights

- Catheter ablation is commonly used and considered a standard technology for treating most atrial and ventricular arrhythmias.

- In the case of atrial fibrillation, catheter ablation is increasingly recommended for patients who are symptomatic and unresponsive to drug therapy.

- Pulsed field ablation has emerged as a promising innovation, offering a nonthermal alternative with potential advantages in safety and efficacy.

- Utilizing temporary mechanical circulatory support may provide increased success rates in high-risk patients with severe heart failure or heart failure with reduced ejection fraction.

## Author details

Shriya Sharma*, Rohan M. Goswami, Juan Leoni and Jose Ruiz
Division of Advanced Heart Failure and Transplant, Mayo Clinic in Florida, USA

*Address all correspondence to: shriyasharmap@gmail.com

## References

[1] Ernst S. Catheter ablation: General principles and advances. Cardiac Electrophysiology Clinics. 2017;**9**(2):311-317. DOI: 10.1016/j.ccep.2017.02.012

[2] Friedman PA. Novel mapping techniques for cardiac electrophysiology. Heart (British Cardiac Society). 2002;**87**(6):575-582. DOI: 10.1136/heart.87.6.575

[3] Hindricks G, Packer DL. Catheter ablation of atrial fibrillation: recent advances and future challenges. Europace: European Pacing, Arrhythmias, and Cardiac Electrophysiology: Journal of the Working Groups on Cardiac Pacing, Arrhythmias, and Cardiac Cellular Electrophysiology of the European Society of Cardiology. 2002;**24**(2):ii1-ii2. DOI: 10.1093/europace/euac035

[4] Parameswaran R et al. Catheter ablation for atrial fibrillation: current indications and evolving technologies. Nature Reviews. 2021;**18**(3):210-225. DOI: 10.1038/s41569-020-00451-x

[5] Calkins H. Catheter ablation to maintain sinus rhythm. Circulation. 2012;**125**(11):1439-1445. DOI: 10.1161/CIRCULATIONAHA.111.019943

[6] Bisbal F, Mont L. New insights on ablation of persistent atrial fibrillation: Evidence from The SARA Trial. Journal of Atrial Fibrillation. 2014;**7**(2):1114. DOI: 10.4022/jafib.1114

[7] Marashly Q et al. Innovations in ventricular tachycardia ablation. Journal of Interventional Cardiac Electrophysiology: An International Journal of Arrhythmias and Pacing. 2023;**66**(6):1499-1518. DOI: 10.1007/s10840-022-01311-z

[8] Guandalini GS et al. Ventricular tachycardia ablation: Past, present, and future perspectives. Clinical Electrophysiology. 2019;**5**(12):1363-1383. DOI: 10.1016/j.jacep.2019.09.015

[9] Al-Khatib SM et al. 2017 AHA/ACC/HRS guideline for management of patients with ventricular arrhythmias and the prevention of sudden cardiac death: Executive summary: A Report of the American College of Cardiology/American Heart Association Task Force on Clinical Practice Guidelines and the Heart Rhythm Society. Heart Rhythm. 2018;**15**(10):e190-e252. DOI: 10.1016/j.hrthm.2017.10.035

[10] Maury P et al. Three-dimensional mapping in the electrophysiological laboratory. Archives of Cardiovascular Diseases. 2018;**111**(6-7):456-464. DOI: 10.1016/j.acvd.2018.03.013

[11] Calkins H. Radiofrequency catheter ablation of supraventricular arrhythmias. Heart (British Cardiac Society). 2001;**85**(5):594-600. DOI: 10.1136/heart.85.5.594

[12] Tracy CM et al. American College of Cardiology/American Heart Association 2006 update of the clinical competence statement on invasive electrophysiology studies, catheterablation, and cardioversion: A report of the American College of Cardiology/American Heart Association/American College of Physicians Task Force on Clinical Competence and Training developed in collaboration with the Heart Rhythm Society. Journal of the American College of Cardiology. 2006;**48**(7):1503-1517. DOI: 10.1016/j.jacc.2006.06.043

[13] Rajak K et al. Extracorporeal membrane oxygenation-impella

(ECPELLA) in a patient with recalcitrant ventricular tachycardia undergoing ablation. Cureus. 2003;**15**(4):e38114. DOI: 10.7759/cureus.38114

[14] Sohns C et al. Catheter ablation in end-stage heart failure with atrial fibrillation. The New England Journal of Medicine. 2023;**389**(15):1380-1389. DOI: 10.1056/NEJMoa2306037

[15] Kotadia ID et al. High-power, short-duration radiofrequency ablation for the treatment of AF. Arrhythmia & Electrophysiology Review. 2020;**8**(4): 265-272. DOI: 10.15420/aer.2019.09

[16] Sun X et al. Efficiency, safety, and efficacy of high-power short-duration radiofrequency ablation in patients with atrial fibrillation. Cardiology Research and Practice. 2021;**2021**:8821467. DOI: 10.1155/2021/8821467

[17] Osorio J et al. Very high-power short-duration, temperature-controlled radiofrequency ablation in paroxysmal atrial fibrillation: The prospective multicenter Q-fficiency trial. JACC. Clinical Electrophysiology. 2023;**9**(4):468-480. DOI: 10.1016/j.jacep.2022.10.019

[18] Reddy VY et al. Pulsed field ablation for pulmonary vein isolation in atrial fibrillation. Journal of the American College of Cardiology vol. 2019;**74**(3): 315-326. DOI: 10.1016/j.jacc.2019.04.021

[19] Bradley CJ, Haines DE. Pulsed field ablation for pulmonary vein isolation in the treatment of atrial fibrillation. Journal of Cardiovascular Electrophysiology. 2020;**31**(8):2136-2147. DOI: 10.1111/jce.14414

[20] Piccini JP et al. Advances in Cardiac electrophysiology. Circulation. Arrhythmia and Electrophysiology. 2022;**15**(12):e009911. DOI: 10.1161/CIRCEP.121.009911

Chapter 12

# Surgical Ablation Techniques

*Daniel L. Beckles*


## Abstract

Atrial fibrillation is the most common arrhythmia affecting millions of people globally. The increasingly aging population and those with established cardiovascular risk factors (i.e., diabetes, obesity, hypertension, heart failure, and sleep apnea) are most susceptible to this arrhythmia and its dreaded complications. Although early detection, primary prevention, and anticoagulation are the most common treatment strategies, newer surgical technologies can halt disease progression, improve quality of life, and decrease mortality. While catheter ablation therapy has proven effective for new-onset paroxysmal atrial fibrillation, minimally invasive and aggressive surgical ablation procedures may offer another option for longstanding atrial fibrillation and recurrent atrial fibrillation that failed catheter ablation.


**Keywords:** atrial fibrillation, ablation, maze procedure, hybrid convergent surgical ablation, left atrial appendage management

## 1. Introduction

Open surgical ablations (SA) started over 40 years ago and were facilitated by the invention of the cardiopulmonary bypass machine, numerous scientific and clinical observational studies, and novel ablation devices [1, 2]. Although age, sex, and genetics are nonmodifiable risk factors for atrial fibrillation (AF), many similar modifiable risk factors for cardiovascular diseases are seen in the general population in patients with AF. In fact, according to the CDC, 47% of the US adult population has at least one risk factor that contributes to heart disease in general [3]. This also explains why AF is the most common complication after open-heart surgery [4]. The preoperative prevalence of AF in patients presenting for cardiac surgery procedures varies depending on the type of procedure, from revascularization for coronary artery disease to valve surgery, and the AF incidence can also increase due to intra-operative and post-operative risk factors [5]. Some modifiable preoperative risk factors include hypertension, diabetes, obesity, smoking, physical inactivity, sleep apnea, alcohol abuse, metabolic syndrome, large left atrial size, and underlying cardiomyopathies [6, 7]. Generally, high oxidative stress and inflammation predispose to AF [8, 9]. Today, the latest guidelines support surgical ablation techniques for AF as a stand-alone procedure or simultaneously with open cardiac surgery to lower morbidity, improve overall survival, and emphasize preoperative risk factor reduction, stroke reduction, and conversion to a normal sinus rhythm [6, 7, 10]. This chapter discusses the surgical treatment of AF.

## 2. Risk stratification for atrial fibrillation

AF is now described in the latest guidelines as a continuous and progressive disease, emphasizing the importance of risk factor modification and lifestyle changes throughout the disease spectrum [6, 7]. The presence of risk factors places patients in a stage 1 (at risk for AF) category out of 4 stages [6, 7]. A multidisciplinary integrated approach to treatment includes patient and family education with expectations, awareness of stroke symptomology, and emphasis on lifestyle modifications with risk factor reduction as a holistic approach to care [6, 7, 10]. Invasive therapies are reserved for failure of medical and risk factor reduction efforts.

Traditional and newer risk calculation models for patients with and without AF risk factors (Stage 1) are used to predict treatment strategies to prevent strokes and their associated mortality in the general population, immediate and long-term post-op follow-up period. The three most used risk calculators are CHARGE-AF, FHS, C2HEST, and CHA2DS2-VASc scores [6, 7]. An elevated risk score is documented to justify initiating anticoagulation therapy for stroke prevention.

The heart team approach is also supported by the latest guidelines, with the cardiac surgeon and electrophysiologist teams utilizing shared knowledge and experience to customize care for each patient's needs using the latest clinical evidence [6]. Atrial fibrillation is a complex disease whose treatment options and strategies are evolving rapidly. The shared goals are to evaluate the risks and benefits of symptom control, efforts to decrease stroke risk, and improve long-term survival and quality of life with maintenance of sinus rhythm [6, 7].

Post-operative atrial fibrillation (POAF) incidence is seen in 10–50% of open cardiac surgery patients [4, 5]. Stroke prevention is one of the significant strategies advances in surgical therapy can offer by directly excluding the left atrial appendage (LAA) from the circulation at the time of surgery since there is a higher risk for bleeding complications if anticoagulation is administered [5–7].

### 2.1 Screening for atrial fibrillation risk factors

Once patients are diagnosed or at risk for AF, they are screened for risk factors from "HEAD2TOES" (**Table 1**) [11]. These risk factors are the first treatment targets

| | Risk factor | Screening tests | Optimization strategy |
|---|---|---|---|
| H | Heart failure | ECHO EF < 40%, BNP > 100, hs-CRP > 2 mg/L | HF meds, colchicine |
| E | Exercise | <150 min/week | Increase walking steps |
| A | Arterial hypertension | BP > 130/80 | Stop salt, DASH diet, and or meds |
| D 2 | Diabetes mellitus 2 | HgbA1c > 6.5%, Fasting Blood Glucose >126 | Mediterranean diet and or meds |
| T | Tobacco use | Smoking history | Cessation |
| O | Obesity | BMI > 30 | Diet and or meds |
| E | Ethanol abuse | >3 drinks/week | Decrease drinking |
| S | Sleep apnea | AHI > 15 | CPAP |

**Table 1.**
*"HEAD2TOES" Adapted and modified from Epidemiology and modifiable risk factors for atrial fibrillation [10].*

| Stage | New terminology | | Plan |
|---|---|---|---|
| 1 | At risk for AF | Presence of risk factors[a] | Reduce risk factors |
| 2 | Pre-AF | Structural or electrical high-risk features[b] | Heightened surveillance |
| 3 | AF | All types of AF | Ablation Treatment |
| 4 | Permanent AF | Failed rhythm control treatments | Medical therapy |

[a]*Risk factors include obesity, lack of physical activity, hypertension, alcohol abuse, diabetes, sleep apnea, genetics, sex and age [6].*
[b]*High-risk features include atrial flutter, atrial enlargement, atrial ectopy, heart failure, coronary artery disease, hypertrophic cardiomyopathy, neuromuscular disorders, and thyroid disease [6].*

**Table 2.**
*New staging for AF recommended by the 2023 ACC/AHA/ACCP/HRS guideline for the diagnosis and management of atrial fibrillation [6].*

and should be addressed and optimized before invasive surgical therapy to reduce surgical morbidity and mortality. There are many classification systems for AF, and the new staging system has now replaced the old system [6].

### 2.2 Stages of atrial fibrillation

The 2023 ACC/AHA/ACCP/HRS Guideline for the Diagnosis and Management of Atrial Fibrillation: A Report of the American College of Cardiology/American Heart Association Joint Committee on Clinical Practice Guidelines provides the latest clinical updates (**Table 2**). The updates included a new staging system for atrial fibrillation and emphasized early rhythm control and continuous risk factor reduction [6].

## 3. Indications for surgical ablation

The 2023 Society of Thoracic Surgeons Clinical Practice Guidelines for the Surgical Treatment of Atrial Fibrillation has updated its recommendations based on the level of evidence (LOE[b]: A, high-quality, B moderate quality, and C, expert opinion, limited data) and classification of recommendations (COR[a]: I, strong benefit and should be performed; IIa, moderate benefit and is reasonable; IIb, unclear benefit and might be reasonable to be performed) summarized in **Table 3** [10]. Also, in 2023, the ACC/AHA/ACCP/HRS Guideline for the Diagnosis and Management of Atrial Fibrillation: A Report of the American College of Cardiology/American Heart Association Joint Committee on Clinical Practice Guidelines was published supporting similar surgical guidelines [6].

In summary, patients with AF have many treatment options that are best assessed and followed by a multidisciplinary heart team approach, including input from an electrophysiologist and a cardiac surgeon [6, 7]. The risks and benefits of each therapy can be customized to offer various medical options, including invasive catheter ablation and surgical ablation recommendations.

For patients with AF and in whom cardiac surgical therapy is indicated, the benefits of surgical ablation and exclusion of the LAA are evident [10].

## 4. Surgical therapy for atrial fibrillation

All surgical treatment options aim to establish normal sinus rhythm (NSR) and decrease stroke risks. Open surgical treatment of atrial fibrillation has evolved

| Recommendations for ALL patients with AF | COR[a] | LOE[b] |
|---|---|---|
| A multidisciplinary heart team approach with treatment planning and long-term follow-up is recommended to optimize patient outcomes. | I | C |
| Recommendations for mitral valve operations with AF | | |
| Surgical Ablation (SA) is recommended for any first-time non-emergent concomitant mitral valve surgery to restore normal sinus rhythm (NSR) and improve outcomes. | I | A |
| Recommendations for ALL other non-mitral valve operations with AF | | |
| Surgical Ablation is recommended for any first-time non-emergent concomitant mitral valve surgery to restore normal sinus rhythm and improve outcomes. | I | B |
| Recommendations for left atrial appendage (LAA) management | | |
| Obliteration of LAA is recommended for ALL first-time, non-emergent cardiac surgery procedures with or without SA to reduce thromboembolic complications. | I | A |
| Recommendation for stand-alone surgical ablation | | |
| Symptomatic AF without structural heart disease refractory to class I/III antiarrhythmic drugs, catheter ablation, or both is reasonable to restore NSR. | IIa | B |
| Recommendations for stand-alone LAA management | | |
| LAA obliteration may be considered as an isolated procedure in patients at high risk for thromboembolic complications and contraindication for oral anticoagulation. | IIb | B |
| Recommendations for patients evaluated for transcatheter valve replacement (i.e., TAVR) with AF | | |
| For patients with low or intermediate surgical risk, surgical valve replacement with SA and LAA occlusion is reasonable for improving long-term outcomes. | IIa | B |

[a]*COR (Classification of Recommendation).*
[b]*LOE (level of Evidence).*

**Table 3.**
*The 2023 society of thoracic surgeons clinical practice guidelines for the surgical treatment of atrial fibrillation [10].*

dramatically with advances in ablation techniques, indications during other surgical procedures, and minimally invasive options.

The gold standard for surgical ablation of AF is the Cox-maze (CM) procedure, pioneered by Dr. James L. Cox, who performed his first procedure in 1987 with the maintenance of a normal sinus rhythm for almost 20 years [12]. The principle of the surgical technique is based on treating the underlying pathophysiology of re-entrant circuits from the pulmonary veins and atrial tissue and halting AF propagation [13]. Initially, the CM procedure involved a cut-and-sew technique on the atrium to create transmural disruption of the re-entrant circuits originating in the pulmonary veins. Today, with the advancement in ablation technologies, the Cox-maze IV procedure can be performed quickly, effectively, and safely with repetitive outcomes [10, 14].

### 4.1 Ablation energy sources and technology

The two most common types of ablation energy used to replace the original cut-and-sew technique with excellent efficacy are cryoablation (freezing) and radiofrequency ablation (heating). Cryoablation uses a malleable wand to safely apply a single cold ablation line (–75C) to the atrial and myocardial tissue to follow the Cox-Maze IV procedure. Radiofrequency (RF) ablation uses radio frequency waves to burn atrial tissue between 2 clamps (bipolar energy) or as a unipolar RF energy source. These energy sources are commonly used for speed, safety, and effectiveness [14, 15].

## 4.2 Surgical ablation techniques

The Cox-maze IV ablation procedure is the most common ablation lesion set used by surgeons over the last two decades. It has proven successful in concomitant, stand-alone, and minimally invasive procedures [14]. **Figure 1** depicts a pictorial drawing of the Cox-maze IV surgical lesions using various energy sources.

The right pulmonary veins are dissected and circulated to accommodate a bipolar RF clamp. Staying closer to the atrial tissue, RF ablation is performed three times and tested for block. Similarly, on the left side, the ligament of Marshall, another source of triggers and drivers of AF, is cauterized, and the left pulmonary veins are encircled with the bipolar Rf clamps and ablated three times until a block is seen [16]. The tip of the LAA is excised, and the RF bipolar clamp is placed inside the LAA and onto the left upper pulmonary vein to complete another ablation line [14, 15]. The base of the LAA is then sized, and an external occlusion device or clip is placed at the base to exclude this lethal organ from circulation and decrease unwanted thromboembolic events. The left atrium can be entered at Sondergaard's Groove to complete the Cox-maze IV procedure, like a mitral valve exposure. On the endocardial left atrial surface, cryoablation or RF ablation can connect the top of the left and right pulmonary veins and the inferior pulmonary veins to complete the "box" lesion set. Next, the coronary sinus (CS) is marked on the epicardial surface, ablated with the cryoprobe, and marked on the endocardial surface, followed by another cryo ablation line from the mitral annulus to the left atrium incision towards the right lower pulmonary vein joining the CS marker [14]. Next, the SVC and IVC snares are tightened in preparation for the right-sided lesions. The retrograde catheter is removed, the right atriotomy is extended anteriorly, this incision is connected to the tricuspid valve annulus with a cryoablation line, and three RF ablations are placed from this incision. Starting at the retrograde insertion towards the SVC, then towards the IVC, and lastly, towards the right atrial appendage tip, and the right atrium is closed, completes the biatrial Cox-maze IV procedure summarized in **Figure 1** [14].

The Cox-maze IV procedure can also be performed minimally invasively without the need for open sternotomy and incorporate as many lesion sets described above

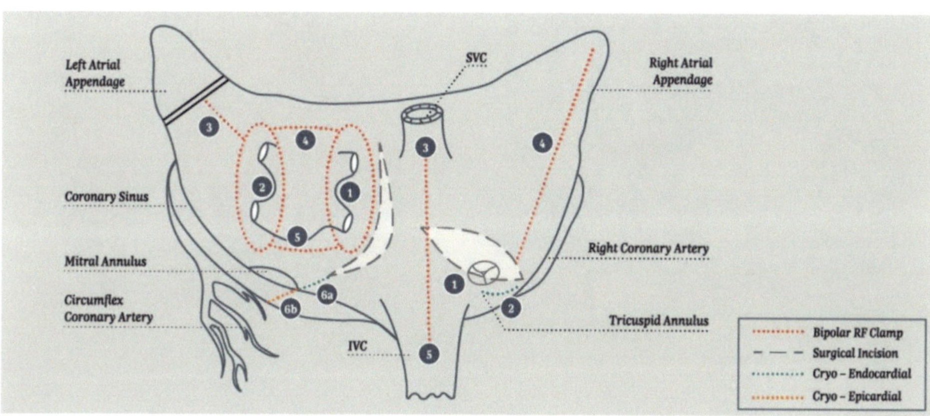


**Figure 1.**
*Cox-maze procedure (used with permission from AtriCure, Inc.).*

using video-assisted thoracoscopic surgery (VATS) technology, similar energy sources, and instruments either unilaterally or bilaterally [2, 14].

One of the most challenging clinical atrial fibrillation patients is those presenting with persistent and long-standing persistent atrial fibrillation, where catheter ablation has poor outcomes. An innovative clinical trial proposed combining the best catheter-based endocardial therapy with the best surgical ablation technology in a minimally invasive fashion named CONVERGE TRIAL (Convergence of Epicardial and Endocardial Ablation for the Treatment of Symptomatic Persistent AF). The former procedure is performed by an electrophysiologist and the latter by a cardiothoracic surgeon. A prospective, randomized, controlled CONVERGE IDE trial compared hybrid AF ablation or a convergent procedure to endocardial catheter RF ablation alone [17]. The trial specifically targeted an unmet need of patients with long-standing persistent atrial fibrillation (LSPAF). The lesion set targets the pulmonary vein and the posterior left atrium, as shown in **Figure 2**.

Results of the CONVERGENT trial were significantly positive, and today, slight modifications were made to the initial hybrid Convergent procedure. Surgery is performed first under general anesthesia with left lung isolation and a left VATS approach to open the left pericardium, ligate the ligament of Marshall, size the base of the LAA, and place an external occlusion device or clip (i.e., AtriClip, AtriCure Inc.) under transesophageal echocardiography guidance [17, 18]. A left chest drain is placed, and next, a subxiphoid approach to the pericardial space is created, and a pericardioscopic evaluation is performed to identify all four pulmonary veins, pre-ablation mapping, initiating epicardial RF ablation using unipolar source (i.e., Epi-Sense, Atricure, Inc.) with systemic anticoagulation. A completion epicardial mapping is performed, and a pericardial drain is placed. During the trial, the second part of the procedure was conducted under the same general anesthesia by an electrophysiologist who performed an endocardial ablation guided by electroanatomical mapping with completion of the pulmonary vein isolation (PVI) using irrigated

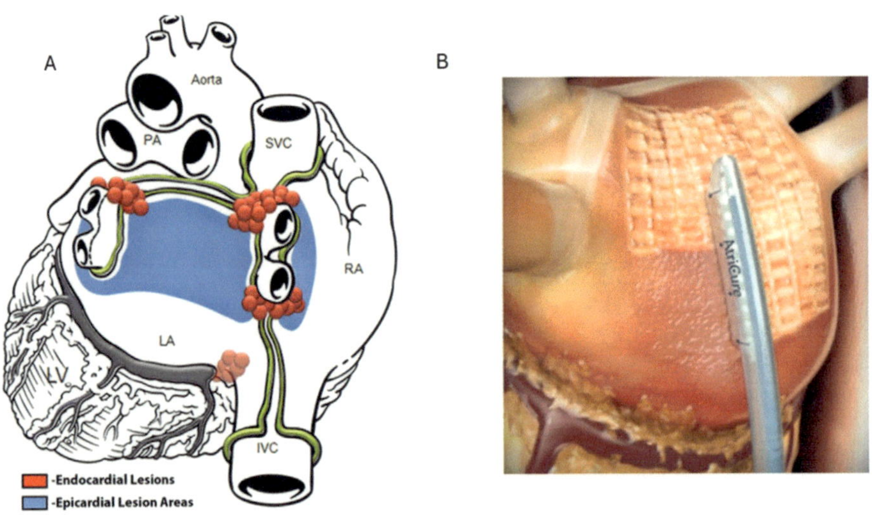


**Figure 2.**
*The CONVERGE trial: (A) Hybrid Convergent arm with surgical ablation lines on the epicardial surface shown in blue, endocardial ablation lines in red and green denote the pericardial reflection, and (B) Epicardial ablation of the left posterior atrium using an RF ablation (used with permission from AtriCure, Inc.).*

RF catheter and created a cavotricuspid isthmus (CTI) line [17, 18]. Today, most Hybrid AF therapy centers perform these procedures separately up to 1–2 months apart to accommodate adequate scar formation at the ablation sites with healing and decreased edema between procedures, thereby providing a better mapping and ablation map in the second procedure. The ease of scheduling, shorter general anesthesia, and shorter EP lab time are also favorable for team efficiency [17, 18].

One of the most well-studied applications of the surgical ablation technique using the Cox-maze procedure is in concomitant open-heart surgery cases where patients with indicated cardiac surgery procedures and have an atrial fibrillation diagnosis undergo surgical correction and a Cox-maze procedure simultaneously [19]. Most of the Cox-maze procedure is performed off-pump and with a beating heart to reduce cross-clamp times, along with surgical correction of the primary cardiac diagnosis. Although recent guidelines support concomitant surgeries with COR level 1 and LOE A, the procedure is underperformed in the USA and worldwide [2, 18, 19]. The 30-day outcomes of surgical ablation in concomitant surgical procedures and on long-term survival were superior, as discussed in the results below [19, 20]. Therefore, more surgical education is needed to establish centers of excellence for treating AF concomitantly using surgical ablation techniques.

### 4.3 Surgical left atrial appendage (LAA) exclusion

The left atrial appendage accounts for most thromboembolic events, and since the advent of the Cox-maze procedure, all surgical ablation approaches for the treatment of AF have excluded the LAA from circulation [2, 13]. Various methods are used for LAA exclusion, including cutting and sewing from the epicardial surface, suturing close to the endocardial surface, and endoscopic stapler devices to the latest, more consistent AtriClip (AtriCure Inc.) The LAA is the source of up to 90% of clots that result in strokes and other thromboembolic complications and has electrical circuits that account for up to 30% of the AF burden [21, 22]. Therefore, one of the most significant advantages of surgical ablations is the safe access and isolation of the LAA from circulation [21].

## 5. Results of surgical ablation

Most published outcome results are relatively small, single-institution studies and show good reproducibility and safety. A 2018 meta-analysis of randomized controlled trials (20 studies, n = 1407) to assess the effect of concomitant surgical AF ablation on post-operative freedom from AF showed that at 12 months, 70% of ablated patients were free from AF [23]. This study also showed no difference in mortality, stroke, pacemaker implantation, or myocardial infarction. There was an increased hospital length of stay for patients who underwent ablation [23]. A retrospective single-center study looking at 15 years of data in patients with atrial fibrillation treated with Cox-maze IV procedure at the time of surgery (concomitant), those with atrial fibrillation but not offered ablation during surgery, and those with no history of atrial fibrillation undergoing surgery [20]. 30-day mortality was similar between all groups, and greater survival was seen for the Cox-maze IV group compared to the untreated AF group. The 10-year survival for the Cox-maze IV group was 62% versus 42% for the untreated atrial fibrillation group. Overall, in selected patients, concomitant treatment of atrial fibrillation at the time of cardiac surgery offers statistically improved long-term survival with no difference in morbidity and mortality [20]. The published results of surgical ablation in randomized and non-randomized trials were reviewed, and the latest STS clinical practice guidelines were summarized using the evidence level and recommendations classification as shown in **Table 3** [10].

## 6. Conclusions

A remains the most common cardiac arrhythmia in the world and leads to significant morbidity and mortality [6]. AF shares similar classic risk factors for cardiovascular diseases, which is the leading cause of death worldwide [3]. The latest guidelines incorporate an aggressive upstream risk factor reduction and define stage 1 as having risk factors only without AF [6]. A holistic multidisciplinary team approach to care is highly recommended [9].

Technological advances over the last three decades have included novel medical therapies, anticoagulation drugs, safer catheter ablation devices, improved surgical ablation devices, and minimally invasive surgical techniques for treating all stages of atrial fibrillation. Unfortunately, no two patients are alike, with a complex array of modifiable and nonmodifiable risk factor combinations. To better access the long-term arrhythmia-free survival of AF patients, accurate documentation and demographics, like most quality databases and reporting structures with monitoring for consistency in techniques and outcomes data, are needed. Surgical ablation techniques have stood the test of time and continue to improve outcomes, survival, and quality of life.

## Author details

Daniel L. Beckles
Ochsner Christus Health, Department of Cardiothoracic Surgery, Lake Charles, LA, USA

*Address all correspondence to: daniel.beckles@Ochsner.org

## References

[1] Hessel EA. A brief history of cardiopulmonary bypass. Seminars in Cardiothoracic and Vascular Anesthesia. 2014;**18**(2):87-100. DOI: 10.1177/1089253214530045

[2] McCarthy PM, Cox JL, Kislitsina ON, Kruse J, Churyla A, Malaisrie SC, et al. Surgery and catheter ablation for atrial fibrillation: History, current practice, and future directions. Journal of Clinical Medicine. 2022;**11**:210. DOI: 10.3390/jcm1101021

[3] CDC. About Heart Disease. [Internet]. 2024. Available from: https://www.cdc.gov/heart-disease/about/index.html

[4] McIntyre WF. Post-operative atrial fibrillation after cardiac surgery: Challenges throughout the patient journey. Frontiers in Cardiovascular Medicine. 2023;**10**:1156626. DOI: 10.3389/fcvm.2023.1156626

[5] Bowdish ME, D'Agostino RS, Thourani VH, Schwann TA, Krohn C, Desai N, et al. Adult cardiac surgery database: 2021Update on outcomes, quality, and research. The Annals of Thoracic Surgery. 2021;**111**:1770-1780. DOI: 10.1016/j.athoracsur.2021.03.043

[6] Joglar J, Chung M, et al. 2023 ACC/AHA/ACCP/HRS guideline for the diagnosis and management of atrial fibrillation: A report of the American College of Cardiology/American Heart Association joint committee on clinical practice guidelines. Journal of the American College of Cardiology. 2024;**83**(1):109-279. DOI: 10.1016/j.jacc.2023.08.017

[7] Hindricks G, Potpara T, et al. 2020 ESC guidelines for the diagnosis and management of atrial fibrillation developed in collaboration with the European Association for Cardio-Thoracic Surgery (EACTS): The task force for the diagnosis and management of atrial fibrillation of the European Society of Cardiology (ESC) developed with the special contribution of the European heart rhythm association (EHRA) of the ESC. European Heart Journal. 2021;**42**(5):373-498. DOI: 10.1093/eurheartj/ehaa612

[8] Nso N, Bookani KR, Metzl M, MD, Radparvar F. Role of inflammation in atrial fibrillation: A comprehensive review of current knowledge. Journal of Arrhythmia. 2021;**37**(1):1-10. DOI: 10.1002/joa3.12473

[9] Dobrev D, Jordi Heijman J, Hiram R, Nattel S, Li N. Inflammatory signaling in atrial cardiomyocytes: A novel unifying principle in atrial fibrillation pathophysiology. Nature Reviews. Cardiology. 2023;**20**:145-167. DOI: 10.1038/s41569-022-00759-w

[10] Wyler von Ballmoos MC, Hui DS, Mehaffey JH, Malaisrie SC, Vardas PN, Gillinov AM, et al. The society of thoracic surgeons 2023 clinical practice guidelines for the surgical treatment of atrial fibrillation. The Annals of Thoracic Surgery. 2024;**27**:S0003-4975(24)00057-2. DOI: 10.1016/j.athoracsur.2024.01.007

[11] Adrian D, Elliott AD, Middeldorp ME, Van Gelder IC, Albert CM, Sanders P. Epidemiology and modifiable risk factors for atrial fibrillation. Nature Reviews Cardiology. 2023;**20**:404-417. DOI: 10.1038/s41569-022-00820-8

[12] Cox JL. The first maze procedure. The Journal of Thoracic and Cardiovascular Surgery. 2011;**141**:1093-1097

[13] Edgerton ZJ, Edgerton JR. History of surgery for atrial fibrillation. Heart Rhythm. 2009;**6**:S1-S4. DOI: 10.1016/j.hrthm.2009.07.047

[14] Martha MO, MMO MG, Barron L, Yates TAE, Christian W, Zemlin CW, et al. The Cox-maze procedure: What lesions and why. JTCVS Techniques. 2023;**17**:84-93. DOI: 10.1016/j.xjtc.2022.11.009

[15] Tzeis S et al. European heart rhythm association/Heart Rhythm Society/Asia Pacific Heart Rhythm Society/Latin American Heart Rhythm Society expert consensus statement on catheter and surgical ablation of atrial fibrillation. EP Europace. 2024;**26**(4):1-107. DOI: 10.1093/europace/euae043

[16] Hwang C, Chen PS. Ligament of Marshall: Why it is important for atrial fibrillation ablation. Heart Rhythm Society. 2009;**6**(12):S35-S40. DOI: 10.1016/j.hrthm.2009.08.034

[17] De Lurgio DB et al. Hybrid convergent procedure for the treatment of persistent and long-standing persistent atrial fibrillation: Results of CONVERGE clinical trial. Circulation. Arrhythmia and Electrophysiology. 2020;**13**:e009288. DOI: 10.1161/CIRCEP.120.009288

[18] De Lurgio DB et al. Atrial fibrillation symptom reduction and improved quality of life following the hybrid convergent procedure: A CONVERGE trial subanalysis. Annals of Cardiothoracic Surgery. 2024;**13**(2):155-164. DOI: 10.21037/acs-2023-afm-15

[19] McCarthy PM, Davidson CJ, Kruse J, Lerner DJ, Braid-Forbes MJ, McCrea MM, et al. Prevalence of atrial fibrillation before cardiac surgery and factors associated with concomitant ablation. The Journal of Thoracic and Cardiovascular Surgery. 2020;**159**:2245-2253. DOI: 10.1016/j.jtcvs.2019.06.062

[20] Musharbash FN et al. Performance of the Cox-maze IV procedure is associated with improved long-term survival in patients with atrial fibrillation undergoing cardiac surgery. The Journal of Thoracic and Cardiovascular Surgery. 2018;**155**:159-170. DOI: 10.1016/j.jtcvs.2017.09.095

[21] Regazzoli D, Ancona F, Trevisi N, Guarracini F, Radinovic A, Oppizzi M, et al. Left atrial appendage: Physiology, pathology, and role as a therapeutic target. BioMed Research International. 2015;**2015**:205013. DOI: 10.1155/2015/205013

[22] Nishimura M, Lupercio-Lopez F, Hsu JC. Left atrial appendage electrical isolation as a target in atrial fibrillation. JACC: Clinical Electrophysiology. 2019;**5**:407-416. DOI: 10.1016/j.jacep.2019.02.00

[23] McClure GR, Belley-Cote EP, Jaffer IH, Dvirnik N, An KR, Fortin G, et al. Surgical ablation of atrial fibrillation: A systematic review and meta-analysis of randomized controlled trials. Europace. 2018;**20**:1442-1450. DOI: 10.1093/europace/eux336

Chapter 13

# Hybrid Ablation: Two-Center Experience

*Alexandr Zotov, Igor Khamnagadaev, Oleg Shelest, Emil Sakharov, Alexandr Glupak, Irina Bulavina, Robert Khabazov, Alexandr Troitsky and Natalya Mokrysheva*

## Abstract

Despite the advantages of thoracoscopic radiofrequency ablation, a significant number of recurrences are observed in patient subgroups with heart failure (both preserved and reduced ejection fraction) and long-standing atrial fibrillation (AF). Our study presents the technical description and results of thoracoscopic ablation in 165 patients, 36 of whom underwent a biatrial ablation scheme. Additionally, 22 patients underwent a hybrid approach, combining thoracoscopic and endocardial ablation. In our study, the most common gap of the epicardial isolation line was the anterior segment of the antral part of the right pulmonary veins, where additional ablation was required in 13 (59.1%) patients. The hybrid approach improves treatment efficacy in persistent AF and high-risk patient groups, demonstrating a favorable safety profile and comprehensive treatment solution.

**Keywords:** hybrid ablation, persistent atrial fibrillation, thoracoscopic ablation, box-lesion, biatrial ablation, persistent AF, long-standing persistent AF

## 1. Introduction

In 1987, James Cox identified macro-reentry waves based on electrophysiological studies and animal experiments, establishing their size and circulation duration in specific atrial locations. This research laid the foundation for the MAZE procedure [1]. Initially, the procedure was performed exclusively under cardiopulmonary bypass, which was associated with numerous complications and was technically demanding. For these reasons, incisions were replaced by forming lines with ablation devices [2].

Today, surgical ablation using radiofrequency and cryo-energy (MAZE-IV) is a safe and effective method for treating atrial fibrillation (AF). It has shown excellent results regardless of the duration of the arrhythmia [3]. The evolution of surgical technologies has allowed for a minimally invasive approach for patients with isolated AF who do not require valve correction or coronary artery bypass grafting.

In 2005, Wolf and colleagues [4] reported the results of minimally invasive video-assisted ablation using radiofrequency energy (VATS), which initiated a new direction in AF surgery. Later, J.R. Doty described the "Galaxy" operation (Gemini-S Ablation and Left Atrial Appendage Excision) [5]. A feature of the procedure is the creation of a complete circular lesion according to the "Box-lesion" scheme due to the design of the electrodes. Resection or clipping of the left atrial appendage (LAA) completes the procedure, eliminating a potential source of thromboembolism.

In our clinic, thoracoscopic treatment of AF using irrigated ablation has been performed since 2017. The total number of patients who underwent thoracoscopic ablation (TA) was 165. At the time of hospitalization, 139 patients had AF recorded on electrocardiography (ECG). The clinical characteristics of the patients are presented in **Table 1**.

All patients underwent coronary angiography and echocardiography before surgery to exclude ischemic and valvular causes of arrhythmia. On the day of surgery, before transporting the patient to the operating room, transesophageal echocardiography was performed to exclude LAA thrombosis. All patients underwent irrigated ablation according to a modified scheme [6]. LAA resection was performed in 163 (98,8%) patients. The average blood loss volume was 150 ml, and in 19,4% of cases, extubation was performed on the operating table. Conversion to mini-thoracotomy was performed in 6 (3,6%) patients due to bleeding during LAA resection. A permanent pacemaker (PPM) was implanted in 3 (1,8%) patients due to the development of sick sinus syndrome. One patient (0,6%) required prolonged noninvasive ventilation due to left diaphragm paresis. During the implementation of the technique, 1 (0,6%) death occurred from multiple organ failures in the postoperative period. The median stay in the intensive care unit was 19.5 hours (16,7; 22,2). At discharge, sinus rhythm was achieved in 155 (93,9%) patients.

| Characteristic | Value |
|---|---|
| Paroxysmal | 21 (12,7%) |
| Persistent | 47 (28,5%) |
| Long-standing persistent | 97 (58,8%) |
| History of arrhythmia, months | 60 (24; 120) |
| CHA2DS2-VASc, points | 2 (2; 3) |
| History of catheter RFA | 42 (25,5%) |
| History of pacemaker implantation | 1 (0,6%) |
| NYHA 0 | 27 (16,4%) |
| NYHA I | 26 (15,8%) |
| NYHA II | 104 (63,0%) |
| NYHA III | 8 (4,8%) |
| LA volume index, ml/m$^2$ | 40,0 (34,8; 46,6) |
| Pulmonary artery pressure, mm Hg | 32,0 (28,0; 39,0) |
| LVEF, % | 57 (53; 60) |
| Number of patients with reduced LVEF | 33 (20,0%) |
| Number of patients with pulmonary hypertension | 58 (35,2%) |
| Number of patients with LA atriomegaly | 113 (68,5%) |

*Description: CHA2DS2-VASc: A clinical prediction rule for estimating the risk of stroke in patients with atrial fibrillation; RFA: Radiofrequency ablation; NYHA: New York Heart Association functional classification, which classifies the extent of heart failure; LA: Left atrium; LVEF: Left ventricular ejection fraction.*

**Table 1.**
*Brief clinical characteristics.*

In the long-term period, 158 (95,7%) patients were examined. The recurrence rate of AF was assessed using Holter monitoring. The median follow-up period was 28,6 months (10,0; 35,6). At the time of follow-up, freedom from AF with thoracoscopic treatment was achieved in 122 (77,2%) patients, and with additional antiarrhythmic therapy and touch-up procedures, it was 139 (88,0%) patients. Most patients showed a regression of heart failure symptoms, confirmed by changes in N-terminal pro-b-type natriuretic peptide levels (NT-proBNP). There was also a significant reduction in the left atrial volume index (LAVI) and an increase in ejection fraction (EF) (**Table 2**). Adverse events included acute cerebrovascular accidents or transient ischemic attacks in 4 (2.5%) patients and PPM implantation in 2 (1.3%) patients. Also, 10 (6,3%) patients had repeated hospitalizations due to progressive HF. There were no deaths associated with cardiovascular events.

Subanalysis revealed a negative trend in the subgroups of patients with long-standing persistent AF, patients with heart failure and reduced EF, and patients with heart failure and preserved EF (**Figure 1**). To identify patients with heart failure and preserved left ventricular EF, the HFA-PEFF (Heart Failure Association Pre-test assessment, echocardiography, and natriuretic peptide, Functional testing, Final etiology) algorithm, developed by the Heart Failure Association of the European

| Characteristic | Before operation | Follow-up | P-value |
|---|---|---|---|
| LA volume, ml | 81,0 (68,5; 95,0) | 74,0 (63,5; 85,5) | 0,005 |
| LA volume index, ml/m$^2$ | 38,8 (34,5; 44,8) | 35,6 (30,0; 42,7) | 0,006 |
| Pulmonary artery pressure, mm Hg | 32,0 (28,0; 38,2) | 32 (26; 39,0) | 0,665 |
| LVEF, % | 56,0 (53; 60) | 60,0 (57; 62) | <0,001 |
| NT-proBNP pg./ml | 602,8 (280,4; 971,2) | 224,2 (140,5; 350,0) | 0,031 |

*Description: LA: Left atrium; LVEF: Left ventricular ejection fraction, NT-proBNP: N-terminal pro b-type natriuretic peptide levels.*

**Table 2.**
*Myocardial remodeling and NT-proBNP dynamics.*

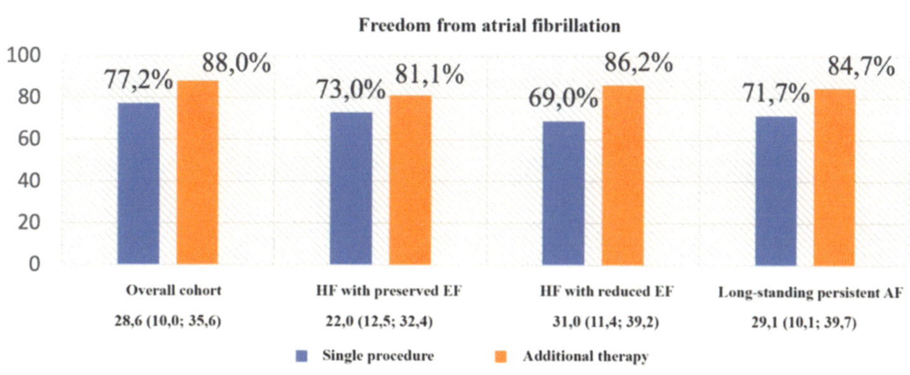


**Figure 1.**
*Freedom from atrial fibrillation in different patient groups. Description: The chart compares the outcomes between a single procedure and additional therapy in the overall cohort, patients with heart failure with preserved ejection fraction (EF), HF with reduced EF, and patients with long-standing persistent AF. The blue bars represent the outcomes for a single procedure, while the orange bars represent the outcomes for additional therapy. The follow-up period is presented as medians and interquartile ranges.*

Society of Cardiology, was used [7]. According to this algorithm, patients scoring five points or more were classified as having confirmed heart failure.

The observed negative trend in freedom from AF in subgroups of patients with long-standing persistent AF, heart failure with preserved myocardial contractility, and heart failure with reduced EF necessitate the modification of the ablation protocol. Considering that in all groups, additional therapy improved treatment outcomes, given the above data and James Cox's recommendations to approximate the minimally invasive ablation scheme to the original MAZE-IV procedure [8], we have implemented additional ablation interventions on the right and left atria (biatrial approach) followed by endocardial ablation (hybrid treatment) to improve surgical outcomes.

## 2. Thoracoscopic stage

The original "GALAXY" procedure consists of several key steps:

- Pericardiotomy, mobilization of the oblique and transverse sinuses, and guidewires placement.

- Circular isolation following the "Box-lesion" scheme.

- Resection of the LAA and verification of conduction block.

In our clinical practice, we use a modified procedure that includes more electrode applications and changes in the curvature of the branches relative to the posterior wall of the left atrium [6]. We perform repeated ablation applications without unclamping to minimize the possibility of gap formation. Ralph J. Damiano Jr.'s group demonstrated the effectiveness of this approach [9]. As mentioned earlier, we use a biatrial ablation scheme in the subgroups of patients with long-standing persistent arrhythmia, heart failure with preserved myocardial contractility, and reduced EF.

The procedure is performed under general anesthesia and double-lumen lung ventilation. The patient is positioned on the operating table in the "supine" position (**Figure 2**).

On the right side of the chest, three thoracoscopic ports are placed in the 3rd, 5th, and 6th intercostal spaces. Carbon dioxide is insufflated into the right pleural cavity through an insufflator at an average rate of 2–5 liters per minute. The optimal pressure

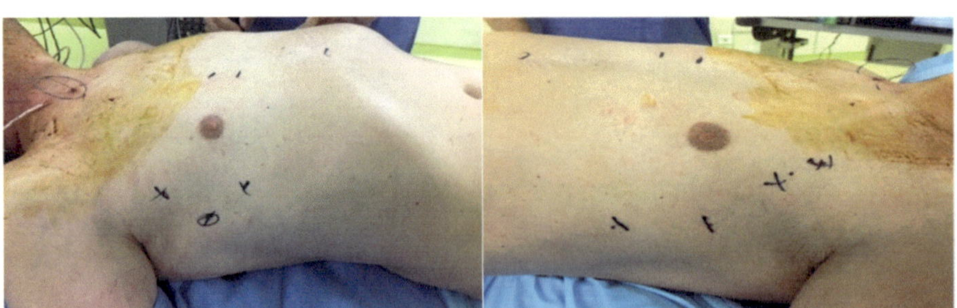

**Figure 2.**
*Patient positioning on the operating table. Description: The patient is positioned lying on their back on the operating table. A marker on the lateral surface of the chest indicates the placement sites for thoracoscopic access.*

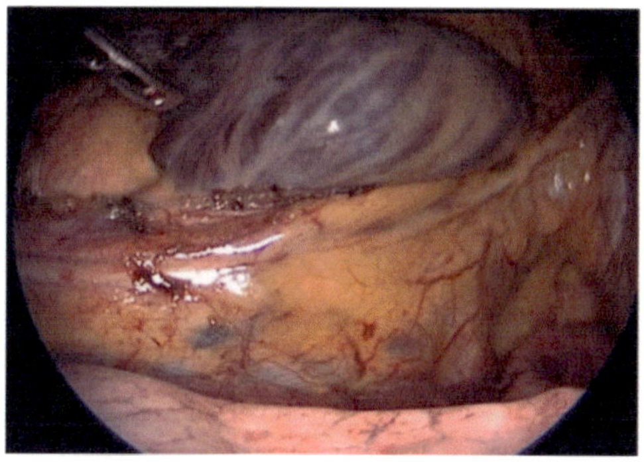

**Figure 3.**
*Right pericardiotomy. Description: Pericardiotomy is performed 1.5 cm above the phrenic nerve, extending until the aorta and inferior vena cava are visualized.*

in the chest cavity for the procedure is approximately 6–8 mm Hg. An endoscope is introduced through the middle port, visualizing the pericardium and the phrenic nerve, after which the pericardium is incised 1.5–2 cm above the nerve (**Figure 3**). The pericardium can be opened with endoscopic scissors or LigaSure instruments. Flexible guidewires are introduced through the lower thoracoscopic port after mobilization of the oblique and transverse sinuses of the pericardium. The first guidewire is passed through the transverse sinus, and the second through the oblique sinus of the pericardium.

The next stage begins with single-lung ventilation of the right lung. On the left side, three thoracoscopic ports are placed in the 3rd, 5th, and 6th intercostal spaces, and $CO_2$ is insufflated. An endoscope is introduced through the port, and the pericardium is visualized similarly. After opening the pericardium below the phrenic nerve, the flexible guidewires are visualized and extracted through the lower thoracoscopic port (**Figure 4**).

Bipolar irrigated ablation begins on the left side. The ablation device is attached to the tips of the guidewires, and the electrode is introduced into the chest. Under thoracoscopic camera control, the open branches of the clamp-electrode are placed in the transverse and oblique sinuses (**Figure 5**).

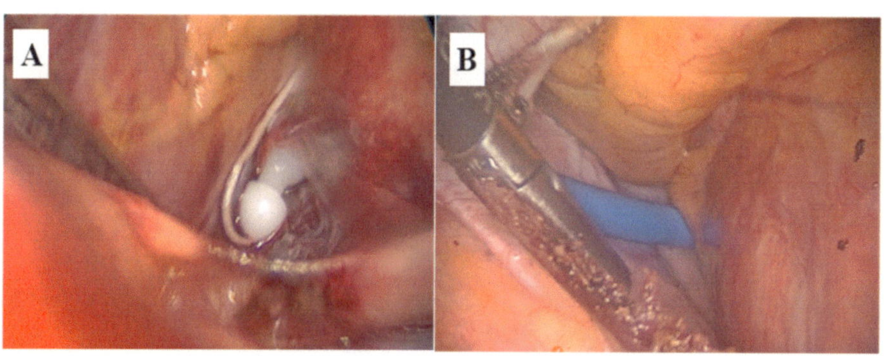


**Figure 4.**
*Flexible guidewires are extracted from the pericardial sinuses. Description: A: Visualization of the flexible guidewire in the transverse sinus at the base of the left atrial appendage. B: Visualization of the flexible guidewire in the oblique sinus of the pericardium.*

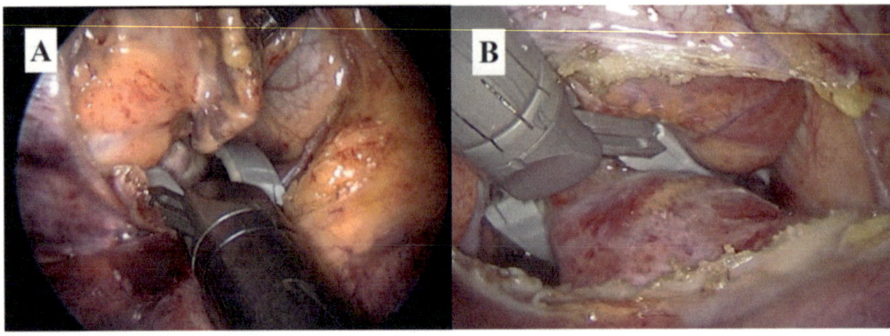


**Figure 5.**
*Ablation electrode installation. Description: The branches of the bipolar radiofrequency clamp are positioned for left (A) and right (B) side ablation.*

The ablation clamp's original design isolates the posterior wall of the left atrium as a single block. At the completion of the bipolar electrode ablation, the lines intersect, forming a "Box-lesion".

The next step includes additional ablation of the right atrium, specifically the cava-caval line and the line along the free wall of the right atrium (**Figure 6**). The final stage entails creating a line to the base of the LAA, followed by resection of the LAA with a stapling device. The stapler is positioned along the base of the LAA. Once a satisfactory position of the stapler is achieved, the LAA is stapled and simultaneously resected (**Figure 7**).

The next step is to perform an exit-block test. The pulmonary veins are stimulated behind the ablation line, and the absence of a response to cardiac stimulation confirms their isolation. After the procedure, drains are placed, and the thoracoscopic ports are closed. The final ablation scheme is presented in **Figure 8**.

In our study, 36 patients underwent a biatrial ablation scheme. The procedure demonstrated an acceptable safety profile, and there were no fatalities in this group of patients. The median duration of stay in the intensive care unit was 17.1 hours (15.5; 19.1). Two (5.5%) patients developed sick sinus syndrome and a permanent pacemaker was implanted in them, while the remaining 34 patients were discharged with sinus rhythm.

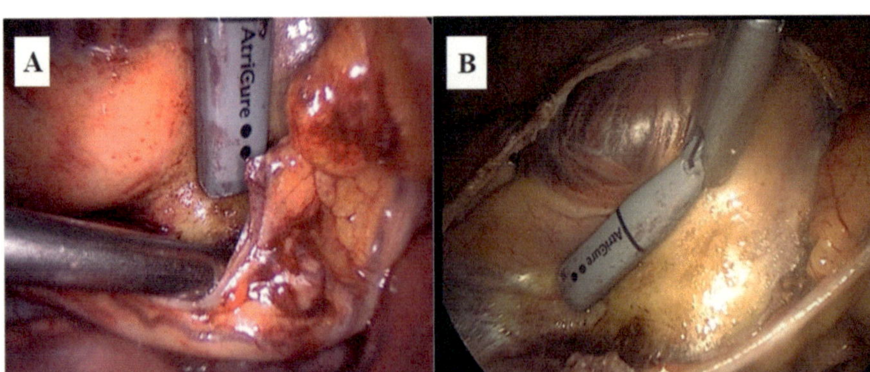


**Figure 6.**
*Stages of biatrial ablation. Description: A: Creation of the line along the lateral wall of the right atrium; B: Creation of the cava-caval line.*

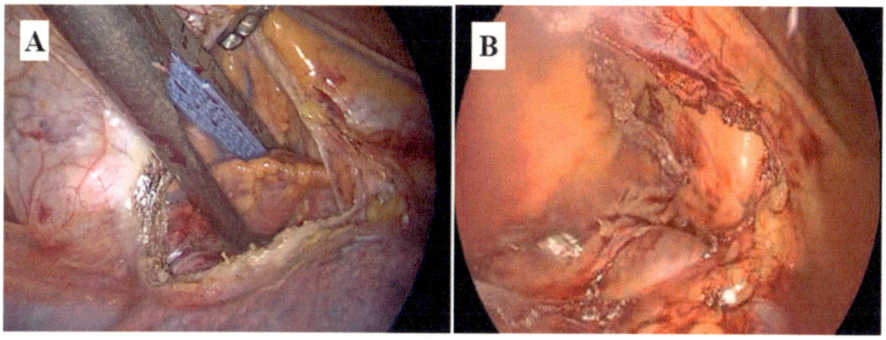


**Figure 7.**
*Stage of left atrial appendage resection. Description: A: Positioning the surgical stapler in the resection area. B: The result of left atrial appendage resection.*

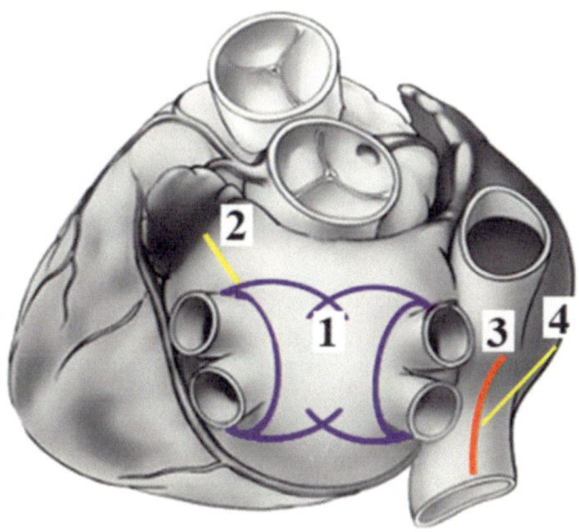


**Figure 8.**
*Biatrial ablation scheme. Description: 1: Box-lesion. 2: Line connecting the ridge and box-lesion. 3: Cava-caval line. 4: Line along the lateral wall of the right atrium.*

## 3. Endocardial stage

The procedure is performed under endotracheal anesthesia. Using ultrasound navigation, puncture and catheterization of the right internal jugular and right femoral veins are performed. Diagnostic electrodes are introduced into the right heart chambers and placed in the coronary sinus and right ventricle. Transseptal catheterization of the LA is performed at the level of the fossa ovalis under transesophageal or intracardiac ultrasound guidance. Systemic heparinization is required at this stage, maintaining an activated clotting time of 300–400 seconds. Rapid ventricular pacing is used to contrast the left atrium and PVs. Next, a three-dimensional reconstruction of the left atrium is performed using high-density mapping. If sinus rhythm or AF is present at this stage, a bipolar map of the LA is created. In the case of reentrant atrial tachycardia, an activation map of the LA is created to identify the critical tachycardia zone. The bipolar and activation maps are overlaid to identify areas of recovered conduction after the TA. In these areas, a series of radiofrequency energy applications are performed—30 W on the anterior wall (ablation index 400), 25 W on the posterior wall of the LA (ablation index 350), and 40 W on the mitral isthmus (ablation index 400). Bidirectional conduction block is verified in the distal pulmonary vein and mitral isthmus. Then, the ablation electrode is moved to the right atrium, and linear ablation of the cavotricuspid isthmus (CTI) is performed (40 W, ablation index 400). A bidirectional conduction block is verified in the CTI area. Endocardial ablation of the mitral isthmus and CTI are performed only in the case of diagnosed peri-mitral or typical atrial flutter (AFL).

Subsequently, control transesophageal or intracardiac echocardiography and control intracardiac electrophysiological study are performed, followed by an attempt to induce atrial tachyarrhythmias using incremental and programmed atrial stimulation. If reentrant atrial tachycardia is induced, the investigation heart chamber's activation map is created, followed by catheter ablation of the critical tachycardia zone.

**Figure 9(A-C)** shows a three-dimensional reconstruction of the LA in a patient with a recurrence of AF and AFL 4 months after TA. In fragments A and B, the results of bipolar mapping of the LA during intracardiac electrophysiological study (EPS) are shown—the posterior wall of the LA and the left pulmonary veins (PVs) are electrically isolated from the LA; in the anterior segment of the right PVs, an area of recovered electrical activity is identified (outlined with a yellow dashed line). After endocardial

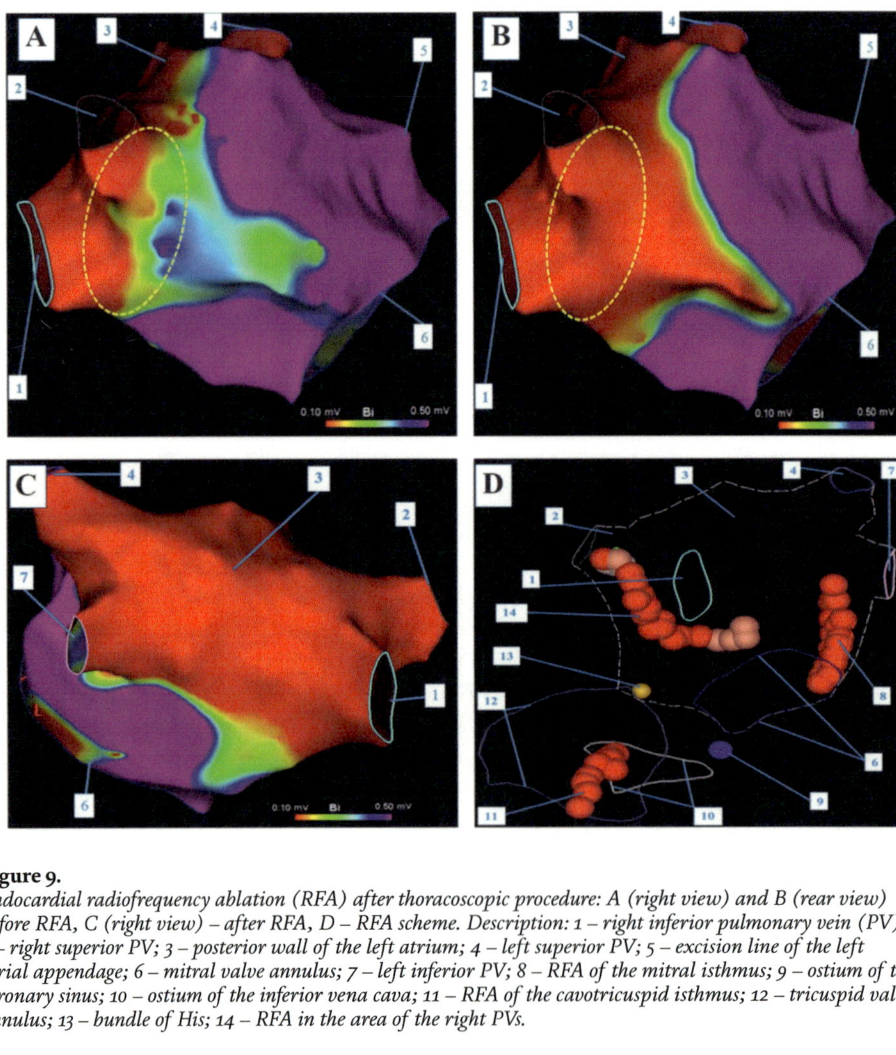


**Figure 9.**
*Endocardial radiofrequency ablation (RFA) after thoracoscopic procedure: A (right view) and B (rear view) before RFA, C (right view) – after RFA, D – RFA scheme. Description: 1 – right inferior pulmonary vein (PV); 2 – right superior PV; 3 – posterior wall of the left atrium; 4 – left superior PV; 5 – excision line of the left atrial appendage; 6 – mitral valve annulus; 7 – left inferior PV; 8 – RFA of the mitral isthmus; 9 – ostium of the coronary sinus; 10 – ostium of the inferior vena cava; 11 – RFA of the cavotricuspid isthmus; 12 – tricuspid valve annulus; 13 – bundle of His; 14 – RFA in the area of the right PVs.*

radiofrequency ablation (RFA), a bidirectional conduction block is achieved in this area, and there is no electrical activity in the pulmonary vein ostia (**Figure 9B**). A schematic of the endocardial RFA applied in this case is shown in **Figure 9D**.

**Figure 9** shows that linear RFA was performed in the anterior segment of the right PVs to restore electrical isolation. The RFA schematic shows endocardial RFA in the mitral isthmus and CTI areas. These interventions were performed due to an intraoperative induction of peri-mitral AFL, followed by a typical AFL.

In the second stage of treatment, 22 patients underwent EPS. The second stage of treatment was aimed at the identification of pulmonary vein reconnection areas after TA. If reconnection areas were detected, segmental catheter RFA was performed with verification of the bidirectional conduction block. In the case of atrial tachycardia detection or induction, mapping was performed, followed by catheter RFA in the critical tachycardia zone.

According to the results of EPS in patients after the previous TA, it was noted that the restoration of electrical activity in the antral part of the PVs occurred in 15 (68.2%) out of 22 patients. In all these cases, the previously performed epicardial interventions were supplemented with endocardial RFA in the identified PV and LA reconnection areas. In 5 (22,7%) out of 22 patients, RFA of the CTI was performed due to the induction of typical AFL during EPS. Additionally, in cases of peri-mitral AF induction, RFA of the mitral isthmus was performed in 6 (27.3%) out of 22 patients (**Table 3**) (**Figure 10**).

It was found that the most common area of PVs and LA reconnection after irrigated TA is the anterior segment of the antral part of the right PVs. Restoration of electrical activity in this area was identified in 13 out of 22 patients (59.1%). Reconnection of PVs and LA was less frequently noted in the lower and posterior segments of the antral part of the right PVs: 8 out of 22 patients (36.4%) and 6 out of 22 patients (27.3%), respectively. Other areas of PV and LA reconnection were

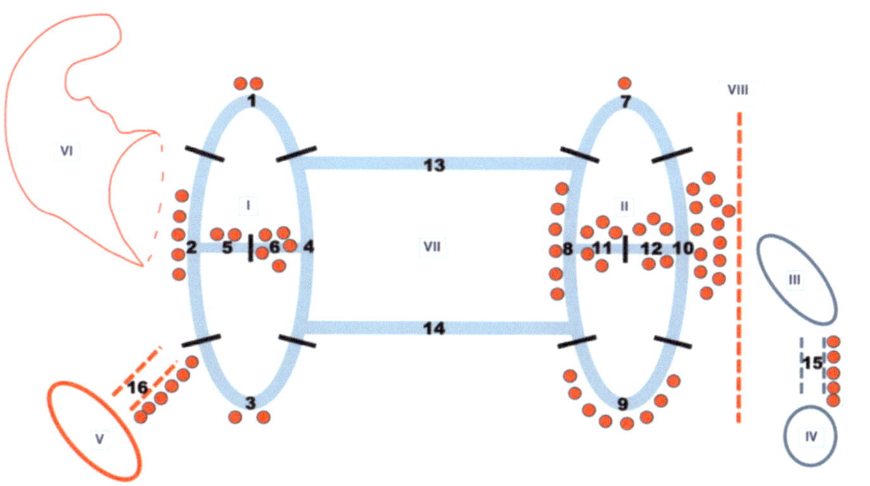


**Figure 10.**
*Areas of reconnection of the pulmonary veins and left atrium after epicardial bipolar irrigated thoracoscopic radiofrequency ablation of the left atrium. Description: Red dots indicate areas in the left atrium where endocardial radiofrequency ablation was performed (each dot corresponds to one patient). Roman numerals indicate the anatomical structures of the atrium. Arabic numerals indicate segments corresponding to the numbers in **Table** 3. I – Antral part of the left pulmonary veins; II – Antral part of the right pulmonary veins; III – Tricuspid valve annulus; IV – Ostium of the inferior vena cava; V – Mitral valve annulus; VI – Left atrial appendage; VII – Posterior wall of the left atrium; VIII – Interatrial septum.*

rarely diagnosed, with the frequency of occurrence not exceeding 22.7% (5 out of 22 patients). In the long-term follow-up period, with a median follow-up of 13 months (11;18), 20 (90,9%) patients were free from supraventricular arrhythmias, as recorded by Holter ECG (**Figure 11**).

| № | Heart segment | Number of patients (%) |
|---|---|---|
| 1 | Upper segment of the antral part of the left PVs | 2 (9,1%) |
| 2 | Anterior segment of the left PVs in the area of the ridge | 5 (22,7%) |
| 3 | Lower segment of the antral part of the left PVs | 2 (9,1%) |
| 4 | Posterior segment of the antral part of the left PVs | 0 (0,0%) |
| 5 | Anterior part of the ridge of the left PVs | 2 (9,1%) |
| 6 | Posterior part of the ridge of the left PVs | 5 (22,7%) |
| 7 | Upper segment of the antral part of the right PVs | 1 (4,5%) |
| 8 | Posterior segment of the antral part of the right PVs | 6 (27,3%) |
| 9 | Lower segment of the antral part of the right PVs | 8 (36,4%) |
| 10 | Anterior segment of the antral part of the right PVs | 13 (59,1%) |
| 11 | Posterior part of the ridge of the right PVs | 5 (22,7%) |
| 12 | Anterior part of the ridge of the right PVs | 5 (22,7%) |
| 13 | Upper segment of the posterior wall of the left atrium | 0 (0,0%) |
| 14 | Lower segment of the posterior wall of the left atrium | 0 (0,0%) |
| 15 | Cavotricuspid isthmus | 5 (22,7%) |
| 16 | Mitral isthmus | 6 (27,3%) |

**Table 3.**
*Types of performed catheter interventions.*

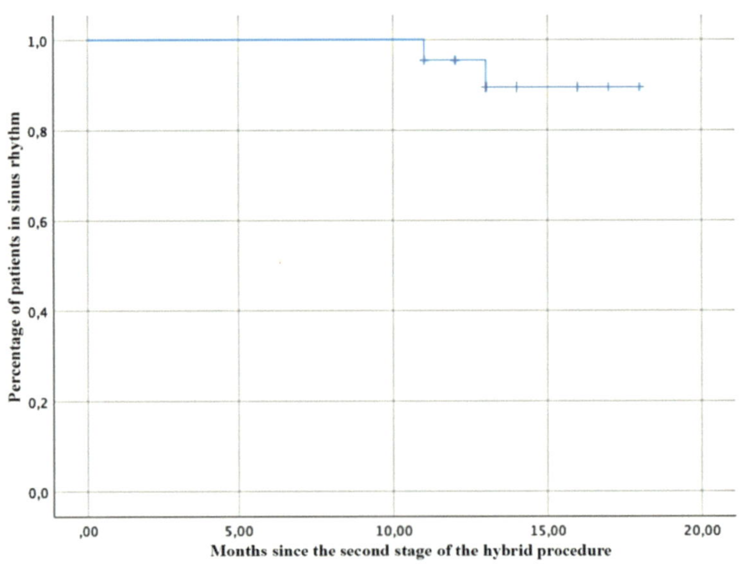


**Figure 11.**
*Kaplan-Meier curve for supraventricular arrhythmias freedom after the second stage of the hybrid procedure.*

## 4. Discussion

Despite TA's benefit and satisfactory safety profile, several issues remain unresolved—the inability to ablate the mitral isthmus zone and the macro-reentry wave circuits in the right atrium. In patients with extensive epicardial adipose tissue, achieving a complete transmural closed ablation line is often impossible, leading to the formation of gaps [9].

Incomplete ablation zones can serve as a source of AF recurrence and may also transform into substrates for atypical AFL. Additionally, no thoracoscopic ablation protocol currently includes interventions in the CTI area [10, 11].

In some cases, these shortcomings lead to AF recurrence, the development of typical and atypical AFL in the postoperative period. These factors have led to the conclusion that a more aggressive surgical strategy is needed, combining the advantages of thoracoscopic and endovascular techniques.

The initial procedures, combining thoracoscopic and catheter ablation, were performed using a single anesthesia. These procedures included isolation following the "Box-lesion" scheme and forming additional lines in the mitral and tricuspid isthmus areas using a catheter method [12, 13].

Pison conducted one of the first studies on hybrid treatment from 2009 to 2010. The authors reported a 92% freedom from AF 1 year after the procedure in patients, among whom 11 had non-paroxysmal arrhythmia. Even then, the authors suggested that the procedure could be performed sequentially in two stages, with the indication being AF recurrence or the appearance of other supraventricular tachyarrhythmias in the delayed period [14].

In 2017, a consensus from European Arrhythmology Societies defined hybrid treatment—it is a pre-planned intervention conducted jointly by interventional arrhythmologists and cardiac surgeons, either simultaneously or in two stages, within no more than 6 months [15]. In 2020, the hybrid procedure was included in the clinical guidelines of the European Society of Cardiology and the European Association for Cardio-Thoracic Surgery for the treatment of AF. It is recommended for patients with symptomatic paroxysmal or persistent arrhythmia refractory to antiarrhythmic therapy and has a class 2A recommendation [16].

In the multicenter HISTORIC-AF study (Historical Control Study to Assess Safety and Efficacy of the Hybrid Procedure in Non-valvular Atrial Fibrillation), the freedom from AF 1 year after the procedure was 88% in patients with non-paroxysmal AF [17]. More recent studies confirm the advantage of the hybrid strategy, showing freedom from AF of about 70–85% in the long-term follow-up period [18–20].

When used separately, the hybrid procedure overcomes the limitations of endocardial and epicardial approaches. Thus, the hybrid approach allows the recreation of the "Maze-IV" ablation scheme using minimally invasive surgical technologies. As a result, there is an increase in effectiveness in treating patients with persistent forms of AF and other groups at high risk of recurrence. Given the absence of the need for cardiopulmonary bypass, this procedure successfully competes with the MAZE-IV operation performed through a mini-thoracotomy approach [21].

The timing between the epicardial and endocardial stages of the operation remains unexplored. Some surgeons perform hybrid interventions using a single anesthesia. For the epicardial stage, it is possible to use the Episense tool (Convergent procedure) or perform the epicardial protocol with thoracoscopic instruments, completing the procedure with catheter intervention in the mitral isthmus zone, ablation of the CTI zone, and additional isolation of the PVs [22, 23].

This approach demonstrates an advantage in the number of hospitalizations, reducing treatment costs. However, during a single procedure, false-positive and false-negative results may arise due to tissue edema, making it difficult to assess the isolation of lines after the epicardial stage [24].

Other teams perform the catheter stage after a 3-month blind period, adhering to the opinion that additional catheter ablations should be performed exclusively in epicardial ablation line gaps, incomplete conduction block, and confirmed typical or atypical AFL [25].

We adhere to a waiting strategy in our clinical practice for the following reasons:

- Firstly, identifying gaps in the primary epicardial ablation line immediately after the intervention, in the presence of inflammation and myocardial edema, is challenging. A time interval is needed for scar tissue formation and stabilization of epicardial ablation zones.

- Secondly, performing a simultaneous procedure increases the duration of the operation and possibly the frequency of postoperative complications.

- Thirdly, not all patients may require a catheter procedure. For these reasons, we perform the hybrid procedure in two stages, waiting for at least 3 months.

Given the long-term results of arrhythmia freedom in patients with heart failure, both with reduced and preserved EF, and with long-standing persistent AF, we currently consider the possibility of hybrid ablation for these patient groups. In our clinical practice, we have started using a modified HFA-PEFF algorithm, which helps identify patients with heart failure and preserved ejection fraction. This algorithm has helped us determine a new group of patients for whom a hybrid approach is necessary.

In our study, the most common gap of the epicardial isolation line was the anterior segment of the antral part of the right PVs. This is due to the anatomical features of this segment, the design features of the electrodes, and the development of epicardial adipose tissue in the Waterston groove. It is challenging to achieve a transmural ablation line in patients with extensive epicardial adipose tissue development and significant atriomegaly. As a result, we destroy the adipose tissue and additionally perform ablation with the MLP electrode (AtriCure) in this zone.

The hybrid approach has demonstrated an acceptable safety profile. In all 22 patients, no complications were registered that affected hospitalization time, leading to the conclusion that this approach is safe for treating patients with AF.

## Acknowledgements

Hybrid treatment was funded by:

Federal Scientific and Clinical Center for Specialized Medical Assistance and Medical Technologies of the Federal Medical Biological Agency - the program of state guarantees of medical care.

Endocrinology Research Centre - Governmental grant (Task, assignment number 123021000043-0).

## Author details

Alexandr Zotov[1], Igor Khamnagadaev[2,3], Oleg Shelest[1*], Emil Sakharov[1], Alexandr Glupak[1], Irina Bulavina[4], Robert Khabazov[1], Alexandr Troitsky[1] and Natalya Mokrysheva[2]

1 Federal Scientific and Clinical Center for Specialized Medical Assistance and Medical Technologies of the Federal Medical Biological Agency, Moscow, Russian Federation

2 Endocrinology Research Centre, Moscow, Russian Federation

3 Veltischev Research and Clinical Institute for Pediatrics and Pediatric Surgery of the Pirogov Russian National Research Medical University, Moscow, Russian Federation

4 Moscow City Clinical Hospital named after V.M. Buyanov, Moscow, Russian Federation

*Address all correspondence to: toshelest@gmail.com

## References


[1] Cox JL, Schuessler RB, D'Agostino HJ Jr, Stone CM, Chang BC, Cain ME, et al. The surgical treatment of atrial fibrillation. II. Intraoperative electrophysiologic mapping and description of the electrophysiologic basis of atrial flutter and atrial fibrillation. The Journal of Thoracic and Cardiovascular Surgery. 1991;**101**:406-426

[2] Tischer TS, Schneider R, Lauschke J, Nesselmann C, Steinhoff G, Bänsch D. Adjunctive surgical atrial fibrillation ablation during cardiac surgery: Real life experiences. Herzschrittmachertherapie & Elektrophysiologie. 2015;**26**(3):291-296. DOI: 10.1007/s00399-015-0379-1

[3] Ad N, Holmes SD, Massimiano PS, et al. Long-term outcome following concomitant mitral valve surgery and Cox maze procedure for atrial fibrillation. The Journal of Thoracic and Cardiovascular Surgery. 2018;**155**:983-994. DOI: 10.1016/j.jtcvs.2017.09.135

[4] Wolf RK, Schneeberger EW, Osterday R, Miller D, Merrill W, Flege JB Jr, et al. Video-assisted bilateral pulmonary vein isolation and left atrial appendage exclusion for atrial fibrillation. The Journal of Thoracic and Cardiovascular Surgery. 2005;**130**(3):797-802. DOI: 10.1016/j.jtcvs.2005.04.005

[5] Doty JR, Archbold JA, Upton RF. Galaxy procedure: A new approach to atrial fibrillation surgery. Innovations. 2010;**5**(5):366-370. DOI: 10.1097/IMI.0b013e3181f87238

[6] Zotov A, Vachev S, Borisov D, Troitskiy A, Khabazov R. Thoracoscopic pulmonary vein and left atrial posterior wall isolation combined with left atrial appendage resection in patients with long-standing persistent atrial fibrillation. Brazilian Journal of Cardiovascular Surgery. 2020;**35**(1):22-27. DOI: 10.21470/1678-9741-2019-0132

[7] Pieske B, Tschöpe C, de Boer RA, et al. How to diagnose heart failure with preserved ejection fraction: The HFA–PEFF diagnostic algorithm: A consensus recommendation from the Heart Failure Association (HFA) of the European Society of Cardiology (ESC). European Heart Journal. 2019;**40**(40):3297-3317. DOI: 10.1093/eurheartj/ehz641

[8] Cox JL, Churyla A, Malaisrie SC, et al. A hybrid maze procedure for long-standing persistent atrial fibrillation. The Annals of Thoracic Surgery. 2019;**107**(2):610-618. DOI: 10.1016/j.athoracsur.2018.06.064

[9] Khiabani AJ, MacGregor RM, Redfearn DP, Massey HT, et al. Bipolar radiofrequency ablation on explanted human hearts: How to ensure transmural lesions. The Annals of Thoracic Surgery. 2020;**110**(6):1933-1939. DOI: 10.1016/j.athoracsur.2020.04.079

[10] Edgerton JR, Edgerton ZJ, Weaver T, Mack MJ. Minimally invasive pulmonary vein isolation and partial autonomic denervation for surgical treatment of atrial fibrillation. The Annals of Thoracic Surgery. 2008;**86**:35-39. DOI: 10.1016/j.athoracsur.2008.03.071

[11] Gillinov AM, Bhavani S, Blackstone EH, et al. Surgery for permanent atrial fibrillation: Impact of patient factors and lesion set. The Annals of Thoracic Surgery. 2006;**82**:502-513; discussion 513. DOI: 10.1016/j.athoracsur.2006.02.030

[12] Mahapatra S, LaPar DJ, Kamath S, Payne J, Bilchick KC, Mangrum JM, et al. Initial experience of sequential surgical epicardial-catheter endocardial ablation for persistent and longstanding persistent atrial fibrillation with long-term follow-up. The Annals of Thoracic Surgery. 2011;**91**(6):1890-1898. DOI: 10.1016/j.athoracsur.2011.02.045

[13] Pak HN, Hwang C, Lim HE, Kim JS, Kim YH. Hybrid epicardial and endocardial ablation of persistent or permanent atrial fibrillation: A new approach for difficult cases. Journal of Cardiovascular Electrophysiology. 2007;**18**(9):917-923. DOI: 10.1111/j.1540-8167.2007.00882.x

[14] Pison L, La Meir M, van Opstal J, Blaauw Y, Maessen J, Crijns HJ. Hybrid thoracoscopic surgical and transvenous catheter ablation of atrial fibrillation. Journal of the American College of Cardiology. 2012;**60**(1):54-61. DOI: 10.1016/j.jacc.2011.12.055

[15] Calkins H, Hindricks G, Cappato R, et al. HRS/EHRA/ECAS/APHRS/SOLAECE expert consensus statement on catheter and surgical ablation of atrial fibrillation: Executive summary. Heart Rhythm. 2017;**14**(10):e445-e494. DOI: 10.1007/s10840-017-0277-z

[16] Hindricks G, Potpara T, Dagres N, Arbelo E, Bax JJ, Blomström-Lundqvist C, et al.; ESC Scientific Document Group. 2020 ESC guidelines for the diagnosis and management of atrial fibrillation developed in collaboration with the European Association for Cardio-Thoracic Surgery (EACTS): The task force for the diagnosis and management of atrial fibrillation of the European Society of Cardiology (ESC) developed with the special contribution of the European Heart Rhythm Association (EHRA) of the ESC. European Heart Journal. 2021;**42**(5):373-498. DOI: 10.1093/eurheartj/ehaa612. Erratum in: Eur Heart J. 2021;42(5):507

[17] Muneretto C, Bisleri G, Badoe N, et al. European prospective multicentre study of hybrid thoracoscopic and transcatheter ablation of persistent atrial fibrillation: The HISTORIC-AF trial. European Journal of Cardio-Thoracic Surgery. 2017;**52**(4):740-745. DOI: 10.1093/ejcts/ezx162

[18] Kim YH, Kim JY, Choi HY, et al. Efficacy and safety of hybrid ablation for atrial fibrillation: A systematic review and meta-analysis. International Journal of Arrhythmia. 2020;**21**(1):22-31. DOI: 10.1186/s42444-020-00035-4

[19] Verma A, Jiang CY, Betts TR, et al. Approaches to catheter ablation for persistent atrial fibrillation. The New England Journal of Medicine. 2015;**372**:1812-1822. DOI: 10.1056/NEJMoa1408288

[20] Berger WR, Meulendijks AM, Limpens J, et al. Long-term outcomes of hybrid thoracoscopic surgical and transvenous catheter ablation of atrial fibrillation: A meta-analysis. European Journal of Cardio-Thoracic Surgery. 2021;**23**(10):1568-1578. DOI: 10.1093/europace/euab156

[21] Ruaengsri C, Schill MR, Khiabani AJ, Schuessler RB, Melby SJ, Damiano RJ. The Cox-maze IV procedure in its second decade: Still the gold standard? European Journal of Cardio-Thoracic Surgery. 2018;**53**(Suppl 1):i19-i25. DOI: 10.1093/ejcts/ezx326

[22] Gulkarov I, Wong B, Kowalski M, Worku B, Afzal A, Ivanov A, et al. Convergent ablation for persistent atrial fibrillation: Single center experience. Journal of Cardiac Surgery. 2019;**34**(10):1037-1043. DOI: 10.1111/jocs.14204. Epub 2019 August 2

[23] Kurfirst V, Mokracek A, Bulava A, et al. Two-staged hybrid treatment of persistent atrial fibrillation: Short-term single-centre results. Interactive Cardiovascular and Thoracic Surgery. 2014;**18**(4):451-456. DOI: 10.1093/icvts/ivt538

[24] On YK, Jeong DS. Updates in hybrid AF ablation: A hybrid approach to surgical epicardial ablation and catheter endocardial ablation in persistent atrial fibrillation. International Journal of Arrhythmia. 2022;**23**:5. DOI: 10.1186/s42444-021-00056-6

[25] van der Heijden CAJ, Weberndörfer V, Vroomen M, Luermans JG, Chaldoupi SM, Bidar E, et al. Hybrid ablation versus repeated catheter ablation in persistent atrial fibrillation: A randomized controlled trial. JACC: Clinical Electrophysiology. 2023;**9**(7 Pt 2):1013-1023. DOI: 10.1016/j.jacep.2022.12.011. Epub 2023 January 18

Chapter 14

# Renal Sympathetic Denervation in Atrial Fibrillation Treatment

*Mustafa Ucar*

## Abstract

Atrial fibrillation (AF) is a chronic and progressive disease. The most common causes of AF are age and hypertension. Treatment is challenging and the main treatment is medical. Despite optimal medical treatment in accordance with guidelines, many patients remain symptomatic. At this stage, catheter ablation-based applications have made a breakthrough in the treatment of AF. Pulmonary vein isolation is the cornerstone of treatment, but pulmonary vein isolation is often not sufficient. Identification of additional isolation sites and targeting these sites has been essential in the treatment of atrial fibrillation. Therefore, new treatment strategies are being sought. While renal sympathetic denervation was initially used in the treatment of resistant hypertension, its efficacy in the treatment of cardiac arrhythmias, including AF, has been established. In this article, we will describe the role of renal sympathetic denervation in the treatment of AF and will not include a comparison with other treatments.

**Keywords:** atrial fibrillation, arrhythmia, renal sympathetic denervation, radiofrequency ablation, electrophysiology

## 1. Introduction

AF is the most common arrhythmia in adults. According to The Global Burden of Disease 2019 study, more than 59 million individuals lived with AF in 2019 [1]. The true prevalence of AF is higher because of many individuals who are not diagnosed until symptoms develop. The prevalence of AF will rise to 15.9 million in 2050 in America and 17.9 million in 2060 in Europe [2, 3]. AF increases the risk of stroke 4–5 fold, the risk of dementia 2 fold, the risk of heart failure 3 fold, and the risk of mortality 2 fold [4]. The most important risk factor is age and its prevalence doubles with each decade above the age of 35 years of age and affected men more than women [5].

AF is a supraventricular tachyarrhythmia with uncoordinated atrial activation and ineffective atrial contraction. Electrocardiogram (ECG) characteristics are irregular R-R intervals when atrioventricular (AV) conduction is present, absence of distinct P waves and fibrillatory waves. AF can be documented by 12-lead ECG, rhythm stripes, etc., but will always require visual confirmation. AF can be categorised as follows: paroxysmal AF (episodes intermittent, terminates in 7 days of onset), persistent AF (that is continuous and sustains for >7 days and requires intervention), long-standing persistent AF (that is continuous for >12 months), and permanent AF (no longer pursue a rhythm control strategy after discussion between patient and clinician) [6].

Due to the complex pathophysiology of the disease, its treatment is also challenging and this subject is beyond the scope of this article. On the other hand, catheter ablation is a method with proven efficacy in the treatment of AF. Pulmonary vein isolation is considered the only catheter ablation method with demonstrated efficacy and is recommended in current guidelines [6]. However, despite PVI, the desired results have not been achieved in most individuals. Therefore, new methods are being investigated and evaluated. Renal sympathetic denervation is one of these methods.

## 2. Cardiac autonomic nervous system

William Harvey has described the relationship between the heart and the nervous system [7]. The autonomic nervous system (ANS) not only regulates the heart rate and hemodynamic changes but also plays a central role in the pathogenesis of cardiac arrhythmias such as AF. The cardiac autonomic nervous system can be divided into intrinsic and extrinsic parts. The extrinsic part fibres provide connections between the heart and the nervous system, whereas the intrinsic part consists of fibres and ganglions once they enter the pericardial sac [8]. Extrinsic ANS includes superior cervical ganglia, cervicothoracic (stellate) ganglia, and thoracic ganglia. İntrinsic ANS includes numerous ganglia, which are organised into complex plexi on the surfaces of the atrias and ventricles. Atrial plexis are located especially around sinus node territory, inferior vena cava-left atrium junction, and pulmonary vein-left atrium junction. Ventricular plexis are located at the origins of major cardiac blood vessels [9, 10].

With neurohormonal activation and neuronal remodelling, inhibition of the parasympathetic system increases, and sympathetic afferent and efferent outputs to the heart increase, resulting in a predisposition for arrhythmias. Sympathetic neuronal activation increases norepinephrine and neuropeptide Y and co-transmitters such as galanin at the cardiac level [11, 12]. Intracellular calcium influx starts with norepinephrine-mediated sympathetic stimulation. In response to transmembrane calcium influx, calcium is released by sarcoplasmic reticulum calcium channels (ryanodine receptors) [13]. Due to the discrepancy in intracellular calcium and action potential, forward sodium/calcium (Na/Ca) exchanger current increases, resulting in early afterdepolarization and triggered activity. This triggered activity plays an important role in the development of AF in the LA-PV region, which is rich in ganglion plexus. Therefore, this region is a target for catheter ablation [14].

## 3. Renal sympathetic system and denervation

Sympathetic activation also activates the renin-angiotensin-aldosterone system. As a result, profibrotic pathways are activated, leading to atrial structural changes. These fibrotic changes lead to proarrhythmogenic electrophysiological abnormalities. For example, angiotensin 2 causes atrial fibroblasts to differentiate into myofibroblasts [15]. Therefore, angiotensin-converting enzyme inhibitors reduce the development of AF.

Denervation of the renal sympathetic nerves results in a systemic effect. The evaluation of the renal arteries and the nerve network surrounding them is based on autopsy studies. Renal sympathetic nerves originate at spinal segments.

T11 to L3 and contain inputs from the thoracic and lumbar splanchnic nerves, aortic plexus, and posterior vagal trunk. Renal sympathetic postganglionic nerves exit

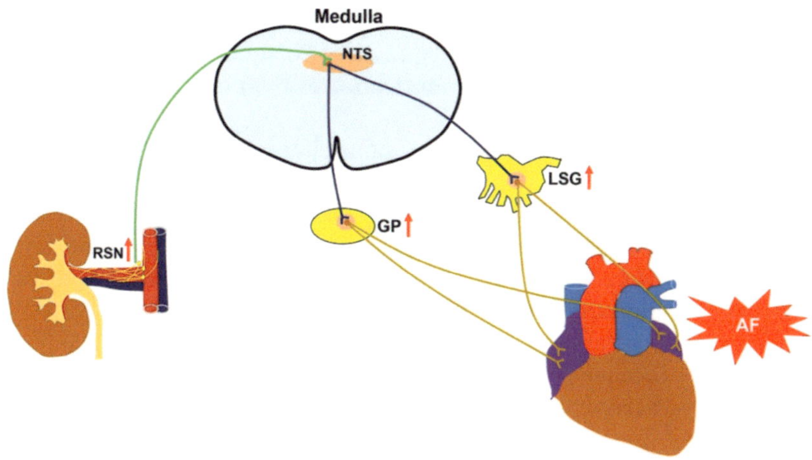


**Figure 1.**
*Activation of the renal sympathetic nerve (RSN) affects nucleus of the solitary tract (NST). NTS neurons increase the nerve activity of atrial ganglionated plexi (GP) and the left stellate (LSG). This activation contributes to the initiation and maintenance of AF.*

the ganglia and enter the hilum side of the kidney near the renal arteries and veins [16]. The renal sympathetic nerves travel through the adventitia of the renal arteries. According to the autopsy data, more than 90% of the renal artery nerve network is within 2 mm of the lumen. In addition, nerves extended 6–7 mm into the lumen, denser nerve networks were observed in the proximal and middle renal arteries, and nerves were found closer to the lumen in the distal part of the vessel [17, 18]. **Figure 1** shows the interaction between renal and cardiac autonomic nerves and its role in the development of AF.

Sympathetic nerve activity affects chronotropy and dromotropy and sympathetic activity plays an important role in development of arrhythmias. As a result, renal sympathetic denervation seems to be a different approach in the treatment of arrhythmias.

Renal sympathetic denervation applications date back to a century ago. The first application of bilateral renal sympathetic denervation for the treatment of essential hypertension was performed in 1934 [19]. Although renal sympathetic denervation remained in the background with the development of antihypertensive drugs, the renal sympathetic system started to be re-examined in the 2000s in uncontrolled hypertensive patients in whom medical treatment was resistant. In 2009, the efficacy and safety of catheter-based renal sympathetic denervation were demonstrated in patients with resistant hypertension. Subsequently, many studies have been presented in this field. As a result of these studies, more data on the renal sympathetic system and neuromodulation have been obtained, and the effects on other cardiovascular diseases, including arrhythmias, have begun to be evaluated [20].

## 4. Renal sympathetic denervation techniques

In the past, especially before the use of antihypertensive agents, aggressive surgical sympathectomy methods were used. However, surgical sympathectomy was associated with serious undesirable consequences such as postural hypotension, hyperhidrosis, sexual dysfunction, and depression. Fortunately, with the introduction of antihypertensive agents and demonstration of their efficacy, surgical methods were abandoned [21].

Nevertheless, despite the widespread use of antihypertensive agents, there is a significant population that remains uncontrolled. In the 2000s, the sympathetic system became of interest again. The effects of catheter-based renal sympathetic denervation on hypertension were finally demonstrated and favourable effects on atrial and ventricular arrhythmias were observed in these patients. As will be discussed later, renal sympathetic denervation in addition to pulmonary vein isolation has been shown to be more effective.

Percutaneous techniques include catheter-based radiofrequency ablation, ultrasonic ablation therapy, and pharmacological ablation mediated by infusion catheters [22].

Ultrasound ablation therapy is performed by generating frictional thermal energy through the interaction of high-frequency environmental ultrasonic waves and surrounding fluids. Fewer complications and ablation of better precise areas are targeted. The currently available ultrasound ablation technology includes the PARADISE Percutaneous Denervation System (ReCor Medical, Ronkonkoma, NY), the TIVUS system (Cardiosonic, Tel Aviv, Israel), and the Kona Surround Sound system (Kona Medical, Bellevue, WA). Clinical data is not yet available.

The pharmacological ablation technique uses catheter guidance systems. Therapeutic agents are injected directly into the adventitial tissue and renal nerve ablation is aimed without injuring the vascular intima and media. This technique has not yet been evaluated in the management of arrhythmias [21].

Another technique in the management of renal denervation-associated arrhythmia is catheter-based radiofrequency ablation. Dedicated systems can be used for radiofrequency ablation as well as standard cardiac ablation systems. Due to pain during renal nerve ablation, the procedure is performed under sedation and analgesia. The procedure starts with aortagraphy with a pigtail catheter and then both renal arteries and accessory arteries, if any, are selectively visualized. If available, real-time 3-dimensional aorta-renal artery maps can be constructed with the use of an ablation catheter and an electroanatomic navigation system. Activated clotting time >250 msec is aimed. Nitrates are applied to prevent vasospasm. Artery diameters >3 mm and <50% stenosis are required for the procedure. In addition, the main segment must be >20 mm for 4 simultaneous radiofrequency ablations. If the main renal artery segment length is below 20 mm, the first branches should be between 3 and 8 mm and the length should be above 20 mm. If the eligibility criteria are not met again, the second branches are evaluated. It should be ablated from distal to proximal without overlap to the extent appropriate for the anatomy. If accessory arteries are present, ablation is also performed [23]. The criterion for success is usually met when the sudden increase in blood pressure of about 15 mm Hg is eliminated or greatly reduced after high-frequency stimulation. Although it is a generally safe procedure, complications that may develop in angiographic procedures can be observed. Complications such as haematoma at the site of intervention, retroperitoneal haemorrhage, trauma to large arteries, renal artery spasm, dissection or rupture, allergy due to the opaque substance used, nephropathy, and bradycardia may develop. In a consensus report published in 2023, it was stated that there was no significant association with renal artery stenosis or deterioration in renal function in the long term [24].

## 5. Renal sympathetic denervation studies and meta-analysis in atrial fibrillation

In the past 10 years, studies evaluating the efficacy of renal sympathetic denervation in the treatment of atrial fibrillation have been published. Studies have shown the effectiveness of renal sympathetic denervation on structural and electrical remodelling and haemodynamic filling pressures in the management of AF.

In this section of the article, some encouraging studies on renal sympathetic denervation in the treatment of AF will be presented.

## 6. The evaluate renal denervation in addition to catheter ablation to eliminate atrial fibrillation (ERADICATE AF)

In the management of AF, perhaps this is the most interesting study evaluating catheter-based renal sympathetic denervation with promising results. The study was a randomized, single-blind, multicentre involving 5 pivot centres in Germany, Russia, and Poland, conducted between April 2013 and March 2018, with follow-up completed in March 2019. A total of 302 patients with hypertension despite taking at least 1 antihypertensive agent and scheduled for catheter ablation because of paroxysmal AF were included in the study. In 148 patients, only pulmonary vein isolation was performed, while 154 patients underwent renal denervation in addition to pulmonary vein isolation. Additional left atrial lesions were not included and a cavotricuspid isthmus ablation was performed only in patients in whom atrial flutter was detected on ECG or atrial flutter was induced during the procedure. Renal denervation was performed using an ablation catheter (3.5-mm tip Thermocool family, Biosense Webster Inc) and an electroanatomic navigation system (CARTO, Biosense Webster Inc). The aim was to place a spiral lesion set in each renal artery. The criterion for success was the elimination of a sudden rise in blood pressure of 15 mmHg. In most patients undergoing renal denervation, a standard irrigated ablation catheter was used, but in selected patients, specifically designed and approved single or multielectrode radiofrequency delivery systems were used. 283 patients completed the trial. Freedom from atrial fibrillation, flutter, or tachycardia at 12 months was observed in 84 of 148 (56.5%) of those undergoing pulmonary vein isolation alone and in 111 of 154 (72.1%) of those undergoing pulmonary vein isolation plus renal denervation (hazard ratio, 0.57; 95% CI, 0.38 to 0.85; $P = 0.006$). Mean systolic blood pressure from baseline to 12 months decreased from 151 to 147 mm Hg in the isolation-only group and from 150 to 135 mm Hg in the renal denervation group (between-group difference, −13 mm Hg; 95% CI, −15 to −11 mm Hg; $P < 0.001$). Procedural complications were similar and the addition of renal denervation to the procedure did not cause any additional risk. The authors concluded that adding renal denervation to standard pulmonary vein isolation significantly increased the likelihood of freedom from atrial fibrillation at 12 months [25].

## 7. Pulmonary vein isolation combined with spironolactone or renal sympathetic denervation in patients with chronic kidney disease, uncontrolled hypertension, paroxysmal atrial fibrillation, and a pacemaker (Kiuchi Study)

This was a single-centre, prospective, longitudinal, randomised, double-blind study. Patients were recruited from January 2014 until June 2015. 69 patients were included in the study and the patients were randomly divided into two groups. 36 patients received spironolactone treatment in addition to pulmonary vein isolation and 33 patients received renal denervation in addition to pulmonary vein isolation. Patients had uncontrolled hypertension, a history of symptomatic paroxysmal AF, chronic kidney disease, and a dual-chamber pacemaker. Patients were followed for 1 year. At 3, 6, 9, and 12 months, pacemaker recordings were analysed for arrhythmias and AF burden. All patients underwent complete PVI using a three-dimensional mapping system (EnSite Velocity; St. Jude Medical) without additional ablation lesion sets or lines. The EnligHTN™ multielectrode renal denervation ablation catheter (St. Jude Medical, St. Paul, MN, USA) was used for renal denervation. At least 8 lesions were performed at the main trunk of bilateral renal arteries. At the end of the 12th month, AF burden was 12% lower in the pulmonary vein isolation plus renal denervation group ($P < 0.0001$). The authors concluded that pulmonary vein isolation plus renal denervation is safe and appears to be superior to pulmonary vein isolation plus spironolactone in BP reduction, augmentation of AF event-free rate, reduction of AF burden, and improvement of renal function [26].

## 8. AFFORD study (atrial fibrillation reduction by renal sympathetic denervation)

This was a single-arm pilot study including 20 patients from Netherlands. Inclusion criteria were met: paroxysmal or persistent AF, hypertension (mean office systolic BP $\geq$ 140 mmHg), use of $\geq$2 antihypertensive drugs, age $\geq$ 18 years, estimated glomerular filtration rate (eGFR) > 45 ml/min/1.73 $m^2$. The EnligHTN™ multielectrode renal denervation ablation catheter (St. Jude Medical, St. Paul, MN, USA) was used for renal denervation. At least 8 successful ablations were aimed at each renal artery. The change in patients' quality of life at the end of the 12th month was also evaluated with the Atrial Fibrillation Effect on Quality of life (AFEQT) questionnaire. AF burden in min/day decreased from a median of 1.39 (0–11) pre-renal denervation to 0.67 (0–31.6) at 6 months ($p = 0.64$) and to 0.94 (0–6.0) at 12 months (pre-renal denervation vs. 12 months; $p = 0.03$). Quality of life improved significantly at both 6 months (+ 11 ± 15 points, $p = 0.006$) and 12 months (+ 10 ± 19, $p = 0.04$) as compared to pre-renal denervation. The authors concluded that renal denervation might be able to decrease AF burden with a positive effect on quality of life. On the other hand, a study was small, and large randomised trials are needed [27].

## 9. A randomised comparison of pulmonary vein isolation with versus without concomitant renal artery denervation in patients with refractory symptomatic atrial fibrillation and resistant hypertension

This was the first meaningful trial evaluating renal denervation. 27 patients with drug-resistant hypertension and paroxysmal or persistent AF were included in the study. All patients were followed for ≥1 year. 14 patients were randomised to pulmonary vein isolation only and 13 patients were randomised to pulmonary vein isolation plus renal denervation. No additional lesion sets or lines were applied in the left atria. Cavotricuspid isthmus ablation was performed only in patients who had an atrial flutter history. Aorta-renal artery maps were reconstructed with the use of the same navigation and catheter used for pulmonary vein isolation. 6 lesions were performed both longitudinally and rotationally from distal bifurcation to the ostium of each renal artery. All patients were treated with antiarrhythmic drugs for 6 weeks after pulmonary vein isolation; these drugs were subsequently withdrawn. At the end of the follow-up, significant reductions in systolic (from 181 ± 7 to 156 ± 5, p = 0.001) and diastolic blood pressure (from 97 ± 6 to 87 ± 4, p = 0.001) were observed in patients treated with PVI with renal denervation without significant change in the PVI only group. Nine of the 13 patients (69%) treated with PVI with renal denervation were AF-free at the 12-month post-ablation follow-up examination versus 4 (29%) of the 14 patients in the PVI-only group (p = 0.033). The authors concluded that renal denervation reduces systolic and diastolic blood pressure in patients with drug-resistant hypertension and reduces AF recurrences when combined with pulmonary vein isolation [28].

## 10. Renal sympathetic denervation as upstream therapy during atrial fibrillation ablation, pilot HFIB studies, and meta-analysis

The data for this study were obtained from HFIB (Adjunctive Renal Denervation to Modify Hypertension and Sympathetic tone as Upstream Therapy in the Treatment of Atrial Fibrillation)-1 (n = 30) and HFIB (Adjunctive Renal Denervation to Modify Hypertension and Sympathetic tone as Upstream Therapy in the Treatment of Atrial Fibrillation)-2 (n = 50) studies. Authors performed a meta-analysis including studies (ERADICATE AF) comparing pulmonary vein isolation alone versus pulmonary vein isolation plus renal denervation up to January 2020 in patients with AF and hypertension [25, 26, 28, 29]. At 24 months, AF recurrence occurred in 53 and 38% of the pulmonary vein isolation and pulmonary vein isolation plus renal denervation groups (p = 0.43) in the HFIB-1 study, respectively, and in 27 and 25% of the pulmonary vein isolation and pulmonary vein isolation plus renal denervation groups (p = 0.80) in the HFIB-2 study, respectively. When combined in a meta-analysis including 6 studies (n = 725), adjunctive renal denervation significantly decreased the risk of AF recurrence (risk ratio [RR]: 0.68; 95% confidence interval [CI]: 0.55 to 0.83; p = 0.0002; $I^2$ = 0%) when compared to pulmonary vein isolation. The authors concluded that HFIB-1 and HFIB-2 studies did not demonstrate a benefit with RSDN as an adjunctive upstream therapy during PVI. However, in the meta-analysis, adjunctive RSDN to PVI appears to be safe and improves clinical outcomes in AF patients with a history of hypertension [30].

On the other hand, the Effect of Concomitant Renal Denervation and Cardiac Ablation on Atrial Fibrillation Recurrence (RDN + AF) Study was designed to evaluate the efficacy of AF ablation alone and the addition of renal denervation to AF ablation. It was a prospective, randomised, nonblinded study performed between May 2014 and July 2016 in Germany. 61 patients were randomised. Patients were randomised 1:2 to either AF-only ablation (n = 22) or renal denervation plus AF ablation (n = 39). All patients received pulmonary vein isolation. Also, additional lesions were performed according to the voltage maps (e.g. mitral annulus, left atrium posterior wall). Renal denervation was performed with 'EnligHTN Renal Denervation System', which is a dedicated system. Freedom from AF recurrence in the renal denervation plus AF and AF-only group measured 61 versus 53% $p = 0.622$ at 12 months and 39 versus 47% $p = 0.927$ at 24 months, respectively. Periprocedural complications occurred in 9/61 patients (15%). The authors concluded that adding renal denervation was not associated with a significant blood pressure reduction or improved rhythm outcome at 12 and 24 months [31].

## 11. Conclusion

AF is a difficult disorder to control and treat due to its complex pathophysiology. Currently, no single treatment modality is sufficient. Although pulmonary vein isolation is the cornerstone of treatment, it may be insufficient in many patients. Renal sympathetic denervation seems promising at this point. However, large randomised controlled trials are needed.

## Conflict of interest

The author declares no conflict of interest.

## Author details

Mustafa Ucar
Medicine School Cardiology Department, Celal Bayar University, Manisa, Turkey

*Address all correspondence to: mucar55555@gmail.com

## References

[1] Roth GA, Mensah GA, Johnson CO, et al. Global burden of cardiovascular diseases and risk factors, 1990-2019: Update from the GBD 2019 study. Journal of the American College of Cardiology. 2020;**76**(25):2982-3021

[2] Miyasaka Y, Barnes ME, Gersh BJ, et al. Secular trends in incidence of atrial fibrillation in Olmsted County, Minnesota, 1980 to 2000, and implications on the projections for future prevalence. Circulation. 2006;**114**(2):119-125

[3] Krijthe BP, Kunst A, Benjamin EJ, et al. Projections on the number of individuals with atrial fibrillation in the European Union, from 2000 to 2060. European Heart Journal. 2013;**34**(35):2746-2751

[4] Benjamin EJ, Chen PS, Bild DE, et al. Prevention of atrial fibrillation: Report from a national heart, lung, and blood institute workshop. Circulation. 2009;**119**(4):606-618. DOI: 10.1161/CIRCULATIONAHA.108.825380

[5] Chugh SS, Havmoeller R, Narayanan K, et al. Worldwide epidemiology of atrial fibrillation: A Global Burden of Disease 2010 Study. Circulation. 2014;**129**(8):837-847. DOI: 10.1161/CIRCULATIONAHA.113.005119. Epub 2013 Dec 17

[6] Joglar JA, Chung MK, Armbruster AL, et al. 2023 ACC/AHA/ACCP/HRS guideline for the diagnosis and management of atrial fibrillation: A report of the American College of Cardiology/American Heart Association Joint Committee on Clinical Practice Guidelines. Circulation. 2024;**149**(1):e1-e156. DOI: 10.1161/CIR.0000000000001193. Epub 2023 Nov 30. Erratum in: Circulation. 2024;149(1):e167. doi: 10.1161/CIR.0000000000001207. Erratum in: Circulation. 2024;149(9):e936. doi: 10.1161/CIR.0000000000001218. Erratum in: Circulation. 2024;149(24):e1413. doi: 10.1161/CIR.0000000000001263

[7] Harvey W. Exercitatio Anatomica de Motu Cordis et Sanguinis in Animalibus. Springfield, IL: Charles C Thomas; 1929

[8] Kapa S, Venkatachalam KL, Asirvatham SJ. The autonomic nervous system in cardiac electrophysiology: An elegant interaction and emerging concepts. Cardiology in Review. 2010;**18**:275-284

[9] Armour JA, Murphy DA, Yuan BX, Macdonald S, Hopkins DA. Gross and microscopic anatomy of the human intrinsic cardiac nervous system. The Anatomical Record. 1997;**247**:289-298

[10] Pauza DH, Skripka V, Pauziene N, Stropus R. Morphology, distribution, and variability of the epicardiac neural ganglionated subplexuses in the human heart. The Anatomical Record. 2000;**259**:353-338

[11] Cauti FM, Rossi P, Sommer P. The sympathetic nervous system and ventricular arrhythmias: An inseparable union. European Heart Journal. 2021;**42**(36):3588-3590. DOI: 10.1093/eurheartj/ehab168

[12] Cauti FM, Capone S, Rossi P, et al. Cardiac sympathetic denervation for untreatable ventricular tachycardia in structural heart disease. Strengths and pitfalls of evolving surgical techniques. Journal of Interventional Cardiac Electrophysiology. 2022. DOI: 10.1007/s10840-022-01404-9

[13] Schotten U, Verheule S, Kirchhof P, Goette A. Pathophysiological mechanisms of atrial fibrillation: A translational appraisal. Physiological Reviews. 2011;**91**:265-325

[14] Haissaguerre M, Jais P, Shah DC, Takahashi A, Hocini M, Quiniou G, et al. Spontaneous initiation of atrial fibrillation by ectopic beats originating in the pulmonary veins. The New England Journal of Medicine. 1998;**339**:659-666

[15] Wachtell K, Lehto M, Gerdts E, Olsen MH, Hornestam B, Dahlof B, et al. Angiotensin II receptor blockade reduces new-onset atrial fibrillation and subsequent stroke compared to atenolol: The losartan intervention for end point reduction in hypertension (LIFE) study. Journal of the American College of Cardiology. 2005;**45**(5):712-719

[16] Barajas L, Liu L, Powers K. Anatomy of the renal innervation: Intrarenal aspects and ganglia of origin. Canadian Journal of Physiology and Pharmacology. 1992;**70**(5):735-749. DOI: 10.1139/y92-098

[17] Atherton DS, Deep NL, Mendelsohn FO. Microanatomy of the renal sympathetic nervous system: A human postmortem histologic study. Clinical Anatomy. 2012;**25**:628-633

[18] Sakakura K, Ladich E, Cheng Q, et al. Anatomic assessment of sympathetic periarterial renal nerves in man. Journal of the American College of Cardiology. 2014;**64**:635-643

[19] Page IH, Heuer GJ. The effect of renal denervation on the level of arterial blood pressure and renal function in essential hypertension. The Journal of Clinical Investigation. 1935;**14**:27-30

[20] Krum H, Schlaich M, Whitbourn R, et al. Catheter-based renal sympathetic denervation for resistant hypertension: A multicentre safety and proof-of-principle cohort study. Lancet. 2009;**373**(9671):1275-1281. DOI: 10.1016/S0140-6736(09)60566-3. Epub 2009 Mar 28

[21] Younis A, Steinberg JS. Renal denervation for patients with atrial fibrillation. Current Cardiology Reports. 2021;**23**:126. DOI: 10.1007/s11886-021-01558-4

[22] Bunte MC, Infante de Oliveira E, Shishehbor MH. Endovascular treatment of resistant and uncontrolled hypertension: Therapies on the horizon. JACC: Cardiovascular Interventions. 2013;**6**:1-9

[23] Katsurada K, Shinohara K, Aoki J, et al. Renal denervation: Basic and clinical evidence. Hypertension Research. 2022;**45**:198-209. DOI: 10.1038/s41440-021-00827-7

[24] Barbato E, Azizi M, Schmieder RE, et al. Renal denervation in the management of hypertension in adults. A clinical consensus statement of the ESC Council on Hypertension and the European Association of Percutaneous Cardiovascular Interventions (EAPCI). European Heart Journal. 2023;**44**(15):1313-1330. DOI: 10.1093/eurheartj/ehad054

[25] Steinberg JS, Shabanov V, Ponomarev D, Losik D, Ivanickiy E, Kropotkin E, et al. Effect of renal denervation and catheter ablation vs catheter ablation alone on atrial fibrillation recurrence among patients with paroxysmal atrial fibrillation and hypertension: The ERADICATE-AF randomized clinical trial. Journal of the American Medical Association. 2020;**323**(3):248-255. DOI: 10.1001/jama.2019.21187. Erratum in: JAMA. 2020;323(9):896. doi:10.1001/jama.2020.1367

[26] Kiuchi MG, Chen S, Hoye NA, Pürerfellner H. Pulmonary vein isolation combined with spironolactone or renal sympathetic denervation in patients with chronic kidney disease, uncontrolled hypertension, paroxysmal atrial fibrillation, and a pacemaker. Journal of Interventional Cardiac Electrophysiology. 2018;**51**(1):51-59. DOI: 10.1007/s10840-017-0302-2. Epub 2017 Dec 20

[27] Feyz L, Theuns DA, Bhagwandien R, Strachinaru M, Kardys I, Van Mieghem NM, et al. Atrial fibrillation reduction by renal sympathetic denervation: 12 months' results of the AFFORD study. Clinical Research in Cardiology. 2019;**108**(6):634-642. DOI: 10.1007/s00392-018-1391-3. Epub 2018 Nov 10

[28] Pokushalov E, Romanov A, Corbucci G, Artyomenko S, Baranova V, Turov A, et al. A randomized comparison of pulmonary vein isolation with versus without concomitant renal artery denervation in patients with refractory symptomatic atrial fibrillation and resistant hypertension. Journal of the American College of Cardiology. 2012;**60**(13):1163-1170. DOI: 10.1016/j.jacc.2012.05.036. Epub 2012 Sep 5

[29] Pokushalov E, Romanov A, Katritsis DG, et al. Renal denervation for improving outcomes of catheter ablation in patients with atrial fibrillation and hypertension: Early experience. Heart Rhythm. 2014;**11**(7):1131-1138. DOI: 10.1016/j.hrthm.2014.03.055

[30] Turagam MK, Whang W, Miller MA, Neuzil P, Aryana A, Romanov A, et al. Renal sympathetic denervation as upstream therapy during atrial fibrillation ablation: Pilot HFIB studies and meta-analysis. JACC: Clinical Electrophysiology. 2021;**7**(1):109-123. DOI: 10.1016/j.jacep.2020.08.013. Epub 2020 Oct 28

[31] Kirstein B, Tomala J, Mayer J, Ulbrich S, Wagner M, Pu L, et al. Effect of concomitant renal denervation and cardiac ablation on atrial fibrillation recurrence—RDN+AF study. Journal of Cardiovascular Electrophysiology. 2023;**34**(1):44-53. DOI: 10.1111/jce.15714. Epub 2022 Dec 1

Chapter 15

# Novel Risk Factors Associated with Occurrence and Recurrence of Atrial Fibrillation

*Yujiao Zhang, Zhan Li, Mei Gao and Yinglong Hou*

## Abstract

In order to improve the integrated management of atrial fibrillation (AF), the control of risk factors is becoming increasingly important as a means of upstream treatment. At present, the risk factors for the occurrence and recurrence of AF mainly include age, smoking, drinking, lack of exercise, hypertension, diabetes, obesity, OSA, etc. However, more and more studies have found that some novel risk factors play an important role in the occurrence and recurrence of AF, such as hyperuricemia, hyperhomocysteinemia, hyperbilirubinemia, nonalcoholic fatty liver disease (NAFLD), dyslipidemia, hypoalbuminemia, autoimmune diseases. In this chapter, we focus on several novel risk factors for AF, which can not only improve our understanding of the pathophysiology of AF but also facilitate the adjustment of clinical strategies to reduce the occurrence and recurrence of AF.

**Keywords:** atrial fibrillation, risk factors, novel, occurrence, recurrence

## 1. Introduction

Atrial fibrillation (AF) is the most common form of tachyarrhythmia, whose incidence and prevalence are increasing. The reasons for this include an aging population, increased obesity, increased hypertension, increased incidence of other cardiovascular diseases, and improved overall survival. AF can increase the risk of death by 1.5–2 times, the risk of stroke by 2.4 times, the risk of cognitive impairment or dementia by 1.5 times, the risk of myocardial infarction by 1.5 times, the risk of sudden cardiac death by 2 times, the risk of heart failure (HF) by 5 times, and the risk of chronic kidney disease by 1.6 times [1]. At present, the treatment of AF still faces a high recurrence rate. Since AF can lead to serious sequelae, it is clear that identifying the risk factors for AF can lead to the early detection of asymptomatic patients. An important way to reduce the increasing burden of AF is to modify the risk factors of AF. At present, a number of risk factors related to the occurrence of AF have been proposed, which can be divided into non-modifiable and modifiable risk factors. Non-modifiable risk factors include genes, sex, and age, while modifiable risk factors can also be divided into environmental factors and chronic public diseases. Environmental factors, including obesity, smoking, alcoholism, and lack of exercise, have received extensive attention [2, 3]. Chronic public diseases mainly include type-2 diabetes, hypertension, and obstructive sleep apnea, all of which are thought to increase the risk of AF [3, 4].

Recent studies have shown that the control of upstream risk factors can reduce the occurrence and recurrence of AF [1]. In clinical practice, the risk factors for AF are not only limited to the above risk factors, and studies have found that many new risk factors can also increase the occurrence of AF and its recurrence rate, including hyperuricemia, hyperhomocysteinemia, hyperbilirubinemia, nonalcoholic fatty liver disease (NAFLD), dyslipidemia, hypoalbuminemia, autoimmune diseases, etc. These new risk factors may increase the occurrence of AF. Our aim is to elucidate the relationship between these new risk factors and AF, and to explore the relevant mechanisms and preventative measures, which not only provides new insights into the mechanism of occurrence and recurrence of AF, but also provides a new way of preventing and controlling AF.

## 2. The relationship between new risk factors and the occurrence and recurrence of AF

### 2.1 Hyperuricemia

Uric acid is the end product of purine catabolism. Hyperuricemia was defined by serum uric acid (SUA) levels of over 7.0 mg/dL for men and 6.0 mg/dL for women [5]. Hyperuricemia is usually caused by the imbalance between production and excretion of uric acid. Hyperuricemia is an independent risk factor for gouty arthritis and kidney stones.

Hyperuricemia was significantly associated with AF. Hyperuricemia can be used as an independent risk factor for AF, regardless of the presence of clinical co-existing diseases such as hypertension, diabetes, dyslipidemia, and chronic kidney diseases [6]. Many studies have confirmed a positive correlation between SUA concentration and AF. A prospective cohort study of 123,238 Chinese patients from 2006 to 2014 found that participants with the highest quintile of serum urate had a 1.91-fold higher risk of AF (HR: 1.91, 95% CI, 1.32–2.76; $P = 0.001$) [7]. A meta-analysis of 31 studies involving 504,958 participants conducted by our team, of which eight were cohort studies, showed that high SUA levels significantly increased the incidence of AF [RR: 1.92, 95% CI: 1.68–2.20, $P < 0.01$]. The results from 29 studies revealed that SUA levels were elevated in patients with AF [SMD: 0.55, 95% CI: 0.43–0.66; $P < 0.001$]. Meanwhile, SUA levels in new onset AF [SMD: 0.24, 95% CI: 0.10–0.38, $P < 0.001$], paroxysmal AF [SMD: 0.52, 95% CI: 0.33–0.72, $P < 0.001$], and persistent AF [SMD: 1.23, 95% CI: 0.98–1.48, $P < 0.001$] were significantly higher than those in patients without AF [5]. A newly published study on the relationship between uric acid and recurrence after the ablation of AF showed that SUA level was significantly higher in persistent AF patients than in paroxysmal AF patients. The presence of post-catheter ablation hyperuricemia was strongly related to the recurrence of AF in persistent AF patients [8]. Our team also investigated the correlation between SUA: creatinine ratio (UCR) and the recurrence of AF after catheter ablation. A total of 233 consecutive patients with symptomatic, drug-refractory AF underwent catheter ablation at our hospital, and the results showed that elevated preoperative UCR is associated with the recurrence of AF after catheter ablation, indicating that UCR is probably a predictive factor for the recurrence of AF [9].

Taufiq reported that SUA promoted Hsp 70 expression by promoting the phosphorylation of Akt and HSF1, thus increasing the Kv1.5 proteins. Therefore, inhibiting the Akt/HSF1-HSP70 pathway may be a new way of treatment for AF patients with hyperuricemia [10]. Elevated SUA concentrations may contribute to the pathophysiology of AF through the activation of xanthine oxidorereductase (XOR), the intracellular accumulation of soluble SUA, or the activation of NLRP3 inflammasome induced by sodium urate (MSU) crystals. XOR is a key enzyme that converts SUA precursors into SUA. In contrast, XOR can also be taken as a source of reactive oxygen species (ROS). The accumulation of intracellular uric acid through UAT (URATv1) induces nicotinamide adenine dinucleotide phosphate (NADPH)-oxidase-dependent ROS production to increase Kv1.5. Uric acid-induced Kv1.5 protein stabilization and hypervelocity delayed rectifier current (IKur) enhancement predisplace AF [11]. Therefore, the use of XOR inhibitors (allopurinol and febuxostat), antioxidants (acetylcysteine, glutathione, coenzyme Q10, folic acid tablets, vitamin C, vitamin E, lipoic acid), UAT inhibitors (such as uracil agents), and inflammasome inhibitors may provide potential strategies to reduce the risk of hyperuricemia-induced AF and control SUA levels [11]. In an *in vivo* study of dogs, the XOR inhibitor allopurinol prevented AF through the left ventricular dysfunction caused by atrial pacing [12]. Allopurinol is a first-line drug for the treatment of gout, and its cardioprotective effects have been shown in observational studies of specific populations to potentially prevent myocardial infarction, stroke, AF, and other cardiovascular diseases. However, the efficacy of febuxostat, a new urico-lowering drug, in the treatment of AF and cardiovascular mortality is still controversial [13].

### 2.2 Hyperhomocysteinemia (Hcy)

Hcy is a sulfur-containing amino acid that is a byproduct of methionine conversion into cysteine. It is not present in the diet, but because of its demethylation, it is a derivative of dietary methionine and becomes an essential intermediate for normal mammalian methionine metabolism [14]. The Hcy metabolic pathway is very important because S-adenosine methionine (SAM) is formed in it. SAM is a donor in various methylation reactions such as DNA methylation and catecholamine production. S-adenosine Hcy is produced by SAM in a transmethylation reaction and hydrolyzed to Hcy and adenosine. Such Hcy can either be methylated into methionine by the folate-dependent reaction with vitamin B12 or catabolized into cysteine in a vitamin B6-dependent pathway. The deficiencies of vitamins and enzymes involved in Hcy metabolism and some pathological conditions can lead to the elevated levels of Hcy in the serum, which is known as hyperhomocysteinemia. Hyperhomocysteinemia can be classified as mild (fasting blood Hcy level of 15–30 μmol/l), moderate (30–100 μmol/l), or severe (>100 μmol/l) [15]. Severe hyperhomocysteinemia is attributed to a genetic condition resulting in enzyme deficiency, including B12 and folate metabolism [16]. Severe hyperhomocysteinemia is rarely observed in the population, while the occurrence of mild and moderate hyperhomocysteinemia is quite common. The cause of mild and moderate hyperhomocysteinemia may be micromutation or deficiency in B6, B9, and B12 [17].

Two large population studies, the Atherosclerosis Risk in Communities (ARIC) and the Multi-Ethnic Study of Atherosclerosis (MESA), showed that, during the 10,106 and 67,613 person-years of follow-up, 85 and 351 AF events were identified, respectively. In the fully adjusted model, a meta-analysis of both studies showed a significant association between homocysteine and AF [HR: 1.27, 95% CI: 1.01–1.61] [18].

In the study conducted by Nasso et al., the Hcy levels in patients with nonvalvular AF were evaluated through prospective observation. It was found that the patients with elevated Hcy levels had a higher frequency of AF recurrence, with a higher recurrence rate reached when Hcy levels exceeded 16 μmol/L (ROC 0.807). This may indicate the importance of medication to correct hyperhomocysteinemia in reducing AF recurrence [19]. Snezhitsky et al. studied the prognostic significance of the relationship among Hcy, atrial structure and function remodeling, and clinical manifestations in patients with paroxysmal and persistent AF, including 75 patients with AF in combination with ischemic heart disease (IHD) and essential hypertension (EH) but without significant changes in myocardial structure. The control group included IHD and EH patients without AF. The results suggest that plasma Hcy level is associated with left atrial size and the recurrence of AF. The patients with Hcy levels in excess of 11 μmol/L had a more frequent recurrence of AF [20]. Wang et al. included 717 patients with and without AF but with acute ischemic stroke. Both Hcy and thyroid dysfunction were associated with AF in the patients with acute ischemic stroke [21]. There was a significant difference in serum Hcy ($P = 0.014$) between patients with and without AF. Furthermore, the difference in serum Hcy ($P = 0.007$) and thyroxine levels ($P = 0.004$) between patients with and without AF was also significant in female subgroups. Two recent meta-analyses have shown a clear relationship between hyperhomocysteinemia and the development of AF. A meta-analysis conducted by Rong et al. showed that the results confirmed that AF patients had higher homocysteine levels than control subjects (SMD: 0.58, 95% CI: 0.09–1.06). Compared to control subjects, homocysteine levels were higher in paroxysmal AF (SMD: 0.45, 95% CI: 0.18–0.72) and persistent AF patients (SMD: 1.21, 95% CI: 0.50–1.92). The pooled analysis suggested that patients with elevated homocysteine levels had a markedly higher risk of AF compared to lower homocysteine levels in the categorical variable (OR: 2.21, 95% CI: 1.16–4.21) and continuous variable analyses (OR: 1.13, 95% CI: 1.00–1.27), respectively. In addition, the pooled analysis indicated that recurrent AF patients had significantly higher homocysteine levels than those without recurrence (SMD: 0.65, 95% CI: 0.42–0.88). The pooled analysis of the categorical variables indicated that elevated homocysteine levels were associated with an increased risk of AF recurrence (OR: 3.81, 95% CI: 3.11–4.68) [22]. Another meta-analysis conducted by Dong et al. also confirmed that the patients with elevated Hcy levels had a higher incidence of AF [23]. Charalampidis et al. included 74 major systematic reviews of clinical and non-clinical data, and the results showed that Hcy level seemed to have predictive value for paroxysmal AF [24]. While some studies have suggested an association between plasma Hcy levels and AF, the causal relationship is unclear. Sun et al. conducted a Mendelian Randomization study to investigate the causal relationship between Hcy and AF. Studies have shown that there is no causal relationship between plasma Hcy level and AF [25].

Studies have shown that plasma Hcy is associated with levels of glutathione peroxidase (GPx)-1, which has been shown to regulate the cardiovascular risk associated with Hcy through its antioxidant properties, suggesting that high levels of Hcy are associated with the induction of vascular oxidative stress [26]. In addition, Hcy-induced oxidative stress leading to cardiac fibrosis has proposed several mechanisms of action, including increased reactive oxygen species, nitrotyrosine, matrix metalloproteinases, and decreased endothelial nitric oxide, to counter PPAR-γ and regulate the Akt/$FoxO_3$ pathway. Studies have also demonstrated an association between high Hcy levels and prolonged QTc intervals and longer QRS intervals [24]. In fact, folic acid supplementation has been demonstrated to effectively reduce plasma levels of Hcy. Folic acid supplementation may reverse cardiac dysfunction by reducing myocardial Hcy levels, and possibly by alleviating oxidative stress and myocardial fibrosis [27].

### 2.3 Hyperbilirubinemia

Serum bilirubin, which is the catabolite heme catabolic pathway, has long been used as a biomarker of liver metabolism and excretion capacity. Bilirubin includes hemoglobin and myoglobin catabolites, combining UDP glucuronosyltransferase and glucuronic acid in the liver, allowing it to be excreted in bile. It is widely considered to be an important indicator of liver injury. In recent decades, bilirubin has been recognized as an important endogenous anti-inflammatory and antioxidant molecule that can influence atherosclerosis through a variety of inhibitory mechanisms, including LDL oxidation, vascular smooth muscle cell proliferation, and endothelial dysfunction [28]. Recent studies have shown that serum total bilirubin levels are associated with the prognosis of patients with coronary heart disease [29, 30]. In clinical studies, the role of bilirubin in AF remains controversial and requires further study.

Previous studies have found that the reduction of bilirubin is associated with the occurrence of atrial fibrillation. One study showed a significant reduction in total, direct, and indirect serum bilirubin levels among AF patients compared to the controls [31]. However, subsequent studies have found a positive correlation between bilirubin levels and the occurrence and recurrence of AF. A cross-sectional study was conducted with a total of 181 participants at a single center in Beijing Anzhen Hospital. The patients with pAF had significantly higher rates of age, left atrial (LA) diameter, hemoglobin (Hb) levels, tissue inhibitor of metalloproteinase-1 (TIMP-1), soluble tumor suppressor-2 (sST2), B-type natriuretic peptide (BNP) and indirect bilirubin (Ibil), mean—hemoglobin concentration (MCHC), and hypertension (HTN) and smoking ($P < 0.05$). Multivariable logistic regression analysis found that age (OR: 1.107, 95% CI: 1.016–1.206, $P = 0.02$) and Ibil level (OR: 2.303, 95% CI: 1.158–4.582, $P = 0.017$) were independent predictive factors of the occurrence of pAF in females [32]. An association was found in another study between the higher levels of bilirubin and recurrence of AF following catheter ablation [33]. The elevated bilirubin level after persistent AF radiofrequency catheter ablation (RFCA) is a common phenomenon associated with AF recurrence 1 year after RFCA [34]. Bilirubin level is positively correlated with LAA thrombosis in AF patients, and it may be an indicator of LAA thrombosis [35]. In a study on the correlation between total bilirubin and ischemic stroke in patients with AF, it was found that total bilirubin level was non-linearly correlated with initial ischemic stroke in patients with AF and that the optimal threshold for total bilirubin to be the lowest risk of ischemic stroke was 17.0 mmol/L [36]. Mendelian randomization studies showed through observational analysis that elevated serum bilirubin levels were associated with an increased risk of AF, while genetically predicted bilirubin levels were not associated with the prevalence of AF. Therefore, the observed association between serum bilirubin levels and AF may be a non-causal one and affected by reverse causality or unmeasured confounding factors [37].

The above studies suggest that AF patients may have elevated bilirubin levels due to oxidative stress and inflammation. Elevated bilirubin levels may be an antioxidant and anti-inflammatory mechanism of self-defense. Bilirubin and related heme oxygenase pathways provide cardiac protection through antioxidant properties in cardiovascular disease, while activated heme oxygenase increases bilirubin levels through heme degradation. According to the current role of bilirubin, studies have shown that spirulina is rich in phycocyanobilin, which is a derivative and homolog of biliverdin. It seems to mimic the effective inhibition of biliverdin and free bilirubin on NADPH oxidase activity, playing an antioxidant role [38].

### 2.4 Nonalcoholic fatty liver disease (NAFLD)

NAFLD is a clinicopathological entity that involves the accumulation of hepatic fat or steatosis without various secondary causes such as alcoholism or viral hepatitis. NAFLD is the leading chronic liver disease, affecting approximately 1.7 billion people worldwide. The disease extends from hepatic steatosis to nonalcoholic steatohepatitis (NASH), and the latter may progress to advanced liver fibrosis, cirrhosis, or hepatocellular carcinoma (HCC). In addition, a large proportion of NAFLD patients have metabolic comorbidities, which significantly increase the risk of cardiovascular disease (CVD) and extrahepatic cancer [39]. NAFLD and its complications are not only a huge health burden in Western countries but also increasingly in Asia. Up until recently, NAFLD was not considered a serious public health problem in China [40]. There are growing evidences that NAFLD is not only negatively associated with atherosclerotic disease, but also affects the electrical system of the heart.

Many studies have explored the association between NAFLD and the risk of endemic and occasional AF. However, the results of these studies are inconsistent. NAFLD was associated with a significantly higher risk of existing and subsequent subclinical AF in the Chinese population [41]. In another study conducted in China, the prevalence and trends in NAFLD were first estimated in 2,083,984 people from national health screening centers. The prevalence of NAFLD increased from 22.75 to 35.58% during the study period, with a higher prevalence found among men and people with high BMI or living in the north. NAFLD was significantly associated with a higher risk of AF. The findings suggest that the prevalence of NAFLD and other metabolic disorders, especially overweight and dysglycemia, is high in the NAFLD population [42]. A meta-analysis of 12 cohort studies was conducted to assess the association between NAFLD patients and the incidence of AF, HF, stroke, and cardiovascular mortality. A total of 18,055,072 patients were followed for 6.26 years on average. The main findings supported that being diagnosed with NAFLD increases the risk of developing AF, HF, cerebrovascular complications, and peripheral vascular disease [43]. The most common comorbidities among the NAFLD patients group included hypertension (38% vs. 24%) and diabetes mellitus (14% vs. 8%). The likelihood of AF (RR: 1.42, 95% CI: 1.19–1.68, $P < 0.001$), HF (RR: 1.43, 95% CI 1.03–2.00, $P < 0.001$), stroke (RR: 1.26, 95% CI: 1.16–1.36, $P < 0.001$), revascularization (RR: 4.06, 95% CI: 1.44, 11.46, $P = 0.01$), and CVM (RR: 3.10, 95% CI: 1.43–6.73, $P < 0.001$) was significantly higher in the NAFLD patients group compared to that of the non-NAFLD group. AF and NAFLD share common risk factors, and individually, both are increasing in incidence and prevalence. Epidemiological evidence, experimental studies, and various randomized clinical trials suggest that there is a link between these two entities and that dyslipidemia, insulin resistance, inflammatory environment, and activation of the renin-angiotensin system may be common pathophysiological mechanisms between AF and NAFLD. The relevant literature suggests that they are associated with pro-inflammatory, pro-oxidative, and atherogenic effects, as well as the pro-fibrotic environment that originates from and leads to both conditions. There are other mechanisms contributing to this, such as the dysregulation of the normal gut flora, the role of the pro-oxidant GGT, and the anatomical complications of obesity. Many drugs used to treat NAFLD have been shown to be effective against AF because they target dyslipidemia (DUR-928, Tropifexor/cenicriviroc, Pradigastat), insulin resistance (DPP-4 inhibitors and GLP-1 analogs, Elafibranor), the inflammatory system, oxidation (Vitamin E, Quercetin, Belapectin), or RAS (ACEI and ARBs) [44]. New experimental drugs developed for NAFLD have the potential to treat AF because they target the components of metabolic syndrome or have anti-inflammatory effects.

### 2.5 Dyslipidemia

Dyslipidemia means the metabolic abnormalities of lipoproteins in the body, mainly including elevated total cholesterol (≥240 mg/mL), elevated low-density lipoprotein cholesterol (≥160 mg/mL), elevated triglycerides (≥200 mg/mL), or decreased high-density lipoprotein cholesterol (<40 mg/mL). Numerous evidences suggest that lipid abnormalities are a risk factor for AF [45, 46].

#### *2.5.1 Triglyceride*

Mourtzinis et al. [47] followed up 51,020 hypertensive patients (baseline without AF) for an average of 3.5 years, with 2389 of them found to develop AF. After adjusting other common risk factors for AF, they found no significant correlation between triglyceride levels and newly developed AF in hypertensive patients. Mora et al. [48] followed up 23,738 individuals for an average of 16.4 years, with 795 cases found to experience AF. The study found no significant correlation between triglyceride levels and the occurrence of AF. However, Alonso et al. [49] conducted a study on 7142 individuals with an average follow-up of 9.6 years and 480 cases experienced AF. Multiple regression analysis showed that high triglyceride levels were an independent risk factor for AF occurrence (HR 1.60, ≥ 2.26 mmol/L vs. ≤ 1.70 mmol/L, $P < 0.001$). In addition, a recent large sample multicenter study was conducted on 366,085 individuals with an average follow-up of 5.4 years, and 27,581 individuals experienced AF. Prior to the start of follow-up, blood lipid levels and three-year blood lipid variability were measured in the enrolled population. The study found that the relationship between triglyceride levels and AF was correlated with gender, with high triglyceride variability being an independent risk factor for AF in males and no significant correlation in females [50].

However, the exact triggering mechanism of AF caused by hypertriglyceridemia remains unclear. Previous experimental studies have shown that consuming more fatty acids in high-fat diet models can cause dysfunction of intracellular sodium-calcium ion exchange transporters, thereby inducing an abnormal level of electrical conductivity [51]. At the same time, the posterior wall of the pulmonary vein is rich in adipose tissue, which contains a large amount of sympathetic and parasympathetic nerves. Consuming a large amount of fatty acids can induce arrhythmia by affecting the function of the autonomic nervous system [52]. The study also confirmed that in high fatty acid mouse models, atrial fibrosis occurred [53, 54]. Further research has shown that a high fatty acid diet can cause abnormal lipid deposition in myocardial tissue, and epicardial adipose tissue can secrete various pro-fibrotic and pro-inflammatory factors, thereby promoting atrial fibrosis [55, 56].

It is known that over 95% of the energy required by myocardial cells is derived from oxidative phosphorylation of mitochondria and that in adult hearts, 50–70% of ATP comes from beta-oxidation of fatty acids, which mainly occurs in mitochondria [57, 58]. Therefore, insufficient energy or reduced energy substrate sources from the decomposition of fatty acids can cause heart failure and impair heart functions [57]. On the contrary, excessive intake of fatty acids in the body can also cause a large-scale breakdown of fatty acids, release excessive ROS, and cause cellular damage leading to pathological conditions [59, 60]. Based on this, the metabolic imbalance of cardiomyocytes in a high triglyceride environment may trigger an oxygen-free radical cascade reaction, which may lead to the occurrence and development of AF. Our study found that the induction rate of AF increased in high-fat diet rat models, and high fatty acids damaged the mitochondria of myocardial cells by affecting mitochondrial morphology and function. By reducing the production of NO in myocardial cells through the CRIF1/SIRT1/eNOS/axis, high fatty acid stimulation could inhibit Nrf2 entering the nucleus and activating P21, which promotes neuronal proliferation in the myocardial microenvironment, thus facilitating the occurrence of AF [61].

#### *2.5.2 Total cholesterol and LDL-C*

Alonso et al. [49] found no significant correlation between total cholesterol and LDL-C levels and the occurrence of AF in a mean follow-up of 9.6 years among 7142 individuals. Lee et al. [50] followed up 366,085 individuals for an average of 5.4 years, with 27,581 individuals experiencing AF. Compared to the low total cholesterol level group (4.42–4.71 mmol/L), a high level of total cholesterol (5.28–5.56 mmol/L) was an independent protective factor for AF and could reduce the risk by 22% ($P < 0.01$). The high LDL-C group (3.17–3.43 mmol/L) had a 19% lower risk of AF compared to the low LDL-C group (2.39–2.65 mmol/L) ($P < 0.01$). Li et al. [62] followed up 88,785 individuals for an average of 7.12 years, among which 328 cases experienced AF. After adjusting other risk factors through multiple regression analysis, high levels of LDL-C (>2.86 mmol/L) were found to be an independent protective factor for the occurrence of AF (HR: 0.60, $P < 0.001$). Canpolat et al. [63] performed cryoballoon ablation on 402 patients with AF and found no significant difference in LDL-C levels between the recurrent group and the non-recurrent group after an average follow-up of 20.6 months. However, a meta-analysis showed that the recurrent group had a significant increase in LDL-C levels after AF ablation compared to the non-recurrent group [64].

The correlation and specific mechanisms between total cholesterol and LDL-C levels and the onset and recurrence of AF are still unclear, and statin drugs developed for the upstream treatment of AF may not be affected solely by lowering cholesterol.

#### *2.5.3 HDL-C*

Li et al. [62] followed up 88,785 individuals for an average of 7.12 years, and 328 cases suffered AF. After adjusting other risk factors through multiple regression analysis, they found no significant correlation between HDL-C levels and the occurrence of AF. However, recent studies have shown a negative correlation between HDL-C levels and the occurrence of AF. Alonso [49] followed up 7142 individuals for an average of 9.6 years, and multiple regression showed that high HDL-C levels independently reduced the risk of AF (HR: 0.64, $\geq$1.56 mmol/L vs. $\leq$1.04 mmol/L, $P < 0.001$). Lopez et al. [65] followed up 13,969 individuals for an average of 18.7 years, among which 1433 cases suffered AF. After adjusting age, gender, and race in multiple regression analyses, they found that HDL-C ≥ 1.55 mmol/L was an independent protective factor for the incidence of AF (HR: 0.63, P < 0.0001). Canpolat et al. [63] performed cryoablation on 402 patients with AF. After an average follow-up of 20.6 months, 95 patients experienced AF recurrence. There was no significant difference in statin between the two groups, and the HDL-C level in the recurrent group was significantly lower than in the non-recurrent group (0.93 mmol/L vs. 1.14 mmol/L, P < 0.001). The absolute value of monocytes/HDL-C was significantly correlated with AF recurrence, and the AF recurrence rate showed a significant increase in the highest quartile array compared to the lowest array (68.4% vs. 7.4%, P < 0.001). In recent years, a large number of studies have shown that the decreased levels and function of HDL-C could increase the risk of AF.

The potential mechanisms may be that the low levels of HDL-C or dysfunctional HDL-C can induce myocardial hypertrophy, increase left ventricular mass, cause cardiac dysfunction, and promote the development of heart failure, all of which can increase the incidence of AF [66–68].

In summary, the correlation between triglyceride level and AF is still unclear. Some studies have shown that high triglyceride level is a risk factor for AF. Numerous experiments have confirmed that low total cholesterol levels, low LDL-C levels, and low HDL-C levels can increase the risk of AF. The potential mechanism of blood lipid levels affecting AF is unknown, and it may be related to oxidative stress, inflammatory response, myocardial remodeling, and membrane stability.

### 2.6 Hypoalbuminemia

Serum albumin (ALB) values were measured in g/L after initial admission, and the reference ranges from 35 to 50 g/L, with any value below 35 g/L considered hypoproteinemia.

Zhao et al. [69] found that ALB levels were lower in the AF group than in the control group (P < 0.05). After multivariable adjustment, ALB was found to be independently negatively associated with AF (OR = 0.935, 95% CI: 0.905–0.965, P < 0.05). ALB levels were positively correlated with serum globulin, total cholesterol, triglyceride, low-density lipoprotein cholesterol, high-density lipoprotein cholesterol, serum apolipoprotein A1, and serum apolipoprotein B levels (P < 0.05), but negatively correlated with serum creatinine levels (P < 0.05). The optimal cutoff value of ALB for predicting AF was 37.25 g/L, the sensitivity was 78.0%, and the specificity was 4.6%. A low ALB level is independently associated with AF. Liao et al. [70] used multivariable Cox hazard regression models to assess the association between albumin and incident AF based on Atherosclerosis Risk in Communities (ARIC) Study. They discovered that during a median follow-up of 25.1 years, 2259 (17.6%) participants developed incident AF. After multiple adjustments, serum albumin was found to be inversely associated with the incidence of AF [HR: 0.90, 95% CI 0.86–0.94, per SD (0.27 g/dL) increase; HR: 0.80, 95% CI 0.71–0.91, Q4 vs. Q1, P < 0.01]. However, in Mendelian Randomization (MR) analysis, they found no evidence for a causal relation between serum albumin level and AF, which is based on the inverse-variance weighted (IVW) method.

ALB is the most important protein in the human serum, and its physiological functions include anti-inflammatory effect, antioxidant effect, anticoagulant effect, anti-platelet aggregation, maintenance of colloid osmotic pressure, and transport of various endogenous and exogenous substances [71–74]. Moreover, previous studies suggest that ALB is rich in mercaptan groups, accounting for about 80% of the total mercaptan of plasma scavenging ROS and nitrogen. Also, it can carry NO, which enables its strong antioxidant stress activity [75, 76]. The increase of ROS may enhance ryanodine receptor activity, increase the release of sarcoplasmic reticulum calcium ions, and shorten atrial action potential time to increase the possibility of AF [77, 78]. Furthermore, under physiological conditions, ALB can selectively inhibit TNF-α-induced upregulation of vascular cell adhesion molecule-1 expression and monocyte adhesion. Therefore, it performs a strong anti-inflammatory function [75, 79, 80]. Accordingly, we postulate that the decrease in ALB levels may be related to the decrease in the anti-inflammatory and antioxidant capacity of the body, which could further result in atrial structural and electrical remodeling, for participation in the pathological process of AF. Focusing on monitoring albumin levels may provide a meaningful perspective on predicting AF.

### 2.7 Autoimmune diseases

Autoimmune diseases are chronic inflammatory diseases caused by the loss of autoimmune tolerance, and they are characterized by the appearance of autoantibodies or autoreactive lymphocytes and the impairment of the inhibitory function of regulatory T cells. Autoimmune inflammation can involve multiple organs, leading to systemic inflammatory damage. In recent years, more and more studies have shown that autoimmune diseases, including rheumatoid arthritis, psoriasis, and so on, can lead to an increased risk of cardiovascular disease in patients [81–83]. AF is one of the common arrhythmias induced by autoimmune diseases, and its mechanism may involve immune system deregulation and inflammatory response [84–86].

Rheumatoid arthritis is a chronic immune-mediated disease that mainly affects human joints and can lead to high-intensity persistent inflammatory reactions outside the joints [87]. The heart is one of the main organs targeted by rheumatoid arthritis, and the risk of AF in patients with rheumatoid arthritis is significantly increased ($P < 0.01$) [88]. The results of the national Danish cohort study performed by Lindhardsen et al. [89] showed that the incidence of AF in rheumatoid arthritis patients was 40% higher than in the general population ($P < 0.01$). Dai et al. [90] concluded that rheumatoid arthritis can participate in various pathophysiological processes including atrial fibrosis, apoptosis, and autophagy of atrial cardiomyocytes, which leads to atrial remodeling by increasing the number of cardiac fibroblasts and the expression of inflammatory factors such as TNF-α and IL-6 in rats, thus inducing the occurrence of AF.

Psoriasis is a common skin disease mediated by chronic immunity. In addition to skin and arthritis manifestations, it is also associated with a variety of cardiovascular diseases [91]. The study conducted by Rhee et al. [92] on the Korean population showed that compared to the patients with mild psoriasis, those patients with severe psoriasis had a significantly increased risk of AF ($P < 0.01$). Tasal et al. [93] reported that chronic inflammation mediated by systemic inflammatory cytokines such as TNF- α may be the most important factor linking psoriasis with AF.

The mechanism of arrhythmia caused by immune system dysfunction may involve (1) the crosstalk between immune cells and fibroblasts or cardiomyocytes, leading to fibrosis and AF; (2) the immune cells directly participating in the electrical remodeling of cardiomyocytes through gap junction with Cx43 to trigger AF; and (3) the immune system that can directly affect the function of specific ion channels on the surface of cardiomyocytes through autoantibodies or inflammatory cytokines, thus leading to AF [94–96].

## 3. Summary

AF is a common clinical disease, and its occurrence is the result of complex and multifactorial effects. In conclusion, aside from the traditional variable risk factors, such as hypertension, diabetes, smoking, alcoholism, hyperuricemia, Hcy, hyperbilirubinemia, MAFLD, dyslipidemia, hypoalbuminemia, autoimmune diseases, etc., are the novel variable risk factors of AF. Through the identification of these variable risk factors, the occurrence of AF can be prevented to a certain extent through the health management of high-risk groups and the promotion of a healthy lifestyle, which plays a significant role in promoting the health of the population and reducing medical costs.

## Author details

Yujiao Zhang, Zhan Li, Mei Gao and Yinglong Hou*
Department of Cardiology, The First Affiliated Hospital of Shandong First Medical University and Shandong Provincial Qianfoshan Hospital, China

*Address all correspondence to: houyinglong@sina.com

## References

[1] Joglar JA, Chung MK, Armbruster AL, et al. ACC/AHA/ACCP/HRS guideline for the diagnosis and management of atrial fibrillation: A report of the American College of Cardiology/American Heart Association joint committee on clinical practice guidelines. 2023;**149**(1):e167

[2] Belbasis L, Mavrogiannis MC, Emfietzoglou M, et al. Environmental factors, serum biomarkers and risk of atrial fibrillation: An exposure-wide umbrella review of meta-analyses. European Journal of Epidemiology. 2020;**35**(3):223-239

[3] Nattel S, Kalman JM, Sanders P. Modifiable risk factors and atrial fibrillation. Circulation. 2017;**136**:583-596

[4] Kirchhof P, Benussi S, Kotecha D, et al. 2016 ESC guidelines for the management of atrial fibrillation developed in collaboration with EACTS. European Heart Journal. 2016;**37**:2893-2962

[5] Wang X, Hou Y, Wang X, et al. Relationship between serum uric acid levels and different types of atrial fibrillation: An updated meta-analysis. Nutrition, Metabolism, and Cardiovascular Diseases. 2021;**31**(10):2756-2765

[6] Kuwabara M, Niwa K, Nishihara S, et al. Hyperuricemia is an independent competing risk factor for atrial fibrillation. International Journal of Cardiology. 2017;**231**:137-142

[7] Li S, Cheng J, Cui L, et al. Cohort study of repeated measurements of serum urate and risk of incident atrial fibrillation. Journal of the American Heart Association. 2019;**8**:e012020

[8] Oseto H, Yamashita S, Tokuda M, et al. The association between hyperuricemia and atrial fibrillation recurrence after catheter ablation. Journal of Arrhythmia. 2024;**40**(3):520-526

[9] Zhang Y, Wang Y, Yang X, et al. Serum uric acid: Creatinine ratio (UCR) is associated with recurrence of atrial fibrillation after catheter ablation. Frontiers in Endocrinology (Lausanne). 2023;**14**:1110102

[10] Taufiq F, Maharani N, Li P, et al. Uric acid-induced enhancements of Kv1.5 protein expression and channel activity via the akt-HSF1-hsp70 pathway in HL-1 atrial myocytes. Circulation Journal. 2019;**83**(4):718-726

[11] Taufiq F, Li P, Miake J, Hisatome I. Hyperuricemia as a risk factor for atrial fibrillation due to soluble and crystalized uric acid. Circulation Reports. 2019;**1**(11):469-473

[12] Sakabe M, Fujiki A, Sakamoto T, et al. Xanthine oxidase inhibition prevents atrial fibrillation in a canine model of atrial pacing-induced left ventricular dysfunction. Journal of Cardiovascular Electrophysiology. 2012;**23**(10):1130-1135

[13] Gupta MK, Singh JA. Cardiovascular disease in gout and the protective effect of treatments including urate-lowering therapy. Drugs. 2019;**79**(5):531-541

[14] Finkelstein JD, Martin JJ. Homocysteine. The International Journal of Biochemistry & Cell Biology. 2000;**32**:385-389

[15] Cesari M, Rossi GP, Sticchi D, et al. Is homocysteine important as risk factor

for coronary heart disease? Nutrition, Metabolism, and Cardiovascular Diseases. 2005;**15**:140-147

[16] Maron BA, Loscalzo J. The treatment of hyperhomocysteinemia. Annual Review of Medicine. 2009;**60**:39-54

[17] Kaplan P, Tatarkova Z, Sivonova MK, et al. Homocysteine and mitochondria in cardiovascular and cerebrovascular systems. International Journal of Molecular Sciences. 2020;**21**:7698

[18] Kubota Y, Alonso A, Heckbert SR, et al. Homocysteine and incident atrial fibrillation: The atherosclerosis risk in communities study and the multi-ethnic study of atherosclerosis. Heart, Lung & Circulation. 2019;**28**:615-622

[19] Nasso G, Bonifazi R, Romano V, et al. Increased plasma homocysteine predicts arrhythmia recurrence after minimally invasive epicardial ablation for nonvalvular atrial fibrillation. The Journal of Thoracic and Cardiovascular Surgery. 2013;**146**:848-853

[20] Snezhitsky VA, Yatskevich ES, Doroshenko EM, et al. Homocysteine as a prognostic marker of atrial remodeling and clinical picture in patients with paroxysmal and persistent forms of atrial fibrillation. Klin Med (Mosk). 2016;**94**:16-22

[21] Wang L, Zhang Y. Role of hyperhomocysteine, thyroid dysfunction and their interaction in ischemic stroke patients with non-valvular atrial fibrillation. Scientific Reports. 2020;**10**:12419

[22] Rong H, Huang L, Jin N, et al. Elevated homocysteine levels associated with atrial fibrillation and recurrent atrial fibrillation. International Heart Journal. 2020;**61**:705-712

[23] Dong XJ, Wang BB, Hou FF, et al. Homocysteine (HCY) levels in patients with atrial fibrillation (AF): A meta-analysis. International Journal of Clinical Practice. 2021;**75**:e14738

[24] Charalampidis P, Teperikidis E, Boulmpou A, et al. Homocysteine as a predictor of paroxysmal atrial fibrillation-related events: A scoping review of the literature. Diagnostics (Basel). 2022;**12**(9):2192

[25] Sun X, Lu Y, Wang Z, et al. No causal association between plasma homocysteine levels and atrial fibrillation: A Mendelian randomization study. Nutrition, Metabolism, and Cardiovascular Diseases. 2021;**31**(2):587-591

[26] Schnabel R, Lackner KJ, Rupprecht HJ, et al. Glutathione peroxidase-1 and homocysteine for cardiovascular risk prediction: Results from the atherogene study. Journal of the American College of Cardiology. 2005;**45**:1631-1637

[27] Li W, Tang R, Ouyang S, et al. Folic acid prevents cardiac dysfunction and reduces myocardial fibrosis in a mouse model of high-fat diet-induced obesity. Nutrition and Metabolism. 2017;**14**:68

[28] Xu XQ, Lv ZC, Liu QQ, et al. Direct bilirubin: A new risk factor of adverse outcome in idiopathic pulmonary arterial hypertension. International Journal of Cardiology. 2017;**228**:895-899

[29] Li XL, Zhao CR, Pan CL, et al. Role of bilirubin in the prognosis of coronary artery disease and its relationship with cardiovascular risk factors: A meta-analysis. BMC Cardiovascular Disorders. 2022;**22**:458

[30] Nilsen DWT, Myhre PL, Solheim S, et al. Total bilirubin yields prognostic

information following a myocardial infarction in the elderly. Antioxidants (Basel). 2023;**12**(6):1157

[31] Demir M, Demir C, Uyan U, et al. The relationship between serum bilirubin concentration and atrial fibrillation. Cardiology Research. 2013;**4**(6):186-191

[32] Sun W, Li H, Wang Z, et al. Clinical and laboratory biomarkers in paroxysmal atrial fibrillation: A single center cross-sectional study. Contrast Media & Molecular Imaging. 2022;**2022**:7012377

[33] Chen SC, Chung FP, Chao TF, et al. A link between bilirubin levels and atrial fibrillation recurrence after catheter ablation. Journal of the Chinese Medical Association. 2019;**82**(3):175-178

[34] Shao JM, Shen B, Zhou ZX, et al. Bilirubin elevation during hospitalization post radiofrequency catheter ablation of persistent atrial fibrillation: Variation trend, related factors, and relevance to 1-year recurrence. Clinical Interventions in Aging. 2024;**19**:817-825

[35] Meng W, Wang L, Fan H, et al. Total bilirubin level is associated with the risk of left atrial appendage thrombosis in patients with non-valvular atrial fibrillation. Global Heart. 2022;**17**(1):90

[36] Liu Y, Wang J, Zeng WZ, et al. Nonlinear relationship between serum total bilirubin levels and initial ischemic stroke in patients with non-valvular atrial fibrillation. The Journal of International Medical Research. 2020;**48**(10):300060520962347

[37] Kim SW, Yang JH, Kweon SS, et al. Association between serum bilirubin and atrial fibrillation: A mendelian randomization study. Korean Circulation Journal. 2023;**53**(7):472-479

[38] Mark F. Practical prevention of cardiac remodeling and atrial fibrillation with full-spectrum antioxidant therapy and ancillary strategies. Medical Hypotheses. 2010;**75**(2):141-147

[39] Cai J, Zhang XJ, Li H. Progress and challenges in the prevention and control of nonalcoholic fatty liver disease. Medicinal Research Reviews. 2019;**39**(1):328-348

[40] Mantovani A, Dauriz M, Sandri D, et al. Association between non-alcoholic fatty liver disease and risk of atrial fibrillation in adult individuals: An updated meta-analysis. Liver International. 2019;**39**(4):758-769

[41] Van Kleef LA, Lu Z, Arfan IM, et al. Liver stiffness not fatty liver disease is associated with atrial fibrillation: The Rotterdam study. Journal of Hepatology. 2022;**77**(4):931-938

[42] Lei F, Qin JJ, Song X, et al. The prevalence of MAFLD and its association with atrial fibrillation in a nationwide health check-up population in China. Frontiers in Endocrinology (Lausanne). 2022;**13**:1007171

[43] Jaiswal V, Ang SP, Huang H, et al. Association between nonalcoholic fatty liver disease and atrial fibrillation and other clinical outcomes: A meta-analysis. Journal of Investigative Medicine. 2023;**71**(6):591-602

[44] Haghbin H, Gangwani MK, Ravi SJK, et al. Nonalcoholic fatty liver disease and atrial fibrillation: Possible pathophysiological links and therapeutic interventions. Annals of Gastroenterology. 2020;**33**(6):603-614

[45] Echahidi N, Mohty D, Pibarot P, et al. Obesity and metabolic syndrome are independent risk factors for atrial fibrillation after coronary artery bypass graft surgery. Circulation. 2007;**116** (11 Suppl):I213-I219

[46] Hajhosseiny R, Matthews GK, Lip GY. Metabolic syndrome, atrial fibrillation, and stroke: Tackling an emerging epidemic. Heart Rhythm. 2015;**12**(11):2332-2343

[47] Mourtzinis G, Kahan T, Bengtsson Bostrom K, et al. Relation between lipid profile and new-onset atrial fibrillation in patients with systemic hypertension (from the Swedish primary care cardiovascular database [SPCCD]). The American Journal of Cardiology. 2018;**122**(1):102-107

[48] Mora S, Akinkuolie AO, Sandhu RK, et al. Paradoxical association of lipoprotein measures with incident atrial fibrillation. Circulation Arrhythmia and Electrophysiology. 2014;**7**(4):612-619

[49] Alonso A, Yin X, Roetker NS, et al. Blood lipids and the incidence of atrial fibrillation: The multi-ethnic study of atherosclerosis and the Framingham heart study. Journal of the American Heart Association. 2014;**3**(5):e001211

[50] Lee HJ, Lee SR, Choi EK, et al. Low lipid levels and high variability are associated with the risk of new-onset atrial fibrillation. Journal of the American Heart Association. 2019;**8**(23):e012771

[51] Berecki G, Den Ruijter HM, Verkerk AO, et al. Dietary fish oil reduces the incidence of triggered arrhythmias in pig ventricular myocytes. Heart Rhythm. 2007;**4**(11):1452-1460

[52] Balcioglu AS, Cicek D, Akinci S, et al. Arrhythmogenic evidence for epicardial adipose tissue: Heart rate variability and turbulence are influenced by epicardial fat thickness. Pacing and Clinical Electrophysiology. 2015;**38**(1):99-106

[53] Kondo H, Abe I, Gotoh K, et al. Interleukin 10 treatment ameliorates high-fat diet-induced inflammatory atrial remodeling and fibrillation. Circulation Arrhythmia and Electrophysiology. 2018;**11**(5):e006040

[54] Shuai W, Kong B, Fu H, et al. MD1 deficiency promotes inflammatory atrial remodelling induced by high-fat diets. The Canadian Journal of Cardiology. 2019;**35**(2):208-216

[55] Kremen J, Dolinkova M, Krajickova J, et al. Increased subcutaneous and epicardial adipose tissue production of proinflammatory cytokines in cardiac surgery patients: Possible role in postoperative insulin resistance. The Journal of Clinical Endocrinology and Metabolism. 2006;**91**(11):4620-4627

[56] Mazurek T, Zhang L, Zalewski A, et al. Human epicardial adipose tissue is a source of inflammatory mediators. Circulation. 2003;**108**(20):2460-2466

[57] Lopaschuk GD, Ussher JR, Folmes CD, et al. Myocardial fatty acid metabolism in health and disease. Physiological Reviews. 2010;**90**(1):207-258

[58] Lopaschuk GD, Belke DD, Gamble J, et al. Regulation of fatty acid oxidation in the mammalian heart in health and disease. Biochimica et Biophysica Acta. 1994;**1213**(3):263-276

[59] Onay-Besikci A, Guner S, Arioglu E, et al. The effects of chronic trimetazidine treatment on mechanical function and fatty acid oxidation in diabetic rat hearts. Canadian Journal of Physiology and Pharmacology. 2007;**85**(5):527-535

[60] Sharma V, Dhillon P, Wambolt R, et al. Metoprolol improves cardiac function and modulates cardiac metabolism in the streptozotocin-diabetic rat. American Journal of

Physiology. Heart and Circulatory Physiology. 2008;**294**(4):H1609-H1620

[61] Zhang A, Li H, Song Q, et al. High-fat stimulation induces atrial neural remodeling by reducing NO production via the CRIF1/eNOS/P21 axi. Lipids in Health and Disease. 2023;**22**(1):189

[62] Li X, Gao L, Wang Z, et al. Lipid profile and incidence of atrial fibrillation: A prospective cohort study in China. Clinical Cardiology. 2018;**41**(3):314-320

[63] Canpolat U, Aytemir K, Yorgun H, et al. The role of preprocedural monocyte-to high-density lipoprotein ratio in prediction of atrial fibrillation recurrence after cryoballoon-based catheter ablation. Europace. 2015;**17**(12):1807-1815

[64] Jiang H, Wang W, Wang C, et al. Association of pre-ablation level of potential blood markers with atrial fibrillation recurrence after catheter ablation: A meta analysis. Europace. 2017;**19**(3):392-400

[65] Lopez FL, Agarwal SK, Maclehose RF, et al. Blood lipid levels, lipid-lowering medications, and the incidence of atrial fibrillation: The atherosclerosis risk in communities study. Circulation. Arrhythmia and Electrophysiology. 2012;**5**(1):155-162

[66] Trieb M, Kornej J, Knuplez E, et al. Atrial fibrillation is associated with alterations in HDL function, metabolism, and particle number. Basic Research in Cardiology. 2019;**114**(4):27

[67] Watanabe H, Tanabe N, Yagihara N, et al. Association between lipid profile and risk of atrial fibrillation. Circulation Journal. 2011;**75**(12):2767-2774

[68] Li ZZ, Du X, Guo XY, et al. Association between blood lipid profiles and atrial fibrillation: A case-control study. Medical Science Monitor. 2018;**24**:3903-3908

[69] Zhao D, Jiao H, Zhong X, et al. The association between serum albumin levels and related metabolic factors and atrial fibrillation: A retrospective study. Medicine. 2022;**101**(44):e31581

[70] Liao LZ, Zhang SZ, Li WD, et al. Serum albumin and atrial fibrillation: Insights from epidemiological and mendelian randomization studies. European Journal of Epidemiology. 2020;**35**(2):113-122

[71] Soeters PB, Wolfe RR, Shenkin A. Hypoalbuminemia: Pathogenesis and clinical significance. Journal of Parenteral and Enteral Nutrition. 2019;**43**:181-193

[72] Paar M, Rossmann C, Nusshold C, et al. Anticoagulant action of low, physiologic, and high albumin levels in whole blood. PLoS One. 2017;**12**:e0182997

[73] Lam FW, Cruz MA, Leung HC, et al. Histone induced platelet aggregation is inhibited by normal albumin. Thrombosis Research. 2013;**132**:69-76

[74] Arques S, Ambrosi P. Human serum albumin in the clinical syndrome of heart failure. Journal of Cardiac Failure. 2011;**17**:451-458

[75] Garcia-Martinez R, Caraceni P, Bernardi M, et al. Albumin: Pathophysiologic basis of its role in the treatment of cirrhosis and its complications. Hepatology. 2013;**58**:1836-1846

[76] Roche M, Rondeau P, Singh NR, et al. The antioxidant properties of serum albumin. FEBS Letters. 2008;**582**:1783-1787

[77] Ziolo MT, Mohler PJ. Defining the role of oxidative stress in atrial fibrillation and diabetes. Journal of Cardiovascular Electrophysiology. 2015;**26**:223-225

[78] Sovari AA, Dudley SC Jr. Reactive oxygen species-targeted therapeutic interventions for atrial fibrillation. Frontiers in Physiology. 2012;**3**:311

[79] Wiedermann CJ. Anti-inflammatory activity of albumin. Critical Care Medicine. 2007;**35**:981-982

[80] Zhang W, Frei B. Albumin selectively inhibits TNF alpha-induced expression of vascular cell adhesion molecule-1 in human aortic endothelial cells. Cardiovascular Research. 2002;**55**:820-829

[81] England BR, Thiele GM, Anderson DR, et al. Increased cardiovascular risk in rheumatoid arthritis: Mechanisms and implications. BMJ. 2018;**361**:k1036

[82] Boehncke WH. Systemic inflammation and cardiovascular comorbidity in psoriasis patients: Causes and consequences. Frontiers in Immunology. 2018;**9**:579

[83] Sun G, Ahlehoff O, Fosbøl EL, et al. Long-term incidence of atrial fibrillation in patients with autoimmune disease. Journal of the American College of Cardiology. 2023;**82**(20):1969-1971

[84] Swirski FK, Nahrendorf M. Cardioimmunology: The immune system in cardiac homeostasis and disease. Nature Reviews. Immunology. 2018;**18**(12):733-744

[85] Lazzerini PE, Laghi-Pasini F, Boutjdir M, et al. Cardioimmunology of arrhythmias: The role of autoimmune and inflammatory cardiac channelopathies. Nature Reviews. Immunology. 2019;**19**(1):63-64

[86] Tilly MJ, Geurts S, Zhu F, et al. Autoimmune diseases and new-onset atrial fibrillation: A UK biobank study. Europace. 2023;**25**(3):804-811

[87] Klingenberg R, Lüscher TF. Rheumatoid arthritis and coronary atherosclerosis: Two cousins engaging in a dangerous liaison. European Heart Journal. 2015;**36**(48):3423-3425

[88] Bacani AK, Crowson CS, Roger VL, et al. Increased incidence of atrial fibrillation in patients with rheumatoid arthritis. BioMed Research International. 2015;**2015**:809514

[89] Lindhardsen J, Ahlehoff O, Gislason GH, et al. Risk of atrial fibrillation and stroke in rheumatoid arthritis: Danish nationwide cohort study. BMJ. 2012;**344**:e1257

[90] Dai H, Wang X, Yin S, et al. Atrial fibrillation promotion in a rat model of rheumatoid arthritis. Journal of the American Heart Association. 2017;**6**(12):e007320

[91] Upala S, Shahnawaz A, Sanguankeo A. Psoriasis increases risk of new-onset atrial fibrillation: A systematic review and meta-analysis of prospective observational studies. The Journal of Dermatological Treatment. 2017;**28**(5):406-410

[92] Rhee TM, Lee JH, Choi EK, et al. Increased risk of atrial fibrillation and thromboembolism in patients with severe psoriasis: A nationwide population-based study. Scientific Reports. 2017;**7**(1):9973

[93] Tasal A, Guvenc TS, Kul S, et al. Atrial conduction abnormalities in patients with psoriasis vulgaris. Kardiologia Polska. 2015;**73**(8):637-643

[94] Lazzerini PE, Capecchi PL, Laghi-Pasini F, et al. Autoimmune channelopathies as a novel mechanism in cardiac arrhythmias. Nature Reviews. Cardiology. 2017;**14**(9):521-535

[95] Lazzerini PE, Capecchi PL, Laghi-Pasini F. Systemic inflammation and arrhythmic risk: Lessons from rheumatoid arthritis. European Heart Journal. 2017;**38**(22):1717-1727

[96] Lazzerini PE, Capecchi PL, El-Sherif N, et al. Emerging arrhythmic risk of autoimmune and inflammatory cardiac channelopathies. Journal of the American Heart Association. 2018;**7**(22):e010595

Chapter 16

# Exercise and Atrial Fibrillation: Friends or Foes?

*Ioana Cristina Daha and Elisabeta Bădilă*


## Abstract

Atrial fibrillation (AF) has an increasing prevalence and is foreseen as a true epidemic in the coming years. Moreover, the presence of AF has a huge impact on the everyday quality of life and also on the prognosis of the affected patients. Lifestyle interventions including exercise-based interventions are an essential component of the guideline-driven Atrial Fibrillation Better Care (ABC) pathway. Nevertheless, physicians are not extensively using this extremely valuable tool in AF prevention, both primary and secondary prevention, because of a lack of knowledge and fear of inducing harm. On the other hand, patients are afraid of experiencing symptoms and lower their physical activity to a "safe" minimum. Therefore, shedding light on this important topic is extremely important. The aim of the chapter is to highlight the bivalent and somehow counterintuitive relationship between exercise and atrial fibrillation with a special focus on exercise prescription in everyday AF patients.


**Keywords:** atrial fibrillation, exercise capacity, cardiac rehabilitation, physical activity, lifestyle intervention, left atrium enlargement, endurance sport, athlete's heart, exercise prescription

## 1. Introduction

Exercising on a regular basis promotes cardiovascular health and prevents cardiovascular mortality and morbidity. Regular exercise prevents the development of cardiovascular risk factors and acute cardiovascular events. Nevertheless, physical activity (PA) prevents certain types of neoplasia and also cognitive disturbances. The beneficial effect of exercise applies to the general population and also to cardiovascular-diseased patients [1]. According to WHO, PA refers to "any bodily movement produced by skeletal muscles that requires energy expenditure." Exercise or exercise training (ET) is PA that is goal-oriented to improve or maintain physical fitness and is structured and repetitive [2]. PA and ET promote multiple favorable cardiac and systemic responses. Exercise-mediated signaling pathways and molecules through reduction of myocardial oxidative stress, vascular responses, promotion of physiological cardiac hypertrophy, and cardiac metabolic adaptations play an active role in exercise-induced cardioprotective role. Exercise-regulated molecules can serve as potential biomarkers with the capability to guide effective and safe exercise training in patients with cardiovascular diseases [3]. In healthy seniors with lifelong ET, four to five exercise sessions/week for at least 30 minutes, throughout adulthood, prevented left ventricular stiffening. The beneficial effect on left ventricular function was regardless of duration, intensity or type of exercise but was not maintained for less than four sessions/week [4]. Beyond being beneficial in healthy subjects, exercise can be prescribed as medicine for multiple cardiovascular diseases. Multiple data showed that exercise training has proven a positive impact on the quality of life and risk of hospitalization in heart failure, coronary artery disease, hypertension and cardiomyopathies [1].

## 2. Exercise and atrial fibrillation

Being physically active is one of the main pillars in AF prevention and treatment. Moderate, regular PA contributes to the control of many predisposing factors for AF like obesity, hypertension and diabetes. Therefore, patients with risk factors for AF or with permanent or non-permanent AF should be encouraged to exercise [1, 5]. Current guidelines recommend regular exercise on a daily basis in order to achieve the reduction of AF duration and burden and also AF-related symptoms severity [6, 7]. Unfortunately, the majority of AF patients do not know and do not meet current guideline recommendations regarding PA, with no difference regarding AF type [8]. Nevertheless, exercise intolerance and dyspnea are common among AF patients and in many patients are not aligned to the objectively measured exercise capacity using cardiopulmonary exercise test [9]. In a cohort of 203 patients with non-permanent AF (age 66 ± 11 years, 40.4% female and 32% in AF), rhythm status at the time of exercise testing (AF or sinus) had no impact on exercise capacity evaluated through VO2peak, but the presence of AF during exercise test was correlated with reduced ventilatory efficiency. Almost 25% of the AF patients had reduced exercise capacity, and this was correlated with increased left ventricular filling pressures and reduced chronotropic response and not with rhythm status [9].

### 2.1 Exercise and atrial fibrillation: left atrium is more than an innocent bystander

Atrial enlargement, left atrium (LA) being the most studied one, occurs either as result of a physiological stimuli (exercise and normal pregnancy) or a pathological one (hypertension, valvular disease, and left ventricular hypertrophy) [10, 11]. The occurrence of AF further increases LA volume [12] and pathological remodeling as "AF begets atrial enlargement and atrial enlargement begets AF" [10], leading to atrial myopathy characterized by fibrosis and inflammation besides LA dilation. Electrical remodeling is underpinned and facilitated by complex structural alteration and mechanical dysfunction of the LA [13]. Atrial strain emerged as a powerful tool to assess the complex LA remodeling and the mechanical dysfunction that often precedes the occurrence of AF. Among 154 consecutive paroxysmal and persistent AF patients (age: 62 ± 10, 26% female), higher cardiorespiratory fitness was independently associated with reduced LA remodeling, higher systolic function (LA ejection fraction and LA strain in the reservoir, conduit and booster phase) together with reduced stiffness of the LA, even after adjusting for age, sex and BMI. Obese subjects had larger LA pointing toward a higher degree of remodeling, but normal mechanical function [13].

Depending on the dose, exercise triggers either adaptive or maladaptive enlargement of the atria. Up to 20% of highly trained athletes display mild atrial enlargement as a physiologic adaptation to exercise. The unique physiology that underpinned atrial dilation during prolonged ET refers to the "dam effect." The highest pressure into the atria is during systole when the atrioventricular valves are closed. During exercise, with the increase of the heart rate, the diastole is shorter and atrioventricular valves are closed for the majority of the time. Blood continues to flow at very high rates into the atria because of the high cardiac output which further increases the pressure [14]. It is important to acknowledge that, despite an increase in the volume, the physiologically dilated LA has a normal function with normal strain and myocardial deformation values [15]. Pathological dilation of the LA is characterized by an abnormal structural, electrical, and metabolic remodeling with a negative impact on atrial function and an increased likelihood for the occurrence of AF [10]. LA dilation is an important, independent predictor for new-onset AF in the general population (hazard ratio [HR]: 1.39; 95% confidence interval [CI]: 1.14–1.68 for each 5-mm increase in LA diameter) [16] and AF recurrence after catheter ablation [17, 18] but not among elite athletes. Between 30 [19] and 70% [20] of professional athletes have an increased volume of LA compared to controls without a proportionally related increase in the prevalence of AF. LA dilation varies with the type of sporting discipline, with endurance athletes having the largest LA and strength athletes having the smallest difference compared to controls [21]. In young elite athletes, LA size increased with the volume of training and LA strain decreased in high-volume trainers in men but not in women. Among athletes, LA dysfunction and structural changes like fibrosis rather than LA enlargement are associated with AF risk [22]. Atrial and especially left atrium remodeling could be seen as an important link between physical activity and atrial fibrillation. During exercise, the pressure in LA is increased, and atrial contraction is increasingly important contributing to a rapid diastolic filling of the left ventricle and further enhancement of cardiac output but also to the physiological, adaptive enlargement of the LA. At rest or at a low level of exercise, the LA pressure returns to normal and there are no structural, electrical, or metabolic changes in LA. By contrast, extreme and persistent endurance exercise induces over time atrial fibrosis and inflammation, creating a favorable milieu for AF occurrence [23]. Of note, recreational endurance training is also associated with an increased likelihood of LA dilation, with a linear dose-effect relationship between the number of training hours and the degree of LA enlargement. In elite endurance athletes, excessive exercise is linked to a higher incidence of AF in middle-aged males but not in female subjects [22]. Moreover, depending on the etiology and the subsequent structural, molecular, signaling and functional alterations, atrial remodeling can reverse or not. In this regard, in-depth knowledge about how to prevent or even reverse advanced structural and functional atrial remodeling could be of utmost importance for AF prevention and treatment either in the general population or among extreme endurance athletes [10].

#### *2.1.1 Best friends: exercise prevents atrial fibrillation*

The majority of data show that AF is less prevalent in physically active persons. According to data from the UK Biobank, low levels of PA or sedentary behavior increased the risk of developing AF. PA was recorded with an accelerometer and self-reported [24]. The most convincing data about the value of PA in the prevention of AF come from the UK Biobank. In 502,635 individuals from the UK Biobank, high cardiorespiratory fitness reduced the risk of AF by 60% among those genetically predisposed to AF [25].

## 2.2 Foes: exercise triggers atrial fibrillation

Athlete's heart is the generic term that defines the totality of cardiovascular adaptations to exercise training [26]. Different training intensity and duration elicits different cardiovascular adaptation responses [27]. The prevalence of AF is increased 5–10-fold in long-term high-intensity endurance sports such as Nordic skiing, marathon running or professional cycling [9] more in men than in women [28, 29]. A number of underlying, predisposing conditions have been proposed. Some of them are shared with the general population (e.g., undiagnosed hypertension, excessive alcohol consumption, and sleep apnea). Issues related to long-term competitive sports include vagotonia, atrial fibrosis, atrial ectopic triggers [30], chronic inflammation and also chronic LA dilation [21]. AF is more prevalent in male subjects, whether they are active or former high performance athletes, and in master athletes engaged in high-intensity endurance sports [1].

### *2.2.1 Underlying mechanism of atrial fibrillation promotion by endurance exercise training*

We do not know the exact mechanism by which endurance training promotes AF. Several mechanisms could be involved like pathological, maladaptive remodeling of the LA that results in permanent structural changes and especially fibrosis of the atrial wall persistent elevated LA pressure, local inflammation, enhanced vagal tone and bradycardia. All the above alterations could overlap a genetic predisposition toward AF [22]. In exercise-trained rats, sustained, high-intensity endurance training for 16 weeks increased the probability of AF occurrence by inducing an atrial arrhythmogenic substrate. The following contributors were identified: autonomic changes with an increase in vagal tone, enlargement of the atria and atrial fibrosis. None of the aforementioned contributors was enough to promote an arrhythmogenic atrial substrate when taken separately, but each of them was necessary when taken together with the other two. Moreover, time was an important issue, especially for the development of atrial fibrosis [31]. Increased vagal tone is a well-known "side-effect" of endurance training. The majority of AF episodes in athletes are in the context of increased vagal tone and bradycardia [32]. Enhancement of vagal tone develops in a couple of weeks after the training program onset but is not enough to trigger AF by itself [33]. The underlying mechanism of bradycardia in athletes is linked to increased vagal tone but could also be due to structural remodeling of the sinoatrial node [34]. Among electrophysiological changes that result in the promotion of AF, the shortening of the atrial refractory period in the context of bradycardia could facilitate re-entry at the atrial level [30].

### *2.2.2 How much exercise is too much*

Exercise-training history over the entire lifespan of more than 2000 hours of vigorous, intensive endurance training is associated with an almost 4-fold increase in AF risk, underlying an important dose-response concept [35]. Of note, the annual training burden of an elite athlete could be over 800 hours [36]. Recreational athletes have more modest volumes but over several years resulting in a slower accumulation of LA pathological remodeling and increased AF risk [30]. Short training periods do not increase AF risk [37]. The pathological LA remodeling and the subsequent increase in AF probability require a prolonged history of high-intensity endurance training both in animal models [31] and in athletes [38].

*2.2.3 Detraining changes*

In animal models, AF susceptibility, heart rate and parasympathetic tone returned to baseline values within 4 weeks of detraining. Structural changes of both atria (dilation and fibrosis) remained significant after 4 weeks from the cessation of exercise training [31]. Data from a clinical study showed that the increase in exercise capacity after 3 months of cardiac rehabilitation in old patients with AF was lost when evaluating the patient after another 3 months of inactivity [39].

## 3. Exercising with atrial fibrillation: which is the best approach?

Exercise prescription is made using the "FIIT" approach: frequency, intensity, time and type. There are two major types of exercise: endurance and resistance or strength. Another classification refers to aerobic and anaerobic exercise. Achieving aerobic fitness is the major goal, since it is correlated with a positive impact on cardiovascular risk factors. Exercise frequency refers to the number of times or the period of time a subject is exercising per week. Intensity is a critical issue when prescribing exercise for achieving aerobic fitness. Aerobic training has two different modalities: continuous and interval training. Different sports train different components of physical fitness and at a different intensity. Besides aerobic exercise and resistance training, other training modalities, like Qi-gong and inspiratory muscle training, were also used in AF patients [40]. Choosing the most convenient exercise modality for each patient is based on the person's maximal exercise capacity, type of sport and personal preferences [1].

The general recommendation from the current guidelines is to encourage patients to engage in regular exercise and remain physically active but also to avoid chronic excessive endurance exercise. The most recent guideline [6] recommended moderate-to-vigorous ET in AF patients, to a target of 210 minutes/week. Patients with AF related to excessive ET are excluded. The goal is to reduce AF-related symptoms, the burden of AF and to increase the maintenance of sinus rhythm. Exercise capacity and quality of life are also improved in both permanent and non-permanent AF. Moreover, each 1 MET increase in cardiorespiratory fitness resulted in increased freedom of AF and decrease of AF recurrence by 9% [41].

Of note, when performing exercise tests for the evaluation of AF patients, we expect an exercise capacity that is 15–20% lower and a peak heart rate that is higher than in patients with sinus rhythm [42]. Evaluating and monitoring exercise intensity in AF patients can be challenging. Irregular and rapid heart rates make the evaluation of exercise intensity based on heart rate rather difficult and imprecise. The Borg rating of the perceived exertion category ratio scale is also not reliable. Breathing frequency monitored with wearable technologies may be an alternative [43, 44].

### 3.1 Exercise-based intervention

In the ACTIVE-AF (An Exercise and Physical Activity Program in Patients With Atrial Fibrillation) study, 120 patients with paroxysmal or persistent symptomatic AF were randomized over 6 months to combined home and supervised aerobic exercise or usual care. Participants in an exercise-based intervention group had fewer AF recurrences (twice as likely to be free from AF at 12 months), but only women experienced decreased symptom severity and improved quality of life [45, 46]. Several other short-duration trials with non-permanent AF and permanent AF patients confirmed the positive impact of aerobic exercise-based intervention on quality of life, AF symptom severity and improvement of the maintenance of sinus rhythm [47, 48]. Exercise habits are of utmost importance. In a population-based cohort study [49], performing exercise any time before or after AF diagnosis versus persistent non-exercising was associated with a lower risk of heart failure and mortality. Energy expenditure of regular moderate exercise 170–240 minutes/week or 1000–1499 MET-minutes/week was necessary to lower the risk in this retrospective study [49]. In HF-ACTION (Heart Failure: A Controlled Trial Investigating Outcomes of Exercise Training), patients with heart failure with reduced ejection fraction, supervised aerobic ET followed by home-based exercise program had a positive impact over exercise capacity and prognosis irrespective of the presence of AF [50]. In obese patients with AF, arrhythmia-free survival time and decreased symptom severity with and without rhythm control strategies were incrementally better with cardiorespiratory fitness improvement ≥2 METs [41]. Patients fear that intensive exercise will induce episodes of AF and adopt a sedentary lifestyle. There is no consensus about the best training modality. Regarding AF burden decrease, high-intensity aerobic exercise is not superior to moderate-intensity exercise and both are safe and do not induce AF episodes in non-permanent AF patients [51]. Moderate-intensity continuous training (MICT) has extensive evidence for enhancing quality of life and exercise capacity in AF patients. Several studies have also shown that MICT decreases symptoms and AF burden [52]. MICT is more efficient in the control of AF than low-intensity continuous training (LICT) [53]. High-intensity interval training (HIIT), which has a well-established positive impact on heart failure and coronary artery disease patients [54], could also be beneficial for AF patients. Animal studies underpinned the value of HIIT in reducing the age-dependent vulnerability to AF [55]. Numerous studies have found comparable efficacy of HIIT to MICT in AF patients. There were no significant differences in symptom control, enhancing exercise capacity and reducing the risk associated with AF [52]. Other studies suggested that HIIT may offer additional benefits over MICT in AF patients including improved endothelial function [56]. However, there is no conclusive data about the safety of HIIT across all spectrum of AF patients. Small studies suggest that HIIT is safe but they included only patients with low risk for cardiovascular events and the results cannot be generalized [52].

### 3.2 Comprehensive care including exercise-based intervention

Exercise-based intervention in AF patients can be delivered either stand-alone, or as a component of a multidisciplinary cardiac rehabilitation (CR) program. After an incident AF episode, the inclusion in a cardiac rehabilitation program was associated at the 18th month's follow-up with lower odds of all-cause mortality, rehospitalization and incident stroke but not with lower odds of heart failure. The association of exercise-based CR with the decrease in all-cause mortality was independent of sex, age, comorbidities and AF subtype [57]. In patients with heart failure with the whole spectrum of ejection fraction, exercise-based CR prevented AF over a 2-year follow-up and was associated with lower mortality, hospitalizations and incident stroke [58]. After AF ablation, CR decreases the recurrence of AF with variable effectiveness and diminished impact in obese and persistent AF patients [59]. As an alternative after rhythm control with catheter ablation, home-based CR is also effective for the control of symptoms, increasing the quality of life and improving exercise capacity, especially if combined with digital technologies [60].

## 4. Conclusion, gaps in knowledge and future directions

Exercise and atrial fibrillation are both friends AND foes. The bivalent relationship is based on a J curve with moderate and probably also moderate-intense exercise being in between as an important tool both in the prevention of the first and subsequent recurrent episodes of AF but also in the treatment of the established disease. Sedentary behavior promotes AF and AF-related poor quality of life. Regular sport is associated with a high probability of LA enlargement but does not induce the structural and functional changes that result in AF promotion. Only high-intensive, excessive endurance training is associated with structural, metabolic and functional maladaptive remodeling of the LA and increases the prevalence of AF. There is a dose-response relationship between the volume of lifetime training history and AF risk with no clear threshold of "upper-safe" especially in male subjects but no risk seems to be associated with exercise intensity based on current guidelines recommendation. Exercise-based intervention in AF patients, irrespective of AF type, either alone or as a part of a complex cardiac rehabilitation program is associated with reduced burden and recurrence of arrhythmia, improved AF-related symptoms and quality of life and, in some studies, lower odds of all-cause mortality. Gaps still exist concerning optimal delivery, modality, intensity, duration and monitoring of exercise programs in clinical practice but also concerning the exact mechanism of AF in athletes.

## Conflict of interest

The authors declare no conflict of interest.

## Author details

Ioana Cristina Daha* and Elisabeta Bădilă
Colentina Clinical Hospital, University of Medicine and Pharmacy "Carol Davila", Bucharest, Romania

*Address all correspondence to: ioana.daha@umfcd.ro

## References


[1] Pelliccia A, Sharma S, Gati S, et al. 2020 ESC guidelines on sports cardiology and exercise in patients with cardiovascular disease. European Heart Journal. 2021;**42**:17-96

[2] Caspersen CJ, Powell KE, Christenson GM. Physical activity, exercise, and physical fitness: Definitions and distinctions for health-related research. Public Health Reports. Mar-Apr 1985;**100**(2):126-131

[3] Chen H, Chen C, Spanos M, et al. Exercise training maintains cardiovascular health: Signaling pathways involved and potential therapeutics. Signal Transduction and Targeted Therapy. 2022;**7**:306

[4] Bhella PS, Hastings JL, Fujimoto N, et al. Impact of lifelong exercise "dose" on left ventricular compliance and distensibility. Journal of the American College of Cardiology. 2014;**64**:1257-1266

[5] Elliott AD, Linz D, Verdicchio CV, et al. Exercise and atrial fibrillation: Prevention or causation? Heart, Lung and Circulation. 2018;**27**:1078-1085

[6] Joglar JA, Chung MK, Armbruster AL, et al. ACC/AHA/ACCP/HRS guideline for the diagnosis and management of atrial fibrillation: A report of the American College of Cardiology/American Heart Association Joint Committee on Clinical Practice Guidelines. Circulation. 2 Jan 2024;**149**(1):e1-e156. DOI: 10.1161/CIR.0000000000001193

[7] Hindricks G, Potpara T, Dagres N, et al. 2020 ESC guidelines for the diagnosis and management of atrial fibrillation developed in collaboration with the European Association for Cardio-Thoracic Surgery (EACTS). European Heart Journal. 2021;**42**:373-498

[8] Way KL, Birnie D, Blanchard C, et al. The physical activity levels and sitting time of adults living with atrial fibrillation: The CHAMPLAIN-AF study. CJC Open. 2022;**4**:449-465

[9] Elliott AD, Verdicchio CV, Gallagher C, et al. Factors contributing to exercise intolerance in patients with atrial fibrillation. Heart, Lung and Circulation. 2021;**30**:947-954

[10] Chen YC, Voskoboinik A, Gerche AL, et al. Prevention of pathological atrial remodeling and atrial fibrillation. Journal of the American College of Cardiology. 2021;**77**:2846-2864

[11] Aaroee M, Tischer SG, Christensen R, et al. Atrial remodelling associated with sporting discipline, sex and duration in elite sports: A cross-sectional echocardiographic study among Danish elite athletes. BMJ Open Sport and Exercise Medicine. 2024;**10**:e001880

[12] Sanfilippo AJ, Abascal VM, Sheehan M, et al. Atrial enlargement as a consequence of atrial fibrillation. A Prospective Echocardiographic Study. Circulation. 1990;**82**:792-797

[13] Mishima RS, Ariyaratnam JP, Pitman BM, et al. Cardiorespiratory fitness, obesity and left atrial function in patients with atrial fibrillation. IJC Heart and Vasculature. 2022;**42**:101083

[14] La Gerche A, Claessen G. Increased flow, dam walls, and upstream pressure. JACC: Cardiovascular Imaging. 2016;**9**:1389-1391

[15] D'Andrea A, Bossone E, Radmilovic J, et al. Exercise-induced atrial remodeling. Cardiology Clinics. 2016;**34**:557-565

[16] Vaziri SM, Larson MG, Benjamin EJ, et al. Echocardiographic predictors of nonrheumatic atrial fibrillation. The Framingham Heart Study. Circulation. 1994;**89**:724-730

[17] Bordi L-L, Opincariu D, Benedek T, et al. Left atrial volume quantified by MSCT predicts emergency hospitalizations for AF and arrhythmia recurrence after catheter ablation. Journal of Cardiovascular Emergencies. 2023;**9**:24-31

[18] Desai D, Suthar N. Left atrial volume to predict the recurrence of atrial fibrillation in patients treated with catheter ablation. Journal of Cardiovascular Emergencies. 2023;**9**:22-23

[19] Iskandar A, Mujtaba MT, Thompson PD. Left atrium size in elite athletes. JACC: Cardiovascular Imaging. 2015;**8**:753-762

[20] Mansencal N, Marcadet D-M, Martin F, et al. Echocardiographic characteristics of professional tennis players at the Roland Garros French open. American Heart Journal. 2007;**154**:527-531

[21] Baggish AL. Athletic left atrial dilation. JACC: Cardiovascular Imaging. 2015;**8**:763-765

[22] Flannery MD, Kalman JM, Sanders P, et al. State of the art review: Atrial fibrillation in athletes. Heart, Lung and Circulation. 2017;**26**:983-989

[23] Peritz DC, Catino AB, Csecs I, et al. High-intensity endurance training is associated with left atrial fibrosis. American Heart Journal. 2020;**226**:206-213

[24] Elliott AD, Linz D, Mishima R, et al. Association between physical activity and risk of incident arrhythmias in 402 406 individuals: Evidence from the UK biobank cohort. European Heart Journal. 2020;**41**:1479-1486

[25] Tikkanen E, Gustafsson S, Ingelsson E. Associations of fitness, physical activity, strength, and genetic risk with cardiovascular disease: Longitudinal analyses in the UK biobank study. Circulation. 2018;**137**:2583-2591

[26] Kyrouac D, Levine BD. Editorial commentary: The athlete's heart: Friend or foe? Trends in Cardiovascular Medicine. 2024;**34**:26-28

[27] Zilio F, Di Fusco SA, Flori M, et al. Physical activity and the heart: From well-established cardiovascular benefits to possible adverse effects. Trends in Cardiovascular Medicine. 2024;**34**:18-25

[28] Andersen K, Farahmand B, Ahlbom A, et al. Risk of arrhythmias in 52 755 long-distance cross-country skiers: A cohort study. European Heart Journal. 2013;**34**:3624-3631

[29] Estes NAM, Madias C. Atrial fibrillation in athletes. JACC Clinical Electrophysiology. 2017;**3**:921-928

[30] Elliott AD, Mahajan R, Linz D, et al. Atrial remodeling and ectopic burden in recreational athletes: Implications for risk of atrial fibrillation. Clinical Cardiology. 2018;**41**:843-848

[31] Guasch E, Benito B, Qi X, et al. Atrial fibrillation promotion by endurance exercise. Journal of the American College of Cardiology. 2013;**62**:68-77

[32] Mont L, Elosua R, Brugada J. Endurance sport practice as a risk factor

for atrial fibrillation and atrial flutter. Europace. 2008;**11**:11-17

[33] Collier SR, Kanaley JA, Carhart R Jr, et al. Cardiac autonomic function and baroreflex changes following 4 weeks of resistance versus aerobic training in individuals with pre-hypertension. Acta Physiologica. 2009;**195**:339-348

[34] D'Souza A, Bucchi A, Johnsen AB, et al. Exercise training reduces resting heart rate via downregulation of the funny channel HCN4. Nature Communications. 2014;**5**:3775

[35] Calvo N, Ramos P, Montserrat S, et al. Emerging risk factors and the dose–response relationship between physical activity and lone atrial fibrillation: A prospective case–control study. Europace. 2016;**18**:57-63

[36] Tønnessen E, Sylta Ø, Haugen TA, et al. The road to gold: Training and peaking characteristics in the year prior to a gold medal endurance performance. PLoS One. 2014;**9**:e101796

[37] Pelliccia A, Maron BJ, Di Paolo FM, et al. Prevalence and clinical significance of left atrial remodeling in competitive athletes. Journal of the American College of Cardiology. 2005;**46**:690-696

[38] Molina L, Mont L, Marrugat J, et al. Long-term endurance sport practice increases the incidence of lone atrial fibrillation in men: A follow-up study. EP Europace. 2008;**10**:618-623

[39] Borland M, Bergfeldt L, Cider Å, et al. Effects of 3 months of detraining following cardiac rehabilitation in patients with atrial fibrillation. European Review of Aging and Physical Activity. 2022;**19**:14

[40] Risom SS, Zwisler AD, Johansen PP, Sibilitz KL, Lindschou J, Gluud C, et al. Exercise-based cardiac rehabilitation for adults with atrial fibrillation. Cochrane Database of Systematic Reviews. 9 Feb 2017;**2**(2):CD011197

[41] Pathak RK, Elliott A, Middeldorp ME, et al. Impact of CARDIOrespiratory FITness on arrhythmia recurrence in obese individuals with atrial fibrillation. Journal of the American College of Cardiology. 2015;**66**:985-996

[42] Keteyian SJ, Ehrman JK, Fuller B, et al. Exercise testing and exercise rehabilitation for patients with atrial fibrillation. Journal of Cardiopulmonary Rehabilitation and Prevention. 2019;**39**:65-72

[43] Nishimura S, Tanaka R, Kamikawa S, et al. Borg's exertion scale did not coincide with ventilatory anaerobic threshold in atrial fibrillation patients with restored sinus rhythm after ablation. Journal of Exercise Rehabilitation. 2024;**20**:83-90

[44] Buckley JP, Terada T, Lion A, et al. Is breathing frequency a potential means for monitoring exercise intensity in people with atrial fibrillation and coronary heart disease when heart rate is mitigated? European Journal of Applied Physiology. DOI: 10.1007/s00421-024-05487-2. Epub ahead of print 4 May 2024

[45] Elliott AD, Verdicchio CV, Mahajan R, et al. An exercise and physical activity program in patients with atrial fibrillation. JACC Clinical Electrophysiology. 2023;**9**:455-465

[46] Verdicchio CV, Mahajan R, Middeldorp ME, et al. Influence of sex on efficacy of exercise training for patients with symptomatic atrial fibrillation: Insights from the ACTIVE-AF randomized controlled trial. European Journal of Preventive Cardiology. 2023;**30**:2006-2014

[47] Malmo V, Nes BM, Amundsen BH, et al. Aerobic interval training reduces the burden of atrial fibrillation in the short term: A randomized trial. Circulation. 2016;**133**:466-473

[48] Oesterle A, Giancaterino S, Van Noord MG, et al. Effects of supervised exercise training on atrial fibrillation: A meta-analysis of randomized controlled trials. Journal of Cardiopulmonary Rehabilitation and Prevention. 2022;**42**:258-265

[49] Ahn H-J, Lee S-R, Choi E-K, et al. Association between exercise habits and stroke, heart failure, and mortality in Korean patients with incident atrial fibrillation: A nationwide population-based cohort study. PLoS Medicine. 2021;**18**:e1003659

[50] Luo N, Merrill P, Parikh KS, et al. Exercise training in patients with chronic heart failure and atrial fibrillation. Journal of the American College of Cardiology. 2017;**69**:1683-1691

[51] Skielboe AK, Bandholm TQ, Hakmann S, et al. Cardiovascular exercise and burden of arrhythmia in patients with atrial fibrillation—A randomized controlled trial. PLoS One. 2017;**12**:e0170060

[52] Wang Y, Wang Y, Xu D. Effects of different exercise methods and intensities on the incidence and prognosis of atrial fibrillation. Trends in Cardiovascular Medicine. 2024;**S1050173824000021**

[53] Morseth B, Graff-Iversen S, Jacobsen BK, et al. Physical activity, resting heart rate, and atrial fibrillation: The Tromsø study. European Heart Journal. 2016;**37**:2307-2313

[54] Wisløff U, Støylen A, Loennechen JP, et al. Superior cardiovascular effect of aerobic interval training versus moderate continuous training in heart failure patients: A randomized study. Circulation. 2007;**115**:3086-3094

[55] Malmo V, Kelly A, Garten KS, et al. Aerobic interval training prevents age-dependent vulnerability to atrial fibrillation in rodents. Frontiers in Physiology. 2018;**9**:206

[56] Kim S, Lee S, Han D, et al. One-year aerobic interval training improves endothelial dysfunction in patients with atrial fibrillation: A randomized trial. Internal Medicine. 2023;**62**:2465-2474

[57] Buckley BJR, Harrison SL, Fazio-Eynullayeva E, et al. Exercise-based cardiac rehabilitation and all-cause mortality among patients with atrial fibrillation. Journal of the American Heart Association. 2021;**10**:e020804

[58] Buckley BJR, Harrison SL, Fazio-Eynullayeva E, et al. Cardiac rehabilitation and all-cause mortality in patients with heart failure: A retrospective cohort study. European Journal of Preventive Cardiology. 2021;**28**:1704-1710

[59] Kurasawa Y, Maeda H, Tamaru T, et al. Safety and effectiveness of exercise-based cardiac rehabilitation for patients with atrial fibrillation following radiofrequency catheter ablation therapy: A systematic review and meta-analysis. Cureus. 2023. DOI: 10.7759/cureus.50476. Epub ahead of print 13 December 2023

[60] Liu T, Tang Z, Cai C, et al. Cost-effectiveness analysis of digital therapeutics for home-based cardiac rehabilitation for patients with atrial fibrillation after catheter ablation. Digital Health;**9**:20552076231211548